T0175821

MUSCULOSKELETAL PHYSICAL EXAMINATION

SECOND EDITION

MUSCULOSKELETAL PHYSICAL EXAMINATION

AN EVIDENCE-BASED APPROACH

Gerard A. Malanga, MD
New Jersey Regenerative Institute
Cedar Knolls, New Jersey
Clinical Professor
Department of Physical Medicine and Rehabilitation
Rutgers School of Medicine
New Jersey Medical School
Newark, New Jersey

Kenneth Mautner, MD
Associate Professor
Department of Physical Medicine and Rehabilitation
Emory University
Atlanta, Georgia

ELSEVIER

ELSEVIER

1600 John F. Kennedy Blvd.
Ste. 1800
Philadelphia, PA 19103-2899

MUSCULOSKELETAL PHYSICAL EXAMINATION:
An Evidence-Based Approach
SECOND EDITION

ISBN: 978-0-323-39623-3

Copyright © 2017 by Elsevier, Inc. All rights reserved.

No part of this publication may be reproduced or transmitted in any form or by any means, electronic or mechanical, including photocopying, recording, or any information storage and retrieval system, without permission in writing from the publisher. Details on how to seek permission, further information about the Publisher's permissions policies and our arrangements with organizations such as the Copyright Clearance Center and the Copyright Licensing Agency, can be found at our website: www.elsevier.com/permissions.

This book and the individual contributions contained in it are protected under copyright by the Publisher (other than as may be noted herein).

Notices

Knowledge and best practice in this field are constantly changing. As new research and experience broaden our understanding, changes in research methods, professional practices, or medical treatment may become necessary.

Practitioners and researchers must always rely on their own experience and knowledge in evaluating and using any information, methods, compounds, or experiments described herein. In using such information or methods they should be mindful of their own safety and the safety of others, including parties for whom they have a professional responsibility.

With respect to any drug or pharmaceutical products identified, readers are advised to check the most current information provided (i) on procedures featured or (ii) by the manufacturer of each product to be administered, to verify the recommended dose or formula, the method and duration of administration, and contraindications. It is the responsibility of practitioners, relying on their own experience and knowledge of their patients, to make diagnoses, to determine dosages and the best treatment for each individual patient, and to take all appropriate safety precautions.

To the fullest extent of the law, neither the Publisher nor the authors, contributors, or editors, assume any liability for any injury and/or damage to persons or property as a matter of products liability, negligence or otherwise, or from any use or operation of any methods, products, instructions, or ideas contained in the material herein.

Previous edition copyrighted 2006.

Library of Congress Cataloging-in-Publication Data

Names: Malanga, Gerard A., editor. | Mautner, Kenneth R., editor.
Title: Musculoskeletal physical examination : an evidence-based approach /
   [edited by] Gerard A. Malanga, Kenneth Mautner.
Description: Second edition. | Philadelphia, PA : Elsevier, [2017] | Includes
   bibliographical references and index.
Identifiers: LCCN 2016022179 | ISBN 9780323396233 (hardback : alk. paper)
Subjects: | MESH: Musculoskeletal System | Physical Examination |
   Musculoskeletal Diseases—diagnosis | Diagnostic Tests, Routine—methods |
   Range of Motion, Articular | Evidence-Based Medicine—methods
Classification: LCC RC925.7 | NLM WE 141 | DDC 616.7/0754—dc23 LC record available at
   https://lccn.loc.gov/2016022179

Content Strategist: Kellie J. Heap/Kayla Wolfe
Content Development Specialist: Lisa Barnes
Publishing Services Manager: Hemamalini Rajendrababu
Senior Project Manager: Beula Christopher
Senior Book Designer: Margaret Reid
Marketing Manager: Melissa Fogarty

Printed in United States of America

Last digit is the print number: 9   8   7   6   5

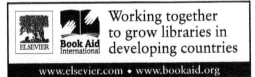

Contributors

Annunziato Amendola, MD
Orthopaedic Surgeon, Duke Orthopaedics, Durham,
   North Carolina

Keith Bengtson, MD
Clinical Director, Hand Rehabilitation, Physical Medicine
   and Rehabilitation, Mayo Clinic, Rochester, Minnesota

Anthony Beutler, MD
Sports Medicine Fellowship Director and Associate
   Professor, Family Medicine, Uniformed Services
   University, Bethesda, Maryland

Amrut Borade, MD
Clinical Research Fellow, Division Of Shoulder Surgery,
   The Johns Hopkins School Of Medicine, Baltimore,
   Maryland
Clinical Research Fellow, Department of Orthopaedic
   Trauma, Geisinger Health System, Danville,
   Pennsylvania

Jay E. Bowen, DO
Assistant Professor, Department of Physical Medicine and
   Rehabilitation, Rutgers—New Jersey Medical School,
   Newark, New Jersey

J. W. Thomas Byrd, MD
Clinical Professor, Department of Orthopaedic Surgery
   and Rehabilitation, School of Medicine, Vanderbilt
   University, Nashville, Tennesee

Larry H. Chou, MD
Medical Director, Sports and Spine Rehabilitation
   Division, Premier Orthopaedic and Sports Medicine
   Associates, LTD, Havertown, Deleware
Clinical Assistant Professor, Department of Physical
   Medicine and Rehabilitation, University of Pennsylvania
   School of Medicine, Philadelphia, Pennsylvania

Matthew J. Fanous, MD
Resident Physician, Physical Medicine and Rehabilitation,
   The Ohio State University Wexner Medical Center,
   Columbus, Ohio

Heather R. Galgon, DO
Attending Physician, Swedish Spine, Sports and
   Musculoskeletal Medicine, Swedish Medical
   Group, Providence Healthcare System, Issaquah,
   Washington

Mederic M. Hall, MD
Assistant Professor, Department of Orthopaedics and
   Rehabilitation, University of Iowa, Iowa City, Iowa

Lisa Huynh, MD
Clinical Assistant Professor, Division of Physical Medicine
   and Rehabilitation, Department of Orthopaedics,
   Stanford University, Redwood City, California

David J. Kennedy, MD
Clinical Assistant Professor, Division of Physical Medicine
   and Rehabilitation, Department of Orthopaedics,
   Stanford University, Redwood City, California

John Kincaid, MD
Nerve Conduction Studies and Needle EMG, Department
   of Neurology, Indiana University, Indianapolis, Indiana

Brian Krabak, MD, MBA, FACSM
Clinical Professor, Department of Rehabilitation,
   Orthopedics and Sports Medicine, University of
   Washington and Seattle Children's Sports Medicine,
   Seattle, Washington

Gerard A. Malanga, MD
New Jersey Regenerative Institute, Cedar Knolls,
   New Jersey
Clinical Professor, Department of Physical Medicine and
   Rehabilitation, Rutgers School of Medicine, New Jersey
   Medical School, Newark, New Jersey

Kenneth Mautner, MD
Associate Professor, Department of Physical Medicine and
   Rehabilitation, Emory University, Atlanta, Georgia

Edward G. McFarland, MD
The Wayne Lewis Professor of Shoulder Surgery
Director, Division of Shoulder Surgery, The Department
   of Orthopaedic Surgery, The Johns Hopkins University,
   Baltimore, Maryland

Matthew S. Mendez-Zfass, MD
Physician, Department of Orthopedic Surgery, Lenox Hill
   Hospital, New York, New York

Kenneth D. Montgomery, MD
Head Team Physician and Chairman, Medical
   Department, New York Jets Football Team
Orthopedic Surgeon, Tri-County Orthopedics, Cedar
   Knolls, New Jersey

Francis G. O'Connor, COL, MC, USA, MD, PhD
Professor and Chair, Military and Emergency Medicine
Associate Director, Consortium for Health and Military
   Performance (CHAMP), Uniformed Services University
   of the Health Sciences, "America's Medical School",
   Bethesda, Maryland

Tutankhamen Pappoe, MD
Medical Director, Pain Management, Phoenix
    Neurological and Pain Institute, Phoenix, Arizona

Joel M. Press, MD
Medical Director, Spine and Sports Rehabilitation Centers,
    Rehabilitation Institute of Chicago
Professor, Physical Medicine and Rehabilitation, Feinberg
    School of Medicine, Chicago, Illinois

Lt Col Ross A. Schumer, MD
Department of Orthopaedic Surgery and Rehabilitation,
    San Antonio Military Medical Center, San Antonio,
    Texas

Jeffrey A. Strakowski, MD
Clinical Associate Professor, Department of Physical
    Medicine and Rehabilitation, The Ohio State University
Associate Director of Medical Education, Physical
    Medicine and Rehabilitation, Riverside Methodist
    Hospital
Director of Musculoskeletal Research, The McConnell
    Spine Sport and Joint Center, Columbus, Ohio

Walter Sussman, DO
Primary Care Sports Medicine Fellow, Department of
    Sporrts Medicine, Physical Medicine and Rehabilitation,
    Emory University, Atlanta, Georgia

Andrew Willis, MD
Faculty, Orthopedic Sports Medicine Fellowship,
    Department of Orthopedic Surgery, Lenox Hill
    Hospital, New York, New York
Attending Orthopedic Surgeon, Department of
    Orthopedic Surgery, Morristown Medical Center,
    Morristown, New Jersey

David N. Woznica, MS, MD
Clinical Instructor, Department of Orthopaedics and
    Rehabilitation, Yale University School of Medicine, New
    Haven, Connecticuit

Foreword

Assessment in musculoskeletal physical diagnosis in the United States is rapidly changing. As the use of advanced diagnostic imaging, including "sports ultrasound," has grown in clinical musculoskeletal care, it has become a tool that far too often is a "go to" resource for the clinician to facilitate a diagnosis. Most seasoned practitioners, however, are well aware that these imaging techniques often confound the assessment effort, and truly have their greatest utility when used in conjunction with point of care physical diagnosis. When I completed my sports medicine fellowship in the early 1990s under the tutelage of Dr. Robert P. Nirschl, which now seems like ancient history, obtaining an MRI was truly a rare event and only used to unravel a diagnostic mystery. In the community where I presently practice, all too often an orthopedic consult or surgical procedure is only contemplated or approved if there is advanced imaging confirmation. As medical assessment is rapidly evolving, so too is medical care delivery and reimbursement. Multiple forces, including the implementation of the Affordable Care Act and the promotion of patient-centered medical care, are calling on clinicians, in particular those who deliver primary care, to optimize diagnosis and treatment at the initial point of medical entry. As clinicians in a brave new world of limited and constrained health-care dollars, we are additionally being challenged to be good stewards of resources and being scrutinized for overuse of diagnostic tests.

As a long-time educator in musculoskeletal medicine, physical examination has been a skill set I have always enjoyed studying, and most importantly, teaching. As an allopathic physician, not trained in manipulation, the physical examination is a foundational skill. The interaction of "laying hands" on a patient after a well-performed history is much more than confirming a diagnosis; it is also an opportunity to assess structure and function. In addition to integrating a clinician's knowledge of functional anatomy and biomechanics is also the need to utilize their skill in assessing a patient's effort and pain. The physical examination also demonstrates to the patient that one is a true practitioner of the medical arts; I have seen far too many patients in consultation where the patient is quick to report that "the last doctor never even bothered to examine me."

In teaching medical students, residents, fellows, and colleagues, I am invariably asked as I demonstrate a Neer test or discuss a Thessaly test just how good the test is. What are the test discriminators such as sensitivity, specificity, and predictive value. We are clearly in the era of evidence-based medicine, and these questions are first and foremost concerns of eager learners. Accordingly, educators and experts in musculoskeletal medicine seek out resources that "answer the mail" in addressing core questions on the validity of the tests we employ in musculoskeletal assessment. As a student myself, I have engaged numerous texts and resources to identify the best information to accurately describe the test and describe its discriminators. Before the first edition of Malanga and Nadler's Physical Examination, there was a clear "gap" in this literature. The first text was an unparalleled entry into the academic arena that offered the reader the original description of all the special tests we incorporate in the clinical examination, as well as a detailed summary of current evidence-based literature to help the end user assess the test's value added. The first edition has literally become one of my favorite resources and one I would frequently recommend to both students and educators. In the years since the first edition, I have had the privilege to engage with Dr. Gerry Malanga at sports medicine meetings, and I always have complemented his contribution to our field. I am thrilled to be a contributing author to this updated edition.

The second edition builds on the success of the first and provides a complete resource for those who administer a musculoskeletal examination. The second edition continues to build and expand on physical examination techniques with up-to-date literature on more recent exam maneuvers such as the Thessaly test and tests for athletic pubalgia. In addition, this edition has gained the resources of some of the experts in the field outside of just PCSM, including notable orthopedic physicians such as Tom Byrd and Ned Amendola. Lastly the video section that precisely explains how to perform the physical examinations has been greatly expanded with many new additional video clips and now will be easier to access from the eBook version, which was not available with the first edition.

In musculoskeletal and sports medicine, many core texts are easily recognized and referred to by the original authors' last names. Examples include **Rockwood and Green's** textbook of fracture care, **DeLee and Drez's** textbook of orthopedic sports medicine. I have no doubt that this resource will emerge, if it has not already done so, as *"the"* resource on evidenced-based physical assessment for the musculoskeletal provider, and quite simply be referred to as **Malanga and Mautner's**. I congratulate Drs. Malanga and Mautner on yet again a wonderful contribution to our discipline because I know this textbook will be an invaluable resource for providers and serve to improve care for thousands of patients and for educators who will instruct the next generation of clinicians.

Francis G. O'Connor, COL, MC, USA, MD, PhD
Professor and Chair
Military and Emergency Medicine
Associate Director
Consortium for Health and
Military Performance (CHAMP)
Uniformed Services University of the Health Sciences
"America's Medical School"
Bethesda, MD

Preface

It has been 10 years since the publication of the first edition of *Musculoskeletal Physical Examination: An Evidenced-based Approach*. Since then, many students, residents, and attending physicians have expressed their gratitude for this type of textbook and its associated videos. Since the initial publication, there has been renewed interest in musculoskeletal physical examination with the development of many additional physical examination maneuvers supported by scientific evidence. The Decade of Bone and Joint has been extended with the knowledge that musculoskeletal conditions are the second most common reason for primary care visits and a major cause of disability and limitation in daily function. In addition, the past decade has seen a greater emphasis on cost-effective and evidence-based medicine with a goal of decreasing unnecessary testing, especially unnecessary imaging studies for musculoskeletal conditions.

This second edition of *Musculoskeletal Physical Examination: An Evidenced-based Approach* is based on the same premise as the first edition: descriptions of how to properly perform various musculoskeletal physical examination maneuvers AND understanding the scientific validity of a "positive" or "negative" test. This edition contains many new physical examination tests that were not previously described at the time of the first edition. We have many new authors of various specialties from Family Practice, Sports Medicine, Physical Medicine, and Rehabilitation as well as Orthopedics. Many additional video clips of physical examination tests have been added to the original set of videos. This edition of the textbook continues to have expanded descriptive photographs and figures, as well as summary tables of the various physical examination tests. The memory and contribution of Dr. Scott Nadler continue to permeate the pages of this new edition as well.

We hope the readers (students, residents, attending physicians, athletic trainers, physical and occupational therapists, etc.) will continue to find this textbook useful in the skillful evaluation of their patients to establish an accurate diagnosis that will facilitate optimal treatment outcomes.

Gerard A. Malanga, MD
Kenneth Mautner, MD

Contents

Video Table of Contents

An Evidence-Based Approach to the Musculoskeletal Physical Examination

Gerard A. Malanga, MD | Kenneth Mautner, MD

Since the publication of the first edition of this textbook, much has changed in the world, including the passing of our dear colleague and coeditor of this textbook, Dr. Scott Nadler. This is not only a great personal loss but also a loss to the many residents and fellows who will never benefit from his teaching skills; still others who will be deprived of his masterful speaking skills; and the medical community in general, which has lost a great mind and researcher.

We are pleased that over the past decade, there appears to be an increased interest in orthopedic physical examination with a great deal of peer-reviewed literature published in orthopedic, rehabilitation, physical therapy, and many other journals and textbooks. New tests have been developed and studied for various orthopedic conditions.[1,2] In addition, a greater emphasis has been placed on education in the performance of the orthopedic physical examination in medical schools and in the related specialty areas of physical medicine rehabilitation; rheumatology; and obviously, orthopedic surgery.

Unfortunately, as noted in the introduction of the first edition of this textbook, there continues to be overemphasis on and increased use of imaging studies such as magnetic resonance imaging (MRI), and recently, musculoskeletal ultrasonography. While these technologies offer incredible resolution of musculoskeletal pathology, the medical literature has clearly demonstrated a significant number of false-positive findings with their use. Moreover, the escalation in the use of MRI and other imaging studies is believed to be due to their indiscriminate use without appropriate indications. It is therefore clear that the appropriate use of imaging studies should require a thorough history and physical examination beforehand.

Overreliance on imaging and other diagnostic studies can additionally result in improper diagnosis and unnecessary treatment. Multiple studies have demonstrated the incidence of MRI abnormalities in normal subjects. This has been reported in the spine,[3] shoulder,[4] knee,[5] and other areas. LaPrade and colleagues[5] noted that 24% of normal individuals have findings consistent with grade II meniscal tears on MRI, and they recommended that clinicians match clinical signs and symptoms with MRI findings before surgical intervention. O'Shea and coworkers[6] noted that the correct diagnosis was made in 83% of patients using the history and physical examination alone in the diagnosis of knee injuries. This, along with the significant findings on MRI in asymptomatic individuals, brings into question the need for MRI or ultrasonography as part of a standard screen for musculoskeletal injury. It also highlights the importance of a properly performed clinical examination.

Musculoskeletal complaints represent some of the most common reasons for patient encounters by primary care physicians.[7] This trend is likely to increase secondary to societal changes in health and fitness, which has led our aging population to be more physically active than in years past. A poor history or physical examination can lead to inappropriate diagnostic testing and will influence patient outcome because treatment may be directed toward abnormal findings on imaging study rather than being based on the patient's complaint and physical exam findings.[8] The history can quickly produce a more discrete differential diagnosis and includes the mechanism of injury; the quality, location, and referral of pain; and the associated functional deficits. The fact that the physical examination is not performed in isolation but rather in conjunction with the history needs to be stressed. The information gained from the history helps focus the physical examination, especially if the physician has a good understanding of the underlying anatomy and biomechanics.

The physical examination of the musculoskeletal system is often limited by a lack of research into the sensitivity and specificity for the disease processes that these tests are used to assess. Sackett and Rennie[9] noted that studies have been limited in regard to the physical exam, though the capability of reporting sensitivity, specificity, and predictive power would be similar to commonly studied laboratory tests. Reliability or reproducibility in regard to the translation of skills between the same or different clinicians at various time points during the course of disease is also poorly defined. Finally, there is no true gold standard by which to assess the validity of the different maneuvers because even reported surgical pathology may be a normal anatomic or age-related change in a variety of disease processes. This does not imply that physical examination maneuvers should be abandoned but rather that they need to be more completely understood and, ultimately, refined. Unfortunately, these issues are not understood by clinicians in various specialties and disciplines, leading to a promulgation of myths rather than facts.

Another issue arises when clinicians fail to recognize the importance of using more than one examination maneuver to make their diagnosis. Andersson and Deyo[10] identified improved sensitivity, specificity, and positive predictive value with the utilization of combinations of tests rather than tests in isolation. This has also been shown in the physical examination of the shoulder[4,7] and other joints. Although this makes the scientific validation of any particular test challenging, it also reinforces the fact that, when properly performed and used in combination, the physical examination can be a powerful clinical tool.[6,11,12] Clearly, improved understanding of the science behind physical examination maneuvers should be part of the evaluation of all clinicians in training and should be initiated at the outset of training rather than after habits have been established and become difficult to change.

Education becomes an important issue when considering musculoskeletal physical examination.[13] Medical students and residents, especially those choosing primary care as a specialty, are poorly trained in the basics of diagnosis and treatment of musculoskeletal problems.[14,15] Freedman and Bernstein examined the basic competency of internal medicine residents and found 78% failed to demonstrate basic competency on a validated musculoskeletal examination with a criterion set by their program directors.[14] These authors had previously noted deficiencies in musculoskeletal knowledge using this same competency examination and noted better scores in residents who had rotated through orthopedics while in medical school.[15] Those who had rotated through rheumatology, physical medicine and rehabilitation, or neurology unfortunately did not have scores significantly different from those who did not rotate in these specialties. Even those who rotated through orthopedics scored lower than the recommended passing score. This suggests that there may be a problem with course content in addition to musculoskeletal exposure in medical school and residency education. Exposure to an outpatient orthopedics or physical medicine and rehabilitation rotation would appear to be beneficial to medical students, residents, and fellows. Mazzuca and Brandt surveyed 271 rheumatology fellows regarding their experience in various aspects of musculoskeletal care; 60% desired more experience in nonoperative sports medicine and indicated that they would have opted for a 3-year fellowship for additional training.[16]

In addition to exposure to musculoskeletal problems, there are issues regarding the knowledge and experience of those who teach these skills. These educators need to have a broad knowledge base, which should include an understanding of the techniques as originally described, test limitations, and educational strategies to relay this information. Overall, the lack of proper training in the diagnosis and treatment of musculoskeletal problems is distressing given the high incidence of patient visits to primary care physicians for musculoskeletal complaints. The simplest route of treatment has been early imaging and referral to a specialist when, in many cases, an appropriate diagnosis based a proper history and physical examination can provide a discrete diagnosis that can be readily treated *without* the need of imaging studies or referral to a specialist.

Proficiency in physical examination skills has not been extensively evaluated. Clinical competency can be measured in many different ways, including the use of traditional multiple choice tests, bedside assessment, and the objective structured clinical examination (OSCE). When a physical examination skill is taught or performed inaccurately, the results are inaccurate information that is communicated to patients and poor examination skills that are disseminated to clinicians in training. Multiple-choice examination questions do not capture the hands-on skills required during physical exam. Bedside evaluation is probably the best assessment of examining skills, but unfortunately, changes in health care leading to increased busywork and patient load have resulted in less time to evaluate these skills at the bedside. Utilizing an OSCE format, Petrusa and associates[17] demonstrated excellent agreement (0.80) in evaluation of resident physical examination skills between patient and faculty evaluators. Utilizing the OSCE to assess interrater reliability of physical examination skills of the ankle, hand, knee, shoulder, and lower back, excellent reliability was demonstrated for examination of the lower back (0.837) and good reliability for the knee (0.582) and hand (0.622), with fair agreement for the ankle (0.460) and shoulder (0.463).[18] Physical examination skills were later compared with the existing gold standard, the board certification examination results, and scores on the test poorly correlated with the physical examination skills of the lower back (0.15) and ankle (−0.64), and only fair agreement was demonstrated with shoulder examination skills (0.44).[18] This tells us that we need better ways to assess examination skills of individuals we are training and that the current means of verifying competency (board certifying examinations) do not currently assess these skills.

Physical examination skills remain a vital part of the art of medicine, which must be supported by as much science as possible. As such, they require proper instruction, practice, and feedback to ensure that they are done correctly. We must take a thoughtful look at the physical exam and ask some important questions. How, why, and what are we doing, and where are we going in regard to the educational needs of those learning these skills? This book was initially undertaken and now has been revised with the goal of improving not only the competency of musculoskeletal physical exam skills but also to assist readers in better understanding the current exams that we perform in order to make them more valuable in the decision-making process. We hope that this text spurs further interest in additional research on the reliability and validity of the existing musculoskeletal physical exam maneuvers, which has increased greatly since the initial publication of this textbook. Potentially, utilizing a scientific approach that is supported by anatomic, biomechanical, and clinical validation, we may be able to develop more sensitive, specific, and reliable tests for the musculoskeletal physical examination. We believe this will lead to better and more cost-effective health care for patients with musculoskeletal conditions.

REFERENCES

1. Karachalios T, Hantes M, Zibis AH, et al. Diagnostic accuracy of a new clinical test (the Thessaly test) for early detection of meniscal tears. *J Bone Joint Surg Am.* 2005;87:955-962.
2. Kim YS, Kim JM, Ha KY, et al. The passive compression test: a new clinical test for superior labral tears of the shoulder. *Am J Sports Med.* 2007;35:1489-1494.
3. Jensen MC, Brant-Zawadzki MN, Obuchowski N, et al. Magnetic resonance imaging of the lumbar spine in people without back pain. *N Engl J Med.* 1994;331:69-73.
4. McFarland EG, Garzon-Muvdi J, Jia X, et al. Clinical and diagnostic tests for shoulder disorders: a critical review. *Br J Sports Med.* 2010;44:328-332.
5. LaPrade RF, Burnett QM, Veenstra MA, et al. The prevalence of abnormal magnetic resonance imaging findings in asymptomatic knees, with correlation of magnetic resonance imaging to arthroscopic findings in symptomatic knees. *Am J Sports Med.* 1994; 22:739-745.

6. O'Shea KJ, Murphy KP, Heekin RD, et al. The diagnostic accuracy of history, physical examination, and radiographs in the evaluation of traumatic knee disorders. *Am J Sports Med.* 1996;24:164-167.
7. Jia X, Petersen SA, Khosravi AH, et al. Examination of the shoulder: the past, the present, and the future. *J Bone Joint Surg Am.* 2009;91(suppl 6):10-18.
8. Solomon DH, Simel DL, Bates DW, et al. The rational physical exam. Does this patient have a torn meniscus or ligament of the knee? Value of the physical examination. *JAMA.* 2001;286:1610-1620.
9. Sackett DL, Rennie D. The science of the art of the clinical examination. *JAMA.* 1992;267:2650-2652.
10. Andersson GB, Deyo RA. History and physical examination in patients with herniated lumbar discs. *Spine.* 1996;21(suppl 24):10S-18S.
11. Ahern MJ, Scultz D, Soden M, et al. The musculoskeletal examination: a neglected clinical skill. *Aust NZ J Med.* 1991;21:303-306.
12. Karpman RR. Musculoskeletal disease in the United States. *Clin Orthop Rel Res.* 2001;385:52-56.
13. Branch VK, Graves G, Hanczyc M, et al. The utility of trained arthritis patient educators in the evaluation and improvement of musculoskeletal examination skills of physicians in training. *Arthritis Care Res.* 1999;12:61-69.
14. Freedman KB, Bernstein J. Educational deficiencies in musculoskeletal medicine. *J Bone Joint Surg.* 2002;84A:604-608.
15. Freedman KB, Bernstein J. The adequacy of medical school education in musculoskeletal medicine. *J Bone Joint Surg.* 1998;80A:1421-1427.
16. Mazzuca SA, Brandt KD. Clinical rheumatology training in an uncertain future: opinions of recent and current rheumatology fellows about an extended fellowship in musculoskeletal medicine. *Arthritis Rheum.* 1994;37:329-332.
17. Petrusa ER, Blackwell TA, Rogers LP, et al. An objective measure of clinical performance. *Am J Med.* 1987;83:34-42.
18. Jain SS, DeLisa JA, Eyles MY, et al. Further experience in development of an objective structured clinical examination for physical medicine and rehabilitation residents. *Am J Phys Med Rehabil.* 1998;77:306-310.

1 Reliability and Validity of Physical Examinations

Heather R. Galgon, DO | Larry H. Chou, MD

INTRODUCTION

In 1880, John Venn, a priest and lecturer in Moral Science at Caius College, Cambridge University, England, introduced and popularized Venn diagrams (Fig. 1.1).[1] Each circle represents a distinct domain that interacts with and is overlapped by other domains. The areas of overlap are more significant than the circles themselves, for within the overlapping areas "truth" can be found. While these diagrams were originally designed as models for mathematics and logic, they can also be used in the philosophy and practice of modern clinical medicine.

The "truth" in medicine represents the underlying diagnosis giving rise to a patient's symptoms and signs. In this version of the Venn diagram, the large circle represents a patient's relevant clinical history. It is the largest of the circles and where the majority of useful information can be found. Partially overlapping the patient's history is a smaller circle representing the physical examination. The exam substantiates findings from the clinical history, but the nonoverlapping area represents its ability to identify issues not uncovered in the patient's history. Last, the smallest circle represents additional clinical testing—whether laboratory, imaging, or electrophysiologic—that can further refine and confirm the true diagnosis denoted by the black dot. The true diagnosis lies within the clinical history, is supported by the physical examination, and is corroborated with other clinical studies.

In modern medicine, the bulk of clinical practice is predicated on the research question and the quality of support by which the question is answered. When critically reviewing the literature, it is paramount to understand these concepts. Indeed, an appreciation of the scientific method is necessary to fully understand the merits and pitfalls of the medical literature such that a conclusion can be properly applied to a specific clinical scenario. This chapter discusses the concepts of *validity* and *reliability,* how they give rise to sensitivity and specificity for diagnostic tests, and how the reported statistics of the various diagnostic tests should be interpreted in the clinical setting.

In contrast to observational cohort, case-control, and cross-sectional studies, the evaluation of diagnostic tests is different. Most observational studies attempt to show an association between the test result (a predictor variable) and the disease. In contrast, diagnostic studies attempt to discriminate between the diseased and the nondiseased. It is insufficient to merely identify an association between the test result and the disease.[2] The concepts of specificity and sensitivity as well as positive and negative predictive value are discussed here.

VALIDITY

Validity represents the truth, whether it is deduced, inferred, or supported by data. There are two types of validity: internal and external.[3] *Internal validity* is the degree to which the results and conclusions from a research study correctly represent the data that were measured in the study. That is, the truth in the study can be correctly explained by the results of the study. However, it is important to recognize that this may not correctly answer the clinical question at hand. While a conclusion can be properly reached based on the available study findings, if the question asked or methods used are incorrect, then meaningful interpretation of the results is suspect. Once internal validity issues are satisfied, then the greater issue is that of external validity.

External validity is the degree to which the internal validity conclusions can be generalized to situations outside of the study. This is the *sine qua non* of meaningful clinical research. That is, can the conclusion of a study that has correctly interpreted its results be used outside of that specific research setting? The variables designed in a study must correctly represent the phenomena of interest. A research study that is so contrived or so artificially oversimplified to a degree that does not exist in the real world clinical setting is of guarded value.

Errors in study design and measurement tools greatly affect validity. How well a measurement represents a phenomenon is influenced by two major sources of error: sampling error and measurement error. In order for a study to be generalizable, the study population needs to parallel the target population. That is, the inclusion criteria for entrance into the study must represent the clinical characteristics and demographics of the population for which the study is intended. The sample size needs to be sufficiently large to avoid bias and increase power (see the following section). It is important to recognize that reporting errors can also occur, though these should be, and often are, identified in the peer review process.

Likewise, measurement errors need to be avoided so that valid conclusions can be drawn from the results. This brings up the concept of the accuracy and precision of a measurement (Fig. 1.2). Accuracy is the degree to which the study measurement reflects the actual measurement. In other words, accuracy represents the validity of the study, whether

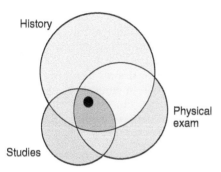

Figure 1.1 Venn diagram.

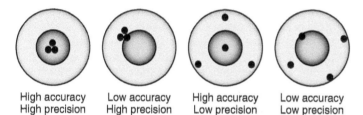

Figure 1.2 Accuracy and precision.

internal or external. Greater accuracy increases the validity of the study.

Accuracy is influenced by systematic errors or bias. Limiting consistent distortion from the observer, subject, or instrument reduces accuracy. Observer distortion is a systematic error on the part of the observer in data gathering or reporting data. Subject bias refers to the consistent distortion of the facts as recalled or perceived by the subject. Instrument bias results from an error in the measurement device, either by malfunctioning or inappropriate usage for a study purpose for which it was not designed. Comparing the measurement to a reference standard best assesses accuracy.

RELIABILITY

Reliability, and the related concept of precision, represents the reproducibility of a test. A test is considered reliable if repeated measurements consistently produce similar results. These results do not need to be compared with a reference standard. Precision refers to the uniformity and consistency of the repeated measurement. It is affected by random error whereby the greater the error, the lower the precision.[4] Standard deviations are typically used to describe precision.

The three primary sources of precision error are observer, subject, and instrument variability. Observer variability is dependent on the observer in gathering data points, whereas subject variability refers to innate differences within the subject population that can contribute to errors. Instrument variability is affected by environmental factors.

Research studies on diagnostic tests are inherently susceptible to random errors.[2] Patients with positive findings may not have the disease by chance alone and vice versa. Because random errors are difficult to control, confidence intervals for sensitivity and specificity should be reported.

Confidence intervals allow for the possibility of random errors given the study's sample size. The ranges of these confidence intervals are perhaps even more important than the actual sensitivity and specificity score.

The degree of concordance between paired measurements is usually expressed as a correlation coefficient (R) or as a kappa statistic (κ). The correlation coefficient is a number between −1 and +1. The absolute value indicates the strength of correlation, where 0 is poor and 1 is high, that is, very precise. Various tests can be used, including the Pearson coefficient, where values are evaluated directly, and the Spearman rank test, where values are placed in rank order and then analyzed.

Reliability measurements need to be observed for test–retest, internal, and interobserver and intraobserver consistency. The test–retest reliability refers to the concordance among repeated measurements on a sample of subjects. Caution must be exercised especially with physical exam maneuvers because the test itself can create errors by factors such as the training effect and learning curve. Internal consistency indicates that separate measures of the same variable will have internal concordance. Intraobserver consistency indicates that repeated measurements by a single observer are reproducible whereas interobserver measurements are reproducible by separate observers of the same event.

Interobserver agreement is often reported as a kappa statistic, which provides a quantitative measure of the magnitude of agreement between observers. For example, the modified scapular assistance test (SAT), as described by Rabin and colleagues,[5] reveals moderate interrater reliability with a kappa coefficient and percent agreement of 0.53 and 77%, respectively, when performed in the scapular plane and 0.62 and 91%, respectively, when performed in the sagittal plane. Based on a higher degree of interobserver agreement, the authors concluded that the modified SAT is more reliable when performed in the sagittal plane.

Precision strongly influences the power of a study.[4] A more precise measurement lends greater statistical power. Power is the probability of rejecting the null hypothesis when it is in fact false. The null hypothesis suggests there is no association between the two variables in question. The power depends on the total number of end-points experienced by a population. By increasing the sample size, the power will increase.[6] This will also decrease the probability that the null hypothesis will be incorrectly accepted.

Validity and reliability are not necessarily linked nor are they mutually exclusive. Although high accuracy and precision are ideal within a given test, unfortunately, this is not often the case. It is possible to have high accuracy yet low precision, and vice versa (Fig. 1.2).

SPECIFICITY AND SENSITIVITY

As mentioned previously, the outcome variable of a diagnostic test is the presence or absence of disease or injury when compared with the ideal reference standard known as the "gold standard." By convention, the gold standard is always positive in patients with the disease and negative in those without the disease. However, in the clinical setting, even the gold standard has its limitations and is not impervious

Table 1.1   Calculating Specificity and Sensitivity

		Disease State	
		Present	**Absent**
Test result	Positive	(a) True positive	(b) False positive
	Negative	(c) False negative	(d) True negative
		(a) + (c) = 100%	(b) + (d) = 100%

to error. Generally, the quality and efficacy of a diagnostic test is obtained by calculating its sensitivity and specificity.

The outcome variable of a diagnostic test falls into one of four situations (Table 1.1):

1. A true-positive result, where the test is positive for the patient who has the disease
2. A false-positive result, where the test is positive but the patient does not have the disease
3. A false-negative result, where the test is negative but the patient has the disease
4. A true-negative result, where the test is negative for the patient who does not have the disease.

Ideally, the best diagnostics tests have no false positives or false negatives. Sensitivities and specificities are unlinked and should not affect one other. It is possible to have any combination of sensitivities and specificities—high sensitivity with high or low specificity, and vice versa. The utility of a test with both low sensitivity and specificity has dubious value.

The sensitivity of a test represents how good it is at identifying disease. Andersson and Deyo[7] used the mnemonic SnNout. If *Sen*sitivity is *high*, a *N*egative test result rules *out* the target diagnosis. It is calculated by the proportion of patients with the disease who have a positive test:

$$\text{Sensitivity} = \text{True positive}/[\text{True positive} + \text{False negative}]$$
$$= (a)/[(a)+(c)].$$

Specificity, on the other hand, represents how good a test is at identifying those patients without disease. Using Andersson's mnemonic, SpPin, if *Sp*ecificity is *high*, a *P*ositive test result rules *in* the target diagnosis. It is calculated as the proportion of patients without the disease who have a negative test:

$$\text{Specificity} = \text{True Negative}/[\text{False positive} + \text{True negative}]$$
$$= (d)/[(b)+(d)].$$

In the chapter on knee examinations (Chapter 9), various physical exam maneuvers are used to assess the integrity of the anterior cruciate ligament (ACL). Using arthroscopy as the gold standard, the Lachman test was 81.8% sensitive and 96.8% specific, and the pivot shift was 81.8% sensitive and 98.4% specific, while the anterior drawer sign was only 40.9% sensitive yet 95.2% specific.[8] With the high sensitivities of the Lachman and the pivot shift test, a negative result on physical examination essentially rules out an ACL tear. Likewise, with the high specificities, a positive finding on the Lachman, pivot shift, and anterior drawer likely rules in the diagnosis. The low sensitivity of the anterior drawer test indicates that it is suboptimal at diagnosing ACL-deficient knees. Although this study was published in 1986, it is unclear why the anterior drawer test is still one of the most beloved tests of the ACL in clinical practice.

POSITIVE AND NEGATIVE PREDICTIVE VALUES

After the specificity and sensitivity of a test have been established, the predictive value of a positive test versus a negative test can be determined if the prevalence of the disease is known. When the prevalence of a disease increases, a patient with a positive test result is more likely to have the disease. It is therefore less likely for that test to represent a false negative. A negative result of a highly sensitive test will probably rule out a common disease. Conversely, however, if a disease is rare, the test must be much more specific for it to be clinically useful.

Predictive values are especially clinically relevant because they utilize information on both the test itself and the population being tested. This introduces the concept of prior probabilities, which is essentially the prevalence of a disease in a single test subject. Prior probability is determined based on the subject's demographics and clinical presentation. Unfortunately, delineating these values on a single subject in order to calculate the positive predictive value in a population of patients is difficult. The calculation for positive predictive value (PV), which is beyond the scope of this chapter, is provided by Bayes theorem:

$$\text{Positive PV} = \text{Likelihood of a true positive}/$$
$$[\text{Likelihood of a true positive} +$$
$$\text{Likelihood of a false positive}]$$

SUMMARY

Correctly analyzing and interpreting conclusions is the cornerstone of modern medical practice. The use of the clinical history, substantiation with the clinical exam, and corroboration with clinical studies to diagnose a patient is predicated on the available scientific studies in the literature. The physical exam requires not only knowledge of how to perform a specific maneuver and its nuances but also knowledge of how the results of a specific test support or challenge a given diagnosis. The reliability and validity of a particular diagnostic exam maneuver will establish the sensitivity and specificity statistics. Understanding the scientific method of a particular study and how its results can be applied to the community at large is critical.

REFERENCES

1. Venn J. On the diagrammatic and mechanical representation of propositions and reasonings. *Philosoph Magazine J Sci S.* 1880;9: 1-18.
2. Browner WS, Newman TB, Cummings SR. Designing a new study. III: Diagnostic tests. In: Hulley SB, Cummings SR, eds. *Designing Clinical Research.* Baltimore: Williams & Wilkins; 1988:87-97.

3. Hulley SB, Newman TB, Cummings SR. Getting started: the anatomy and physiology of research. In: Hulley SB, Cummings SR, eds. *Designing Clinical Research*. Baltimore: Williams & Wilkins; 1988:1-11.

4. Hulley SB, Cummings SR. Planning the measurements: precision and accuracy. In: Hulley SB, Cummings SR, eds. *Designing Clinical Research*. Baltimore: Williams & Wilkins; 1988:31-41.

5. Rabin A, Irrgang JJ, Fitzgerald GK, et al. The intertester reliability of the Scapular Assistance Test. *J Orthop Sports Phys Ther*. 2006; 36:653-660.

6. Hulley SB, Gove S, Browner WS, et al. Choosing the study subjects: specification and sampling. In: Hulley SB, Cummings SR, eds. *Designing Clinical Research*. Baltimore: Williams & Wilkins; 1988: 18-30.

7. Andersson GB, Deyo RA. History and physical examination in patients with herniated lumbar discs. *Spine*. 1996;21(suppl 24): 10S-18S.

8. Katz JW, Fingeroth RJ. The diagnostic accuracy of ruptures of the anterior cruciate ligament comparing the Lachman test, the anterior drawer sign, and the pivot shift test in acute and chronic knee injuries. *Am J Sports Med*. 1986;14:88-91.

2 Sensory, Motor, and Reflex Examination

Jeffrey A. Strakowski, MD | Matthew J. Fanous, MD | John Kincaid, MD

INTRODUCTION

The neurologic examination is an integral component of any musculoskeletal assessment. Determining the relative integrity of the neurologic system is an important step toward arriving at a proper diagnosis and ultimately appropriate management. Neurologic and musculoskeletal injuries can often mimic each other, and the symptoms from the patient's history are not always reliable and specific. Objective findings from appropriately performed sensory, motor, and reflex testing can provide clarity for differentiating these categories of conditions. When a neurologic deficit is present, integration of the results of the different techniques of sensory, motor, and reflex testing should be used to localize the lesion to the extent possible. Additional diagnostic testing should be considered when further clarification of the clinical examination is needed.

SENSORY EXAMINATION

The sensory examination is often the most challenging and time-consuming portion of the neurologic evaluation. When assessing a sensory disturbance, the examination should always be performed in the context of a detailed history, including the nature, distribution, and pattern of onset. Sensory complaints can be characterized by positive or negative symptoms. Examples of positive symptoms include spontaneous sensations such has tingling or shocking. Paresthesias are examples of positive symptoms and are described as tingling or pins and needles occurring spontaneously. Symptoms like this arising from nonnoxious stimuli are termed *allodynia*. Examples of negative symptoms include the lack of normal cutaneous sensation in a certain distribution or inability to identify the location of a body area in space. *Numb, dead, woody,* or *leathery* are terms used by patients to report negative symptoms.

The role of formal sensory testing is to establish objective evidence of the function of the sensory system. Subjective reports of sensory disturbance have less specificity and frequently less accuracy for establishing and localizing a sensory deficit. By contrast, diagnostic certainty is substantially improved by establishing sensory deficit in a specific distribution. It is also clinically useful to determine if the distribution of complaint is the same as the actual sensory deficit. With this in mind, the examiner should make every effort to be consistent in examination technique and to demonstrate reproducibility in the findings.[1] All sensory testing requires cooperation from the patient; however, it should be performed in a manner that minimizes subjectivity from both the patient and the examiner. Actions to improve reliability include confirming the patient understands the test, shielding the examination from the patient's line of site, and repeating the testing. Using tools such as Semmes-Weinstein monofilaments can add objectivity to the evaluation when needed.[2]

Sensory testing is not considered highly sensitive for a neurologic deficit.[3] It has been postulated that at least 50% of the sensory fibers of a peripheral nerve must be dysfunctional before a consistent clinical deficit is detectable. The sensory studies should always be used within the context of the motor and reflex examination as well. The extent of the sensory testing employed should usually be based on the context of the other examination findings.

Sensory deficits can occur as a result of CNS or peripheral nerve system injuries. Light touch and pin prick assessments are the most commonly used tests. Two-point discrimination can be valuable for assessment of both central and peripheral nerve lesions. Techniques to assess multiple sensory pathways are more frequently used in CNS lesions and include light touch, pressure, pain, temperature, vibration, and proprioception.[4] A detailed knowledge of the sensory pathways is needed to reliably localize a lesion to the peripheral versus CNS insults. A detailed discussion of this anatomy is beyond the scope of this chapter. Peripheral nerve lesions should be differentiated between root level, plexus, main nerve trunk, or distal branch level. Knowledge of the dermatome patterns and peripheral nerve cutaneous patterns can help distinguish these potential lesion sites (Fig. 2.1; Video 2-1). The distribution of sensory disturbance can help localize the source of the insult. Sensory loss in the pattern of a dermatome suggests a radicular lesion, whereas a mononeuropathy will have a deficit limited to a peripheral nerve main trunk or one of its branches.[5,6] When the pattern extends beyond a single nerve but remains in peripheral nerve patterns, a plexopathy or polyneuropathy is considered. Generalized, length-dependent neuropathies often produce a "stocking-glove" pattern. In this condition, the distal zone of maximum deficit gradually merges with a zone of less diminished sensation, and then into a region of normal sensation. When a generalized neuropathy is present, the examiner should be vigilant for focal neuropathies superimposed on a more generalized neuropathy. Identifying superimposed lesions requires appropriate history taking and often detailed side-to-side comparisons.

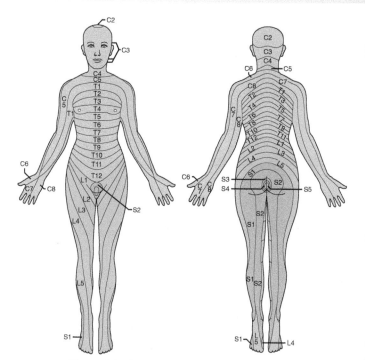

Figure 2.1   Illustration of the dermatome map.

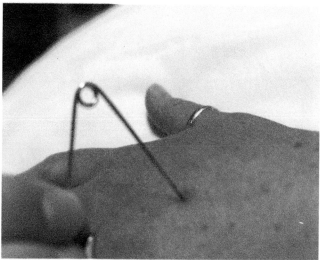

Figure 2.2   Demonstration of the use of a safety pin to assess pain sensation.

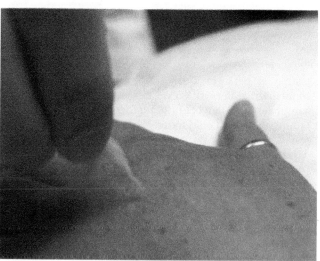

Figure 2.3   Demonstration of the use of a cotton wisp to assess light touch.

Spinal cord pathology should be considered when a sensory impairment is seen in a distribution below a specific dermatomal level. Loss of sensation of the upper limbs and/or upper portion of the truncal area with sparing of the lower limbs or sacral sparing should raise the suspicion of an expanding intraspinal mass. The converse of this, with predominantly lower limb sensory loss, can be seen in the presence of a syrinx.[7] Sensory disturbance on an entire side of the body suggests a central nervous system (CNS) lesion. Concomitant sensory loss on the same side of the face localizes the lesion to above the level of the pons. Sensory examination findings that do not follow physiologic boundaries can be suggestive of nonorganic etiology. Facial sensory disturbances that cross midline, as in a perioral pattern, can be associated with anxiety.

Distinguishing whether the sensory loss is across all modalities or selective can be useful to help determine the source of the deficit. For example, temperature and pain sensation are transmitted along small-diameter nerve fibers and then to the spinothalamic tract. Vibration perception is transmitted via large-diameter, heavily myelinated nerve fibers and then to the dorsal column–medial lemniscus tracts. Selective loss of sensation in these modalities can aid in localization of the lesion and in understanding its mechanism.[8]

Sensory function can be divided clinically into primary and secondary (aka cortical) modalities. Primary modalities include light touch, pressure, pain, temperature, proprioception, and vibration sense. Cortical modalities require the synthesis and integration of the input from the primary modalities. This includes modalities such as two-point discrimination, stereognosis, and graphesthesia. Damage at the level of the parietal lobe can cause impairment of the secondary modalities when the primary modalities are intact. The best screening tests for sensory abnormality in a typical musculoskeletal examination are pain and light touch. The screening for pain sensory function is the use of a safety pin to lightly prick the regions of concern (Fig. 2.2). The patient is asked whether the pinprick feels sharp in the affected area and typically in the same location of the opposite limb. While the examiner uses both the sharp and dull portion of the safety pin, the patient, with eyes closed, is asked to report whether the sensation is sharp or dull. A cotton wisp can be used to test light touch. The patient, with eyes closed, is asked to report when the cotton is felt (Fig. 2.3).

Cortical sensory function can be evaluated with two-point discrimination, stereognosis, and graphesthesia. Two-point discrimination is performed by using two points, such as the tips of an unfolded paper clip to touch two closely separated locations on the skin.[9,10] The patient's eyes should be closed, and he or she asked ask if he or she can feel one or two points[11] (Fig. 2.4). Stereognosis testing is performed by asking the patient to identify a familiar object, such as a key or coin placed in the palm of the hand. Graphesthesia

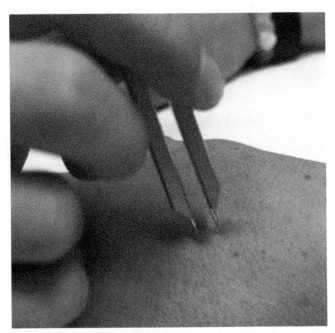

Figure 2.4 Demonstration of the use of calipers to assess two-point discrimination.

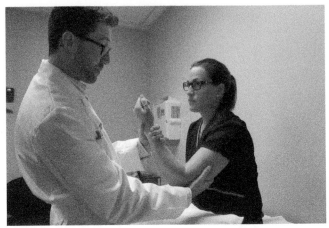

Figure 2.5 Demonstration of the technique of manual muscle testing.

testing is performed by asking the patient to identify numbers that are written on the palm. Temperature sense can be tested with a cold tuning fork or with test tubes containing warm and cold water. When cold sensation is being tested, the body part must be normally warm.[12]

Joint position sense is tested by moving the terminal phalanx of a patient's finger or toe up or down a few degrees. If the patient cannot identify these tiny movements with eyes closed, similar testing should be performed on the larger joints such as the metacarpal phalangeal joint or wrist. The body part being tested should be grasped on the sides rather than the dorsal or ventral aspect to prevent the patient from using pressure cues to detect movement.

To test vibration sense, the examiner places a finger under the patient's distal interphalangeal joint and presses a lightly tapped 128-cycle tuning fork on top of the joint. The patient detects the vibration and then notes its extinction about the same time as the examiner, who feels it through the patient's digit.[13] The age and size of the patient should be considered when assessing abnormalities of vibration sense.[14] Devices designed to improve quantitative measurement of vibration sensation can also be used.[15,16]

PROVOCATIVE MANEUVERS

Provocative maneuvers for eliciting sensory symptoms are notoriously nonspecific for reliably distinguishing true neurologic deficit, but they can sometimes provide clinical clues to the source of pain complaints. An example of this is a patient with chronic pain such as fibromyalgia, whose complaints of paresthesias are magnified by muscle palpation. Tender or "trigger" points in muscle can lead to reporting sensations described as paresthesias but are not related to an identifiable neurologic deficit.

Other maneuvers can potentially lead to dynamic nerve compression and provide clinical clues that contribute to

localization of the source of a pain generator, but they are not specific for either neurologic deficit or nerve entrapment. Examples include the Spurling test in cervical radiculopathy, Adson test in thoracic outlet entrapment, and Phalen sign in median nerve entrapment at the carpal tunnel. Techniques of this nature can potentially produce neurologic or neurologic-like symptoms, but they cannot be expected to alter the sensory examination.

Tapping over a suspected focal peripheral neuropathy to reproduce neuritic symptoms and assess for sensitivity is a frequently cited technique and has been termed the *Tinel sign*. Tinel originally described this technique as a method to determine the location of recovery of regenerating axons after trauma. In his description, the presence of the sign at the location that was being tapped was indicative that the nerve had regenerated to that position.[17,18] Localized sensitivity can develop over an area of peripheral nerve injury; however, percussion over a normal peripheral nerve in a superficial location will also induce pain and paresthesias. The use of this technique should not be considered reliable confirmation of a focal entrapment neuropathy.

MOTOR EXAMINATION

The role of motor testing is to assess the patient's strength. Reports of weakness are not always due to a true motor deficit. Some complain of weakness when they are actually referring to fatigue, malaise, or incoordination. Strength testing is not the same as power, which refers to the rate of performing work. Manual muscle testing is the most commonly used technique for testing strength. With manual muscle testing, the strength of specific muscle groups is tested against resistance, and one side of the body is compared with the other. It is performed by providing a counterforce on a specific point on the limb against the patient's best effort[19] (Fig. 2.5; Video 2-2).

There are a variety of different classification systems for grading manual muscle testing. Most are based on the Medical Research Council 0–5 scale[20] (Table 2.1).

There have been significant modifications of this format by many authors. Most of these scales give ordinal data. This

Table 2.1   Medical Research Council 0–5 Scale

Objective Grade	Qualitative Description	Observation	Range of Motion
5	Normal	Antigravity plus full resistance	Full range of motion
4	Diminished	Antigravity plus some resistance	Full range of motion
3	At least antigravity	Antigravity only	Full range of motion
2	Poor	Gravity omitted	Full range of motion
1	Trace	Evidence of activation	Partial range of motion
0	No activation	No evidence of activation	n/a

n/a, not applicable.

means the values are on an arbitrary numerical scale where the exact numerical quantity has no significance beyond its ability to establish a ranking over the other values. Some of the modifications have been created to provide a designation between these ordinal measures.

In the Medical Research Council scale, the grades of 0, 1, and 2 are tested in a position that minimizes the effect of gravity. This is performed while having the patient's contraction perpendicular to gravitational force. Grades of 3, 4, and 5 are tested with the contraction against gravity. One difficulty with the higher grades in this system is that gravity has more impact on heavier limbs or body regions compared with smaller areas. An example is testing hip flexion in a supine position in comparison with toe extension. Detecting subtle weakness in strong muscles with relatively short lever arms such as the gastroc-soleus complex can also be challenging with manual testing.

Another difficulty with the comparison of higher grades between different examiners is the relative subjectivity of the assessment. Distinguishing mild weakness can be dependent on multiple factors. This includes the size, age, fitness level, and general health of the patient.[21,22] It also can be potentially affected by those same factors in the examiner.[23,24] Other factors can complicate the assessment including orthopedic conditions that preclude full range of motion and other sources of pain or psychological factors that might limit full effort.

Some authors have presented other manual muscle testing protocols in an effort to minimize some of these limitations. Daniels and Worthingham proposed a more functional grading system by testing motion that uses all of the agonists and synergists involved in a particular motion.[25] Kendall and McCreary proposed testing a specific muscle rather than a motion for strength.[26] This method requires a considerably higher skill level with detailed knowledge of anatomy and kinesiology. Regardless of the method used, challenges of subjectivity and variability of patient effort remain.

It is best to use a grading system for motor testing that will be understood by other practitioners who might also be caring for the patient. It is therefore preferable to use a highly reproducible, easily performed examination. A consistent method of performing the examination is necessary for reproducible results.[27]

The testing should be explained to the patient in simple terms to invoke optimum cooperation. In the presence of asymmetric weakness, the testing should first be performed on the uninvolved or less involved side. This helps to properly gauge the contralateral strength and establish that the patient understands the directions for the involved side.

The limbs being examined should first be assessed for passive motion limitations such as joint deformity or joint or muscle contracture. Any orthopedic limitation affecting normal motion should be noted and accounted for when considering strength.

Each muscle group or limb motion should be tested in a consistent fashion. Differences in the point of application of the resistive force will result in varying assessments of strength.[28] Shorter lever arms provide higher strength against the same resistance as longer lever arms. The application of resistance should be as distal as possible from the axis of movement on the moving segment without crossing another joint. The patient should be positioned comfortably on a firm surface with the limb in the correct testing position. The correct testing position ensures that the muscle fibers are correctly aligned. Resistance is applied in a direction opposite the muscle's rotary component and at right angles to the line of the pull of the muscle fibers. The resistance should be applied gradually to give the patient sufficient time to provide resistance. The proximal segment that uses counterpressure to the examiner's resistance should be stabilized to avoid unnecessary movement or muscle substitution. It can be beneficial to place some stronger muscles in a position of mechanical disadvantage when investigating subtle weakness. For example, when assessing strength of the triceps brachii, place the elbow in 90 degrees of flexion instead of full extension, thus limiting the resistance of the extended joint.

When the patient demonstrates that he or she can move the area of interest through full range of motion against gravity, then resistance is applied. If the patient is unable to oppose gravity, then the test movement is positioned in a direction, usually in the transverse plane, to minimize the influence of gravity. Some recommend that the test be repeated up to three times for consistency to determine the muscle strength grade.[29] Manual muscle testing for weakness should include not only muscles in a pattern of the various myotomes, but consideration should also be given to the pattern of peripheral nerves and their branches when appropriate.

OTHER MEASUREMENT TOOLS

Motor testing can be better quantified by use of various measurement tools. A method of strength testing using dedicated measuring devices such as dynameters, strain gauges, and other apparatus is called dynamometry. There are tools available that provide both isometric and isokinetic assessments.[30,31] Isometric testing provides information about force production with a specific, fixed joint angle.

Isokinetic testing measures torque across a joint as it moves through its range of motion.[32,33]

Advantages of testing with these tools include providing interval data with a continuous scale of grades in contrast to the more limited ordinal scale used with conventional manual muscle testing. For this reason, quantitative motor testing with dynamometry typically provides better information for subtle changes in strength that would not be reliably reflected in manual muscle tests.[34,35] Dynamometry is also useful for greater reproducibility in clinical trials. Disadvantages of motor assessment with dynamometry include a relative limitation of muscle groups that can be reliably tested.[36] Follow-up testing by another clinician would require that the clinician also have the same tools available. Additionally, some of the tools for testing, particularly for isokinetic assessment, can be relatively expensive.[37]

FUNCTIONAL MEASURES

Functional assessments are also an important component of motor testing both as a screening test and for identifying deficiencies that might not be evident with routine motor testing. Isolation of specific muscles is often challenging because they generally work in conjunction with synergistic and antagonist muscles.[38] Additionally, the components of the motor cortex represent movements rather than contractions of individual muscles.[39] Assessments of gait or active shoulder motion are examples of complex motor evaluations that can serve as a screen for underlying weakness. Tests such as single leg squats or toe raises can demonstrate side-to-side asymmetry in strength that might not be evident with routine manual muscle testing.

EXAMINATION OF REFLEXES

Reflex testing assesses both sensory and motor pathways and is considered one of the more objective components of the neurologic evaluation.[40] The commonly used reflexes are known as muscle stretch reflexes, or they are sometimes referred to as myotatic reflexes. The muscle stretch reflex is a muscle contraction that occurs in response to stretching of the muscle.[41] This monosynaptic reflex provides regulation of skeletal muscle length in healthy individuals and can be used for diagnostic assessment.[42]

When a muscle lengthens, receptors within the muscle fibers called muscle spindles are activated. This causes afferent sensory neuron depolarization, which travels through the dorsal root ganglion into the spinal cord and synapses with alpha motor neurons in the anterior horn of the spinal cord.[43] This leads to depolarization of the alpha motor neurons at the same and adjacent spinal levels, causing the muscle fibers to contract and resist the stretch (Fig. 2.6). At the same time the reflex is activated, other neurons cause the antagonistic muscle to relax. The entire cascade serves to maintain the muscle at a constant length.

The term *deep tendon reflex* does not accurately reflect the mechanism of this phenomenon. The reflex's response begins with stretch responsive receptors in the muscle fibers, not tendon. Additionally, some reflexes, such as the jaw jerk reflex, do not involve tendon at all. Therefore, the use of this term is discouraged.

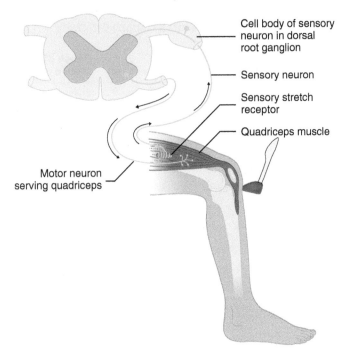

Cell body of sensory neuron in dorsal root ganglion

Sensory neuron

Sensory stretch receptor

Quadriceps muscle

Motor neuron serving quadriceps

Figure 2.6   Illustration of the reflex arc.

The clinical muscle stretch reflex is performed by rapidly striking the tendon of the muscle of interest (Fig. 2.7; Video 2-3). The rapid stretch on the tendon transmits the mechanical impulse to the muscle spindle, activating the reflex. In healthy patients, the response in the form of muscle contraction is seen within 25 milliseconds of the muscle stretch impulse.[44] Muscle stretch reflexes can be performed with either a reflex hammer or with a manual technique. There are various types of reflex hammers available, and the type for clinical use generally is a result of personal preference.[45] (Fig. 2.8). The author's recommendation is to use a manual technique to remove an additional barrier between the patient and the examiner. This is performed by striking the tendon of interest with slightly curved and rigidly held long and ring fingers (Fig. 2.9). This method also alleviates the need to keep track of a reflex hammer.

With whatever technique is used, a short, sharp blow is applied to a tendon, with the muscle of interest kept in minimal extension. The hand that is not responsible for the tendon tap should be held on the muscle being tested. This allows the examiner to feel the muscle response instead of relying only on visual perception to assess for contraction. The patient should be properly positioned and kept as relaxed as possible. Muscle stretch reflexes can be inhibited by anxiety and tension.[46] It is often helpful to use facilitation by placing tension on the tendon of the antagonist muscle or even distraction by having the patient contract muscles in other limbs.[47-49]

Muscle stretch reflexes are affected by the supraspinal CNS. This is done by influencing gamma motor neurons, which regulate the sensitivity of the muscle stretch reflex by tightening or relaxing the fibers within the muscle spindle.[50-52] Common muscle stretch reflexes tested include the jaw jerk (CN V), biceps brachii (C5–C6), brachioradialis (C5–C6), extensor digitorum (C6–C7), triceps brachii

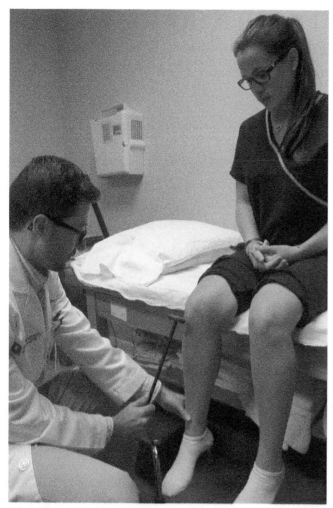

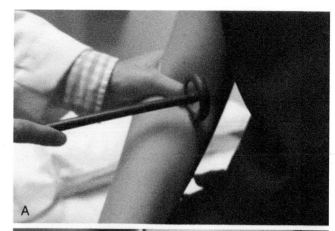

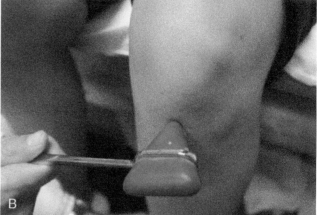

Figure 2.8 Demonstration of the use of different reflex hammers for eliciting muscle stretch reflexes. **A,** Babinski reflex hammer. **B,** Taylor hammer.

Figure 2.7 Demonstration of the technique for eliciting the muscle stretch reflex. In this case, the quadriceps reflex is elicited by briskly striking the patellar tendon, with the patient's knee in a relaxed and flexed position.

(C7–C8), quadriceps (ie, patellar) (L3–L4), semimembranosus (L5, S1), and gastrocnemius (aka Achilles or ankle) (S1, S2).[53] Side-to-side comparisons should always be used with these reflexes to assess for variations.

The most frequently used grading system for muscle stretch reflexes is that of the National Institute of Neurological Disorders and Stroke (NINDS) scale.[54] This is a 5-point scale that ranges from 0 to 5. Zero represents an absent reflex and is virtually always considered abnormal.[55,56] Other values are defined as follows: A score of 1+ represents a diminished reflex and might be normal or abnormal; 2+ represents normal reflexes; 3+ represents a brisk reflex and might be normal or abnormal; 4+ represents a brisk reflex with the presence of clonus, a series of involuntary muscular contractions and relaxations; and 4+ is always considered abnormal.

Consideration should be given to the age of the patient when interpreting reflexes.[57] Individuals without neurologic deficit will experience a decline in reflex response with aging.[58,59] Multiple other factors can influence muscle stretch reflexes, including endocrine changes, medica-

tions, diseases, and drugs.[60-62] The findings should always be used in clinical context. The diagnostic specificity of clearly abnormal reflexes is relatively good, but the presence of normal reflexes does not exclude a neurologic deficit.[63]

PATHOLOGICAL REFLEXES

CLONUS

Clonus is a series of involuntary rhythmic muscle contractions elicited by a rapid passive stretching of a muscle. It is due to a lesion in descending motor neurons and is often associated with increased muscle stretch reflexes and spasticity.[64,65] Clonus is most commonly seen at the ankle but can be found at the ankle, knee, wrist, jaw, or elbow.[66] Clonus can be seen in virtually any muscle group and generally repeats with a frequency of 5 to 8 Hz.[67]

PLANTAR REFLEX

The plantar reflex is a reflex elicited when the sole of the foot is stroked, often with a blunt instrument (Fig. 2.10). In normal adults, the reflex causes flexion of the hallux (Fig. 2.11). An abnormal response, also known as the Babinski sign, named after Joseph Babinski,[68,69] is an extension of the hallux (Fig. 2.12). An abnormal plantar reflex can represent dysfunction of the pyramidal tract. It can sometimes be the

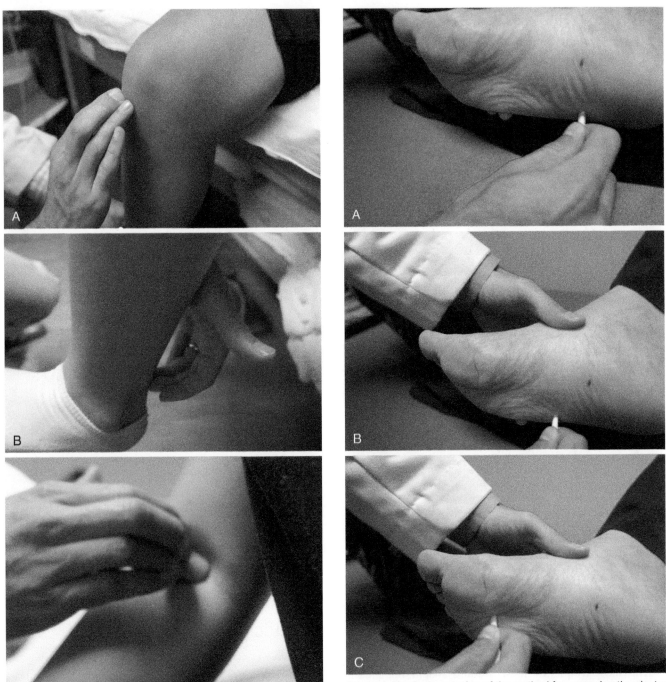

Figure 2.9 Demonstration of the manual technique for eliciting muscle stretch reflexes without a hammer. The fingers are tapped briskly on the tendon. **A,** Patellar. **B,** Achilles. **C,** Biceps Brachii.

Figure 2.10 Demonstration of the method for assessing the plantar reflex. The lateral side of the foot is stroked from the heel along a curve to the area of the metatarsal pads. The progression of movement is shown in **A, B** and **C.**

first and only indication of a CNS lesion. The initial response of the toe should be carefully observed when the reflex appears abnormal. Normal withdrawal with extension of the toes can occur by the patient after the reflex is complete.

HOFFMAN'S REFLEX

Hoffman's reflex (aka finger flexor reflex) is performed by tapping or flicking the terminal phalanx of the long or ring finger. The Hoffman's sign is a positive test that is demonstrated by reflexive flexion of the terminal phalanx of the thumb with this maneuver (Fig. 2.13, Video 2-4). Unlike the Babinski sign, the Hoffman's sign can be seen in normal adults that are naturally somewhat hyperreflexic. The finding more likely represents upper motor neuron pathology when it is an acute onset or unilateral. Hoffman's sign should be interpreted within the context of other neurologic signs and is not considered a good screening test in asymptomatic individuals.[70,71] The mechanism is

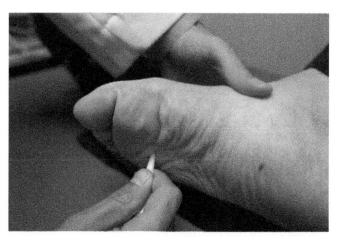

Figure 2.11 Demonstration of the plantar reflex in a normal adult. Note the flexion of the toes after the sole of the foot is stroked.

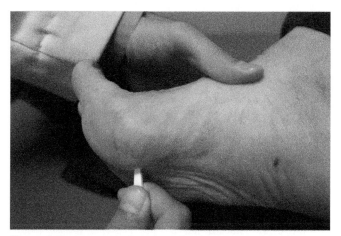

Figure 2.12 Demonstration of an abnormal plantar reflex (Babinski sign) with extension of the hallux after the foot is stroked.

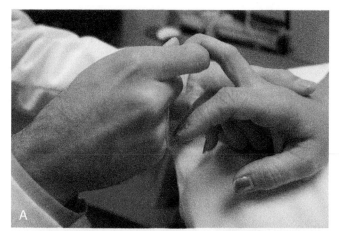

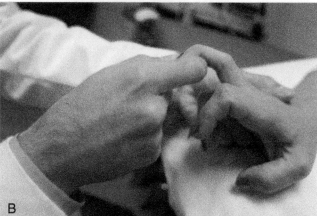

Figure 2.13 A, Demonstration of testing of Hoffman's reflex. **B,** A position of rapid flexion of the terminal phalanx of the thumb occurs in a positive test.

different between the Hoffman's reflex and the plantar reflex. Hoffman's reflex is a monosynaptic muscle stretch reflex, and the plantar reflex is more complicated and not completely understood.[72]

CONCLUSION

The sensory, motor, and reflex examinations should all be performed and integrated to help localize a neurologic deficit to the extent possible. The underlying basis or source of the deficit is more frequently obtained from a detailed history, but the extent of the deficit is obtained from a properly performed physical examination. The history and physical examination should be used to create a differential diagnosis that should guide appropriate use of any additional diagnostic testing. The practitioner should resist relying on imaging and other testing without first creating the proper context with the history and physical examination. Each examination technique has limitations of specificity and sensitivity, but when taken together, sensory, motor, and reflex tests are invaluable components of the neurologic examination.

REFERENCES

1. Dyck PJ, O'Brien PC, Kosanke JL, et al. A 4, 2, and 1 stepping algorithm for quick and accurate estimation of cutaneous sensation threshold. *Neurology.* 1993;43:1508-1512.
2. Bell-Krotoski J. Advances in sensibility evaluation. *Hand Clin.* 1991;7:527-546.
3. Bell-Krotoski J, Weinstein S, Weinstein C. Testing sensibility, including touch-pressure, two-point discrimination, point localization, and vibration. *J Hand Ther.* 1993;6:114-123.
4. Gruener G, Dyck PJ. Quantitative sensory testing: methodology, applications, and future directions. *J Clin Neurophysiol.* 1994;11: 568-583.
5. Inouye Y, Buchthal F. Segmental sensory innervation determined by potentials recorded from cervical spinal nerves. *Brain.* 1977; 100:731-748.
6. Mazurek MT, Shin AY. Upper extremity peripheral nerve anatomy: current concepts and applications. *Clin Orthop Relat Res.* 2001; 383:7-20.
7. Freeman C, Okun MS. Origins of the sensory examination in neurology. *Semin Neurol.* 2002;22:399-408.
8. Dyck PJ, Dyck PJ, Larson TS, et al. Patterns of quantitative sensation testing of hypoesthesia and hyperalgesia are predictive of diabetic polyneuropathy: a study of three cohorts. Nerve growth factor study group. *Diabetes Care.* 2000;23:510-517.
9. Finnell JT, Knopp R, Johnson P, et al. A calibrated paper clip is a reliable measure of two-point discrimination. *Acad Emerg Med.* 2004;11:710-714.
10. Lundborg G, Rosén B. The two-point discrimination test—time for a re-appraisal? *J Hand Surg [Br].* 2004;29:418-422.
11. Dellon AL, Mackinnon SE, Crosby PM. Reliability of two-point discrimination measurements. *J Hand Surg [Am].* 1987;12(Pt 1):693-696.

12. Dyck PJ, Zimmerman I, Gillen DA, et al. Cool, warm, and heat-pain detection thresholds: testing methods and inferences about anatomic distribution of receptors. *Neurology.* 1993;43:1500-1508.

13. Huizing EH. The early descriptions of the so-called tuning-fork tests of Weber, Rinne, Schwabach, and Bing. II. The "Rhine Test" and its first description by Polansky. *ORL J Otorhinolaryngol Relat Spec.* 1975;37:88-91.

14. Burns TM, Taly A, O'Brien PC, et al. Clinical versus quantitative vibration assessment: improving clinical performance. *J Peripher Nerv Syst.* 2002;7:112-117.

15. Gerr FE, Letz R. Reliability of a widely used test of peripheral cutaneous vibration sensitivity and a comparison of two testing protocols. *Br J Ind Med.* 1988;45:635-639.

16. Deng H, He F, Zhang S, et al. Quantitative measurements of vibration threshold in healthy adults and acrylamide workers. *Int Arch Occup Environ Health.* 1993;65:53-56.

17. Tinel J. *Nerve Wounds. Symptomatology of Peripheral Nerve Lesions Caused by War Wounds.* London: Bailliere, Tinall and Cox; 1918.

18. Spinner M. *Injuries to the Major Branches of Peripheral Nerves of the Forearm.* With a translation of J. Tinel's original "Fourmillement" paper by Emanuel B. Kaplan, MD. 2nd ed. Philadelphia: W.B. Saunders Company; 1978:6-13.

19. Lilienfeld AM, Jacobs M, Willis M. A study of the reproducibility of muscle testing and certain other aspects of muscle scoring. *Phys Ther Rev.* 1954;34:279-289.

20. Medical Research Council. *Aids to the Investigation of the Peripheral Nervous System.* London: HMSO; 1975.

21. Jaric S. Muscle strength testing: use of normalisation for body size. *Sports Med.* 2002;32:615-631.

22. Vanpee G, Hermans G, Segers J, et al. Assessment of limb muscle strength in critically ill patients: a systematic review. *Crit Care Med.* 2014;42:701-711.

23. Mulroy SJ, Lassen KD, Chambers SH, et al. The ability of male and female clinicians to effectively test knee extension strength using manual muscle testing. *J Orthop Sports Phys Ther.* 1997;26:192-199.

24. Lu TW, Hsu HC, Chang LY, et al. Enhancing the examiner's resisting force improves the reliability of manual muscle strength measurements: comparison of a new device with hand-held dynamometry. *J Rehabil Med.* 2007;39:679-684.

25. Daniels K, Worthingham C. *Muscle Testing Techniques of Manual Examination.* 5th ed. Philadelphia: W.B. Saunders; 1986.

26. Kendall FP, McCreary EK, Provance PG. *Muscles: Testing and Function.* Baltimore: Williams & Wilkins; 1993.

27. Florence JM, Pandya S, King WM. Intrarater reliability of manual muscle test (Medical Research Council scale) grades in Duchenne's muscular dystrophy. *Phys Ther.* 1992;72:115-122, discussion 122-126.

28. Barbic S, Brouwer B. Test position and hip strength in healthy adults and people with chronic stroke. *Arch Phys Med Rehabil.* 2008;89:784-787.

29. Symons TB, Vandervoort AA, Rice CL, et al. Reliability of a single-session isokinetic and isometric strength measurement protocol in older men. *J Gerontol A Biol Sci Med Sci.* 2005;60:114-119.

30. Emery CA, Maitland ME, Meeuwisse WH. Test-retest reliabilty of isokinetic hip adductor and flexor muscle strength. *Clin J Sport Med.* 1999;9:79-85.

31. Gaines JM, Talbot LA. Isokinetic strength testing in research and practice. *Biol Res Nurs.* 1999;1:57-64.

32. Osternig LR. Isokinetic dynamometry: implications for muscle testing and rehabilitation. *Exerc Sport Sci Rev.* 1986;14:45-80.

33. Baltzopoulos V, Brodie DA. Isokinetic dynamometry. Applications and limitations. *Sports Med.* 1989;8:101-116.

34. Bohannon RW. Manual muscle test scores and dynamometer test scores of knee extension strength. *Arch Phys Med Rehabil.* 1986;67:390-392.

35. Dekkers KJ, Rameckers EA, Smeets RJ. Upper extremity strength measurement for children with cerebral palsy: a systematic review of available instruments. *Phys Ther.* 2014;94:609-622.

36. Visser J, Mans E, de Visser M, et al. Comparison of maximal voluntary isometric contraction and hand-held dynamometry in measuring muscle strength of patients with progressive lower motor neuron syndrome. *Neuromuscul Disord.* 2003;13:744-750.

37. El Mhandi L, Bethoux F. Isokinetic testing in patients with neuromuscular diseases: a focused review. *Am J Phys Med Rehabil.* 2013;92:163-178.

38. Kannus P. Isokinetic evaluation of muscular performance: implications for muscle testing and rehabilitation. *Int J Sports Med.* 1994;15(suppl 1):S11-S118.

39. Ropper A, Samuels M, Klein J. *Adams and Victor's Principles of Neurology.* 10th ed. New York: McGraw-Hill Education Medical; 2014.

40. Paulson GW. Reflexes and neurologists. *Clin Neurol Neurosurg.* 1992;94(suppl):S133-S1366.

41. Louis ED, Kaufmann P. Erb's explanation for the tendon reflexes. Links between science and the clinic. *Arch Neurol.* 1996;53:1187-1189.

42. Litvan I, Mangone CA, Werden W, et al. Reliability of the NINDS Myotatic Reflex Scale. *Neurology.* 1996;47:969-972.

43. Morita H, Petersen N, Christensen LO, et al. Sensitivity of H-reflexes and stretch reflexes to presynaptic inhibition in humans. *J Neurophysiol.* 1998;80:610-620.

44. Burke D, Gandevia SC, McKeon B. Monosynaptic and oligosynaptic contributions to human ankle jerk and H-reflex. *J Neurophysiol.* 1984;52(3):435-448.

45. Marshall GL, Little JW. Deep tendon reflexes: a study of quantitative methods. *J Spinal Cord Med.* 2002;25:94-99.

46. Dick JP. The deep tendon and the abdominal reflexes. *J Neurol Neurosurg Psychiatry.* 2003;74:150-153.

47. Bussel B, Morin C, Pierrot-Deseilligny E. Mechanism of monosynaptic reflex reinforcement during Jendrassik manoeuvre in man. *J Neurol Neurosurg Psychiatry.* 1978;41:40-44.

48. Burke D, McKeon B, Skuse NF. Dependence of the Achilles tendon reflex on the excitability of spinal reflex pathways. *Ann Neurol.* 1981;10:551-556.

49. Rossi-Durand C. The influence of increased muscle spindle sensitivity on Achilles tendon jerk and H-reflex in relaxed human subjects. *Somatosens Mot Res.* 2002;19:286-295.

50. Polus BI, Patak A, Gregory JE, et al. Effect of muscle length on phasic stretch reflexes in humans and cats. *J Neurophysiol.* 1991;66:613-622.

51. Gregory JE, Wood SA, Proske U. An investigation into mechanisms of reflex reinforcement by the Jendrassik manoeuvre. *Exp Brain Res.* 2001;138:366-374.

52. Enríquez-Denton M, Morita H, Christensen LO, et al. Interaction between peripheral afferent activity and presynaptic inhibition of ia afferents in the cat. *J Neurophysiol.* 2002;88:1664-1674.

53. Felsenthal G, Reischer MA. Asymmetric hamstring reflexes indicative of L5 radicular lesions. *Arch Phys Med Rehabil.* 1982;63:377-378.

54. Manschot S, van Passel L, Buskens E, et al. Mayo and NINDS scales for assessment of tendon reflexes: between observer agreement and implications for communication. *J Neurol Neurosurg Psychiatry.* 1998;64:253-255.

55. Bowditch MG, Sanderson P, Livesey JP. The significance of an absent ankle reflex. *J Bone Joint Surg Br.* 1996;78:276-279.

56. Vrancken AF, Kalmijn S, Brugman F, et al. The meaning of distal sensory loss and absent ankle reflexes in relation to age: a meta-analysis. *J Neurol.* 2006;253:578-589.

57. O'Keeffe ST, Smith T, Valacio R, et al. A comparison of two techniques for ankle jerk assessment in elderly subjects. *Lancet.* 1994;344:1619-1620.

58. Kamen G, Koceja DM. Contralateral influences on patellar tendon reflexes in young and old adults. *Neurobiol Aging.* 1989;10:311-315.

59. Chandrasekhar A, Abu Osman NA, et al. Influence of age on patellar tendon reflex response. *PLoS ONE.* 2013;8(11):e80799.

60. Moreau L, Philbert M. [Modifications in the Achillean reflexogram under the influence of quick-acting barbiturates]. [Article in French] *Ann Endocrinol (Paris).* 1968;29(6):781-798.

61. Shafer RB, Nuttall FQ. Achilles reflex in thyroid disorders: a 10-year clinical evaluation. *Am J Med Sci.* 1972;264(4):313-317.

62. Dry J, Leynadier F, Pradalier A, et al. [Changes in Achilles tendon reflex under influence of nonendocrine factors]. [Article in French] *Sem Hop.* 1976;52:1697-1401.

63. Stam J. [Physical diagnostics—tendon reflexes]. [Article in Dutch] *Ned Tijdschr Geneeskd.* 1999;143:848-851.

64. Wallace DM, Ross BH, Thomas CK. Motor unit behavior during clonus. *J Appl Physiol.* 2005;99(6):2166-2172.

65. Rossi A, Mazzocchio R, Scarpini C. Clonus in man: a rhythmic oscillation maintained by a reflex mechanism. *Electroencephalogr Clin Neurophysiol.* 1990;75:56-63.

66. Uysal H, Boyraz I, Yağcıoğlu S, et al. Ankle clonus and its relationship with the medium-latency reflex response of the soleus by peroneal nerve stimulation. *J Electromyogr Kinesiol.* 2011;21:438-444.

67. Boyraz I, Uysal H, Koc B, et al. Clonus: definition, mechanism, treatment. *Med Glas (Zenica).* 2015;12:19-26.

68. Bassetti C. Babinski and Babinski sign. *Spine.* 1995;20:2591-2594.

69. Furukawa T. [Joseph Babinski's contribution to neurological symptomatology]. [Article in Japanese] *Brain Nerve.* 2014;66:1279-1286.

70. Grijalva RA, Hsu FP, Wycliffe ND, et al. Hoffmann sign: clinical correlation of neurological imaging findings in the cervical spine and brain. *Spine.* 2015;40:475-479.

71. Tejus MN, Singh V, Ramesh A, et al. An evaluation of the finger flexion, Hoffman's and plantar reflexes as markers of cervical spinal cord compression—A comparative clinical study. *Clin Neurol Neurosurg.* 2015;134:12-16.

72. Hoffmann G, Kamper DG, Kahn JH, et al. Modulation of stretch reflexes of the finger flexors by sensory feedback from the proximal upper limb poststroke. *J Neurophysiol.* 2009;102:1420-1429.

3 Physical Examination of the Cervical Spine

Lisa Huynh, MD | David J. Kennedy, MD

INTRODUCTION

The annual prevalence of neck pain is estimated to range between 30% and 50%,[1] and nearly half of all individuals will experience neck pain in their lifetime.[2] History and physical examination can provide important clues in determining the etiology of symptoms. Many specialized provocative tests have been described for physical examination of the neck and cervical spine. These tests are routinely performed by clinicians with varying experience and skill. This may lead to error in both the technique and the interpretation of findings.

Several key principles exist in examination of the cervical spine: (1) The exam should be systematic to avoid missing key steps. (2) Generally, exam maneuvers should be done in a stepwise manner so that less painful movements are performed first and most painful movements are completed last; this ensures the least amount of pain carryover, which may confound exam findings. (3) Of crucial concern for any examination of the cervical spine is the ability to differentiate pathologies that merely cause pain from those that adversely affect sensitive neural tissues associated with the cervical spinal cord and its nerve roots.

This chapter provides a comprehensive overview of the physical examination of the cervical spine. For each test, the original description, currently performed technique, reliability, validity, and clinical significance are discussed, based on a comprehensive search of the existing literature. The goal is not necessarily to learn every examination maneuver performed for neck pain but rather to understand the limitations, reliability, and scientifically proven validity of some of the commonly used tests.

INSPECTION

Inspection should begin by noting the position of the head in relation to the line of gravity, which passes through the external auditory meatus; odontoid process; the cervical, thoracic, thoracolumbar, and lumbosacral spine; and the sacral promontory. One should carefully assess not only the upper cervical region but also the relative curvature of the thoracolumbar and lumbosacral spines because the relative positioning of the cervical spine may be influenced by the curvature below. The forward-head position can also be the direct cause of the loss of cervical motion. Caillet[3]

reported a 25% to 50% loss of head rotation with a forwardly protruded head and a significant increase in the gravity-induced weight of the head brought on by this postural abnormality. The forward-head posture thus increases the work requirements of the capital and cervical musculature. Additional features associated with damage to the neural structures may be noted by observation/inspection, including limb muscle atrophy, clumsiness, and balance problems on gait.

PALPATION

Palpation is a common component of cervical spine evaluation. It should be systematic and focus on palpation of the midline spinous processes, the paraspinal musculature, and the underlying zygapophyseal joints (z-joints), as well as the associated cervical spinal musculature. Studies have addressed the accuracy of palpation in identifying the structure or level of the spine and interexaminer reliability. In a study of 69 patients, experienced anesthesiologists were asked to identify the C7 spinous process by palpation, which was then compared with fluoroscopy.[4] The C7 level was chosen because it was believed to be the most prominent and easiest level to identify. The physicians in this study were only able to correctly identify the C7 spinous process 47.9% of the time when compared with fluoroscopy. This was increased to 77.1% with the addition of neck flexion-extension. Additional concerns with the reliability of the cervical spine palpatory examination have been highlighted in a systematic comprehensive review of the literature, which showed overall poor interexaminer reliability for all palpation.[5] Reviewers also found that the level of clinical experience did not improve the reliability in that experienced clinicians fared no better than students in terms of palpatory reliability. Segmental range of motion as assessed by palpation was also found to have very low reliability. Additionally, palpation for soft tissue had very low reliability in all regions tested. Reviews of the literature on manual palpation of trigger points have shown poor reproducibility; however, the majority of studies had poor methodological quality.[6]

Studies on the validity of palpation in the cervical spine are lacking. In 1995, Sandmark and Nisell[7] found in a study of 75 patients with self-reported pain that palpation over the facet joints was the most appropriate screening to corroborate self-reported neck dysfunction. This was based on a reported sensitivity of 82% and a specificity of 79%, in which a single-blinded physiotherapist performed palpation over the cervical z-joints on subjects with and without neck pain.[7] Subjects were then instructed to answer "yes" or "no" if pain had been elicited. Unfortunately, additional studies that compare a palpatory examination to known cervical spine pathology are few; thus, evaluation of the validity of this test is limited.

Collectively, palpation appears to have low interrater reliability and not even perfect intrarater reliability. It also fails to identify the correct target tissue in a significant percentage of cases. However, it still has utility in determining anatomic regions of pain and establishing rapport with the patient. Additionally, studies have shown that palpation is useful for assessing for hypersensitivity to pain and other nonorganic causes of pain. Sobel and associates[8] reported that pain with light touch or pinching of the skin over the cervical region or complaints of widespread tenderness with local palpation in the cervical or upper thoracic region were associated with nonorganic disease. Therefore palpation remains a standard part of the examination, and to accomplish these numerous goals, clinicians must have a thorough understanding of both structural and functional anatomy.

RANGE OF MOTION

The amount of motion that occurs between contiguous vertebrae in the cervical spine is dictated mainly by the anatomic orientation of the z-joints. Paired superior and inferior articular processes project from each pedicle–lamina junction. The superior articular processes of each vertebra articulate with the inferior articular processes of the next higher vertebra to form hyaline cartilage–covered synovial z-joints. These joints are true synovial joints with hyaline cartilage, synovial lining, and a joint capsule that encloses the joint space. They are also known sources of pain because mechanoreceptors and nociceptors richly innervate each cervical zygapophyseal joint. The z-joint capsule for the subatlanto-axial zygapophyseal joints are generally sufficiently lax to permit gliding movements of the facet joints in planes compatible with their facing direction.[9] The atlantooccipital (AO) and atlantoaxial (AA) joints are not true z-joints. True joints extend from C2/C3 to the C7/T1 level. Biomechanical studies have identified flexion and extension motion of the AO joint to be approximately 13 degrees. Lateral bending motion at the AO joint averages 8 degrees with negligible rotation. The AA joint articulates at three locations creating a medial atlantodental and two lateral AA joints.[9] Rotation is the key movement of the AA joint, which averages 47 degrees and is limited by the lateral atlantoaxial joint capsule and the opposite alar ligament. The AA joint accounts for 50% of the total rotation of the cervical spine.[10] There are 10 degrees of total flexion and extension at the AA joint with a negligible amount of lateral bending. Distal to C2, the superior articular processes of the z-joints are oriented in a posterior and superior direction, at a 45-degree angle from the horizontal plane. Flexion and extension are greatest at the C5/C6 and C6/C7 interspaces, where they amount to 17 degrees and 16 degrees, respectively.[11] Lateral bending and rotation of the five lower cervical z-joints tend to be most extensive at the C3/C4 and C4/C5 levels, averaging 11 to 12 degrees.[7]

In a clinical setting where spinal instability is not a concern, range of motion should ideally be initially assessed actively with the patient standing or in a seated posture. This can proceed to passive range of motion in the supine position if an abnormality is identified. By splitting the range of motion exam into active and passive components, the practitioner can assess for a true restriction with a firm end feel versus those reductions in range that are due to pain.

When specific measurements are needed, a goniometer is placed at the external auditory meatus for flexion and extension, at the top of the head for rotation, and at the nares for side-bending (Fig. 3.1). Cervical flexion has been identified to range between 54 and 69 degrees, with extension ranging between 73 and 93 degrees.[12-14] Youdas and coworkers[15] identified extension to range between 20 and 74 degrees with a mean of 52 degrees in patients older than 90 years and a range of 61 to 106 degrees with a mean of 86 degrees in patients between 11 and 19 years. Lateral bending ranged between 11 and 38 degrees, while rotation ranged between 26 and 74 degrees in those older than 90 years. In patients between 11 and 19 years, lateral bending ranged between 30 and 66 degrees, whereas rotation ranged between 50 and 94 degrees. Intraclass correlation coefficients range from 0.84 to 0.95 for intratester reliability of goniometric assessment, and the intertester reliability ranged between 0.73 and 0.92.[16]

Some studies have suggested that diminished range of motion is related to cervical pathology and physical impairment.[17] However, diminished range of motion may also be found in the asymptomatic population. It is well known that motion of the cervical spine decreases with age due to degenerative changes, which are not always symptomatic.[18,19]

NEUROMUSCULAR EVALUATION

The neuromuscular screen is perhaps the most important portion of the examination and should be performed on all patients with neck complaints. The comprehensive neuromuscular examination should include a detailed motor examination (Table 3.1), assessment of reflexes (Table 3.2), and possibly a sensory examination (Table 3.3). The results of these tests should be considered in the context of the patient's complaints and in conjunction with the remainder of the examination.

CERVICAL SPINE TESTS THAT PROVIDE OR RELIEVE PAIN

SPURLING NECK COMPRESSION TEST

Spurling and Scoville first described the Spurling neck compression test, also known as the foraminal compression test, neck compression test, or quadrant test, in 1944 as "the most important diagnostic test and one that is almost pathognomonic of a cervical intraspinal lesion."[20] Their observations were based on the presentation of 12 patients with "ruptured cervical discs" verified during surgery in 1943 at

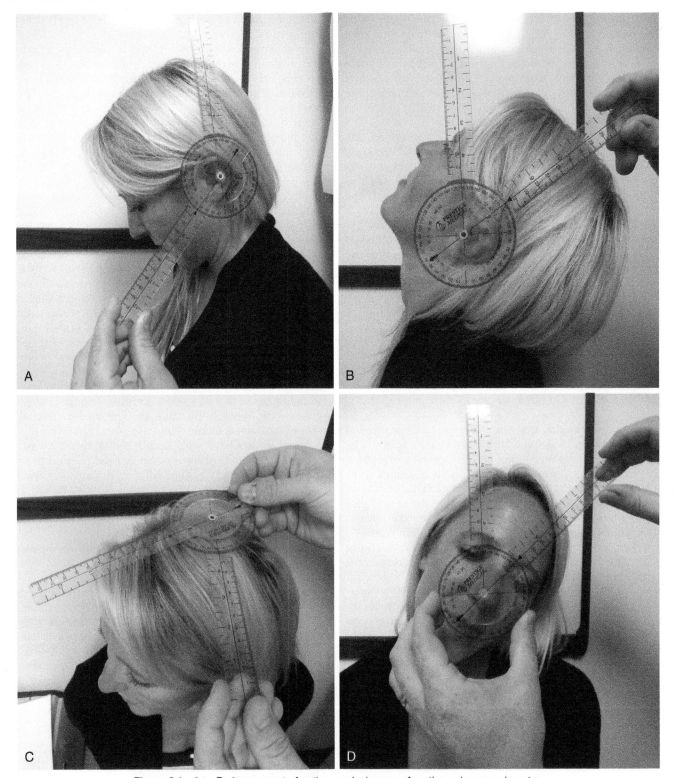

Figure 3.1   A to D, Assessment of active cervical range of motion using a goniometer.

Walter Reed Army Hospital. They originally described "the neck compression test" as follows:

> Tilting the head and neck toward the painful side may be sufficient to reproduce the characteristic pain and radicular features of the lesion. Pressure on the top of the head in this position may greatly intensify the symptoms. Tilting the head away from the lesion usually gives relief (Video 3-1).

Since originally described, several modifications of this test have been suggested. Anekstein and associates[21] performed a prospective study of 67 patients to assess ability of six variations of the Spurling test to reproduce symptoms of cervical radiculopathy. The variations included (1) lateral bending and compression; (2) lateral bending, rotation, and compression; (3) extension and compression; (4)

Table 3.1   Motor Examination

Spine Level	Nerve	Muscle	Testing
C5/C6	Axillary	Deltoid	Arm abducted to the side
C5/C6	Musculocutaneous	Biceps	Elbow flexion
C5–C7	Radial	Triceps	Elbow extension
C6/C7	Median	Pronator teres	Pronation of extended forearm
C6/C7	Radial	Extensor carpi radialis	Wrist extension
C8/T1	Ulnar	Abductor digiti minimi	Abduction of the fifth digit

Table 3.2   Reflex Examination

Spine Level	Reflex
C5/C6	Biceps
C5/C6	Brachioradialis
C6/C7	Pronator teres
C7/C8	Triceps

Table 3.3   Sensory Examination

Spine Level	Sensation
C3	Supraclavicular fossa
C4	Tip of acromion
C5	Lateral epicondyle
C6	Thumb
C7	Middle digit
C8	Fifth digit

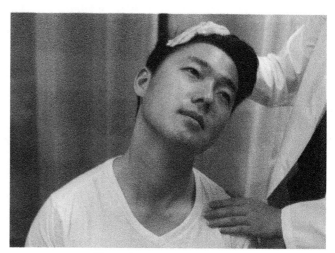

Figure 3.2   Spurling maneuver.

extension and lateral bending; (5) extension, lateral bending, and compression; and (6) extension, rotation, and compression. Results found that maneuvers 5 and 6 were associated with the highest elicited pain and paresthesia, respectively.[21] Methodological flaws in this study prevent conclusive recommendations. Some authors advocate performing the components of the test in a staged manner and halting with the onset of radicular symptoms, preferably reproducing the patient's presenting symptoms.[22-24] Radicular symptoms are described as pain or paresthesias occurring distant from the neck, in the distribution of a cervical spinal nerve root. Currently, this test is performed by extending the neck and rotating the head and then applying downward pressure on the head (Fig. 3.2). The test is considered positive if pain radiates into the limb ipsilateral to the side at which the head is rotated.[25]

Viikari-Juntura[26] conducted a prospective study assessing the interexaminer reliability of common tests performed in the clinical examination of patients with neck and radicular pain. Two blinded expert examiners, who were trained together in the identical performance of the clinical tests, independently examined 52 patients referred for cervical myelography. The neck compression test was performed with each patient in both supine and sitting positions. The patient's neck was passively flexed laterally and slightly rotated ipsilaterally, and the head was then compressed with approximately 7 kg of pressure. A positive test result was considered to be the appearance or aggravation of pain,

numbness, or paresthesias in the shoulder or upper extremity. For the sitting position, κ values ranged from 0.40 to 0.77, which was considered to be "fair to excellent," and the proportion of specific agreement was found to be 0.47 to 0.80, which was also considered to be "fair to excellent." For the supine position, κ values ranged from 0.28 to 0.63, which was considered to be "poor to good," and the proportion of specific agreement was found to be 0.36 to 0.67, which was also considered to be "poor to good." The author concluded that this test has good reliability when performed in the sitting position. This is one of the only studies in the literature assessing interexaminer reliability for the Spurling neck compression test and other provocative test maneuvers of the cervical spine. However, the results are analyzed according to the area of symptom radiation (eg, "right shoulder or upper arm," "right forearm or hand," "left shoulder or upper arm," "left forearm or hand"), instead of classifying the test result as positive or negative. This fragments statistical analysis and makes interpretation difficult.

In 1989, Viikari-Juntura and coworkers[27] published a prospective study assessing the validity of the Spurling neck compression test in diagnosing cervical radiculopathy, along with the axial manual traction and shoulder abduction tests. Forty-three patients who presented for myelography were interviewed and examined before performing the procedure. The Spurling neck compression test was performed with the patient sitting as previously described.[26] The criterion standard used was myelography combined with neurologic exam findings. Based on the study population's myelographic and clinical findings, statistical analysis was performed only for cervical roots C6 to C8. Sensitivity ranged from 40% to 60% and specificity was 92% to 100%. The authors concluded that the test has high specificity but low sensitivity.[26] The results are presented in a manner making interpretation difficult.[26,27]

Tong and Haig[28] reported a sensitivity of 30% and specificity of 93% utilizing electrodiagnostic studies as a criterion standard in 224 patients. Sandmark and Nisell[7] reported a specificity of 92%, sensitivity of 77%, positive predictive value of 80%, and negative predictive value of 91%. However, their study used neck pain symptoms as the criterion standard, and the Spurling neck compression test was considered to be positive if neck pain, not radicular symptoms, was produced. This interpretation is inconsistent with the original and commonly accepted descriptions of the Spurling sign. Because of these methodological issues, the results should be viewed cautiously. Uchihara and associates[29] reported a sensitivity of 28% and a specificity of 100%. However, the criterion standard used was spinal cord deformity on magnetic resonance imaging (MRI) in 65 patients.

In summary, there are few methodologically sound studies that assess the interexaminer reliability, sensitivity, and specificity of the Spurling neck compression test. The literature appears to indicate high specificity but low sensitivity for this test.

SHOULDER ABDUCTION TEST

In 1956 Spurling was reported to have first described the shoulder abduction test, also known as the shoulder abduction relief sign and Bakody sign.[30] In a review on the examination maneuver, Davidson and coworkers[30] described Spurling's initial description as follows: "raising the arm above the head sometimes brings relief of radicular symptoms caused by cervical intervertebral disc pathology." The shoulder abduction relief test is currently described as: "active or passive abduction of the ipsilateral shoulder so that the hand rests on top of the head, with the patient either sitting or supine [Fig. 3.3]. Relief or reduction of ipsilateral cervical radicular symptoms is indicative of a positive test (Video 3-2)."[24] History alone may predict a positive test result because patients often describe raising their arms to alleviate radicular symptoms.

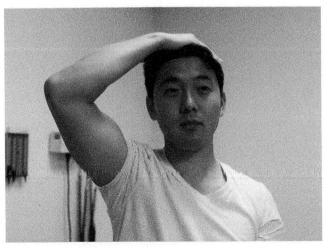

Figure 3.3 Hyperabduction test.

Davidson and associates[30] described 22 patients who presented with severe cervical radicular pain, sensory and motor symptoms, initially unresponsive to outpatient measures. All were found to have large lateral extradural lesions on myelography. Fifteen (68%) of these patients experienced relief of their radicular symptoms with ipsilateral shoulder abduction. The authors hypothesized that reduced nerve root tension is the most likely cause for symptom relief with shoulder abduction. They concluded that the shoulder abduction relief sign is indicative of nerve root compression and predictive of an excellent response to surgical treatment.

Beatty and colleagues[31] described this sign to be indicative of radiculopathy secondary to cervical disc pathology but not from cervical spondylosis. Ellenberg and Honet[23] described the shoulder abduction relief sign as helpful in distinguishing cervical radiculopathy from shoulder pathology, when present. In their experience, the sign is "frequently not present" with cervical radiculopathy, though no statistical data were presented.

Viikari-Juntura[26] prospectively studied the interexaminer reliability of the shoulder abduction relief test in 31 patients with radicular pain, paresthesias, or numbness. It was performed in the seated position with the patient instructed to "lift" the hand above the head. The decrease or disappearance of radicular symptoms indicated a positive test. Kappa scores were poor to fair and ranged from 0.21 to 0.40. The proportion of specific agreement was fair to good, ranging from 0.57 to 0.67. Overall, the test's reliability was described as "fair." Viikari-Juntura and coworkers[27] later investigated the validity of the shoulder abduction relief test on 22 patients. Sensitivity ranged from 43% to 50%, and specificity ranged from 80% to 100%. The authors concluded that the test is highly specific for cervical radiculopathy with low sensitivity.

Similar to the Spurling maneuver, the literature seems to indicate high specificity with low sensitivity for the shoulder abduction relief test. However, the only available prospective study examined a small number of subjects for this test. The only investigation of interexaminer reliability concluded the test to be "fair." Interestingly, incorporation of the abduction maneuver into a nonsurgical treatment program is reported as beneficial for patients with a positive test result.[32]

NECK DISTRACTION TEST

The neck distraction test is also described as the axial manual traction test. The origin of this maneuver is uncertain, but it is well described in the current literature:

> To perform the distraction test, the examiner places one hand under the patient's chin and the other hand around the occiput, then slowly lifts the patient's head. The test is classified as positive if the pain is relieved or decreased when the head is lifted or distracted, indicating pressure on nerve roots that has been relieved (Video 3-3).[24]

This test is commonly performed in the supine position in the presence of radicular symptoms (Fig. 3.4). A positive test result is indicated by relief or lessening of the radicular symptoms and is thought to indicate cervical radiculopathy caused by discogenic pathology.[26,27,33] Viikari-Juntura[26]

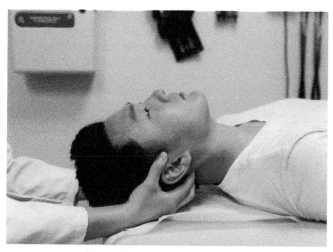

Figure 3.4 Neck distraction test.

concluded that the interexaminer reliability of the neck distraction test is "good." In his prospective study, a traction force of 10 to 15 kg was applied to 29 subjects. Kappa values ranged from 0.50 to 0.71. Using the same examination technique in a 1989 study, Viikari-Juntura and others[27] reported a specificity of 100% and a sensitivity of 40% to 43%. The authors concluded that the axial manual traction test has low sensitivity but is highly specific for radicular pain, and neurologic and radiologic signs of radiculopathy from cervical disc disease. No other studies of interexaminer reliability or validity are reported in the literature.

LHERMITTE SIGN

What is now referred to as the Lhermitte sign was first described by Marie and Chatelin in 1917 at a meeting of the Centres of Military Neurology in Paris.[34] They described "transient 'pins and needles' sensations traveling the spine and limbs on flexion of the head" in some patients with head injuries. It was believed that these symptoms were caused by positional pressure on cervical nerve roots.[35] In 1918 Babinski and Dubois[36] described a patient with a Brown–Sequard syndrome who reported sensations of "electric discharge" upon flexing the head, sneezing, or coughing. They attributed the symptom to the presence of an intramedullary lesion. Lhermitte first wrote on this topic in 1920 when he further elaborated on the symptom's origin in patients with "concussion of the spinal cord."[1] He attributed these symptoms to posterior and lateral column pathology in the cervical spinal cord.[34,37] Lhermitte attributed the "electric discharge" symptoms to demyelination of cervical spinal cord segments and believed this to be an early finding in multiple sclerosis.[37]

The Lhermitte test is currently described as being performed in a variety of ways. It is most commonly described as passive cervical flexion to end range with the patient seated (Fig. 3.5). A positive test result is indicated by the presence of an "electric-like" sensation down the spine or in the extremities (Video 3-4). This is described to occur with cervical spinal cord pathology from a wide variety of conditions, including multiple sclerosis, spinal cord tumor, cervical spondylosis, and radiation myelitis.[23,25,33] The test is also

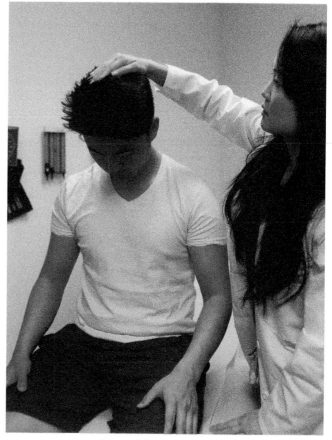

Figure 3.5 Lhermitte sign.

currently described as performed in the following manner, although different from the previous descriptions:

> The patient is in the long leg sitting position on the examining table. The examiner passively flexes the patient's head and one hip simultaneously, with the leg kept straight. A positive test occurs if there is a sharp pain down the spine and into the upper or lower limbs; it indicates dural or meningeal irritation in the spine or possible cervical myelopathy.[24]

No reports investigating the interexaminer reliability of Lhermitte sign could be found in the literature. There are two studies describing the validity of Lhermitte sign, although both have methodological flaws. Sandmark and Nisell[7] reported a sensitivity of 27%, specificity of 90%, positive predictive value of 55%, and negative predictive value of 75% for the active flexion and extension test, which partly resembles Lhermitte test. Uchihara and coworkers[29] reported a high sensitivity and less than 28% specificity, although exact percentages are difficult to discern.

Lhermitte sign was originally described anecdotally, and experience with this test continues to be primarily based on anecdotal observation.

HOFFMANN'S SIGN

The origin of what is now described as Hoffmann's sign remained controversial through the late 1930s until a medical student named Otto Bendheim found a reference to the reflex in a paper written by Hans Curschmann on uremia in 1911.[38] In 1916, Keyser published a paper suggesting the name "Hoffmann's sign" be dropped for "digital reflex" after an extensive search failed to identify the origin of the reflex.[38,39] The sign is attributed to Johann Hoffmann, professor of neurology at Heidelberg, Germany, in the late 19th and early 20th centuries, a pupil of Erb. Hoffmann was reported to demonstrate the sign routinely in lectures and clinics, although he did not discuss it through publication.[38,40] Hoffmann's assistant, Hans Curschmann, who became professor of medicine at the University of Rostock, Germany, described the reflex in the literature in 1911 and named it Hoffmann's sign.[40,41] In 1908, Jakobson described a similar sign, independently and after Hoffmann. Jakobson tapped the distal radius instead of snapping the nail.[38] In 1913, Tromner described the reflex as well.[42,43] In response to an inquiry, Dr. Curschmann later wrote:

> The finger phenomenon mentioned by me originates from Johann Hoffmann, Professor of Neurology at Heidelberg (died 1919). I learned it while his pupil and assistant from 1901 to 1904. He demonstrated it in his classes and clinics as a sign of hyperreflexia of the upper extremity. So far as I know he never published it.[40,41]

Hoffmann's sign was originally described as follows (Fig. 3.6):

> The test is performed by supporting the patient's hand so that it is completely relaxed and the fingers partially flexed. The middle finger is firmly grasped, partially extended, and the nail snapped by the examiner's thumb nail. The snapping should be done with considerable force, even to the point of causing pain. The sign is present if quick flexion of both the thumb and index finger results. Finger nails other than the middle one are sometimes selected for the snapping. The sign is said to be incomplete if only the thumb or only the fingers move (Video 2-4).[41]

There continues to be disagreement as to whether the sign is present if only the thumb flexes.[44,45] Keyser described the test result to be positive "if definite flexion of either the thumb or one or more fingers results."[39]

The clinical significance of Hoffmann's sign has been long disputed.[41,44,46] There are three general views of the meaning of this reflex. One theory is that Hoffmann's sign is a "pathologic sign, indicating pyramidal tract involve-

ment."[44] A second, popular view is that it "indicates pyramidal-tract involvement" but that, owing to its frequent presence in other conditions, "its clinical value is doubtful."[44] Finally, many "do not consider the Hoffmann sign as pathologic or of any clinical value."[44] In 1929, Pitfield observed the sign to be inconsistent in individual patients and to be frequently present in patients with cardiovascular disease.[46] He devised a scale classifying the degree in which the response follows the nail snapping into four groups, "plus 1" to "plus 4." Pitfield also described a maneuver to reinforce or negate if absent as follows:

> The upper arm is encircled by the cuff of a blood pressure apparatus; this is blown to 300 mm; if then the prone hand is examined by snapping the nail an apparently absent reflex will become positive and faint ones will be exalted to a plus three or four. After releasing the pressure and removing the cuff, it sometimes can be noted that a condition of exultation will persist for some minutes, the reflex being more active than it was before compression.[46]

Denno and Meadows[47] described "the dynamic Hoffman's sign" as a modification to assist in the diagnosis of early spondylotic cervical myelopathy. This is performed by "multiple active full flexion to extension of the neck" before performing the Hoffman's sign maneuver as originally described. Echols[41] examined 2017 students at the University of Michigan and observed a Hoffmann's sign in 159 using the lenient criteria of any suggested flexion of the index finger, the thumb, or both. After 4 months, 153 were re-examined, and 32 patients no longer demonstrated the sign, 68 had an "incomplete Hoffmann's sign" with flexion of only one or more fingers, and 53 had a "true Hoffmann's sign" with flexion of both the thumb and index fingers in response to snapping the middle finger, the ring finger, or both. Of the 53 students with "true Hoffmann's signs," only 33 had no history of prior head injury or other central nervous system pathology. The incidence of a "true Hoffmann's sign" was 2.62%, the incidence of an "incomplete Hoffmann's sign" was 3.37%, and the incidence of an unexplained "true Hoffmann's sign" was 1.63%. Echols concluded that "the (true) Hoffmann sign almost always indicates a disturbance of the pyramidal pathway" and "the significance of an incomplete Hoffmann's sign is still unsettled." It should be noted that 62% of the patients with true Hoffman's signs in Echols' study (33/53) were unexplained.

In 1946, Schneck published a preliminary report of a 2.5% to 3% incidence of Hoffmann's sign in more than 2500 subjects in the military.[45] No history or physical examination findings consistent with neurologic disease were elicited in the majority of subjects tested. Madonick[44] noted the overall incidence of Hoffmann's sign to be 2.08% in a study of 2500 patients without neurologic disease, and the sign was more frequent with advancing age. The incidence was 0.7% in those aged 0 to 19 years, 1.2% in those 20 to 39 years, 3.4% in those 40 to 59 years, and 4% in those older than 60 years. The question remained as to whether the Hoffmann sign was due to a functional disturbance of the pyramidal tract or indicated a state of increased muscle tone.

Sung and Wang[48] prospectively evaluated 16 asymptomatic patients with a positive Hoffmann's reflex using cervical radiographs and MRI. Fourteen of 16 (87.5%) cervical spine radiograph were abnormal with spondylosis, and all 16 MRIs

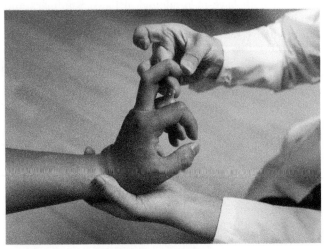

Figure 3.6 Hoffmann's sign.

were interpreted as abnormal with spondylosis and cord compression in 15. The authors concluded that "the presence of a positive Hoffman's reflex was found to be highly associated with the presence of a cervical spine lesion causing neural compression." Imaging studies or further evaluation is not recommended, as the cohort studied remained asymptomatic, with continued yearly follow-up. The small number of subjects and lack of a control group makes strong conclusions pertaining to this study difficult.

Glaser and associates[49] reported a sensitivity of 58%, specificity of 78%, positive predictive value of 62%, and negative predictive value of 75% in a study of 124 patients presenting with cervical complaints. Imaging of the cervical spinal canal for evidence of cord compression with computed tomography (CT) or MRI was used as the criterion standard. When only results of the patients with cervical spine MRIs were evaluated using blinded neuroradiologists, the sensitivity was 33%, specificity was 59%, positive predictive value was 26%, and negative predictive value was 67%. The authors concluded that the Hoffman's sign "without other clinical findings" is not a reliable test to screen for cervical spinal cord compression. This retrospective study is useful despite its methodological flaws.

More recently, Grijalva and coworkers[50] performed a retrospective validity study investigating the relationship between Hoffman's sign and radiographic evidence of cervical spine and brain pathology, with similar diagnostic values as prior studies. Of the 91 patients with a positive Hoffman's sign, 35% were found to have severe cervical cord compression and/or myelomalacia. Forty-seven of the 91 patients had brain imaging studies, of which 10% had positive findings. Of the 80 patients in the negative Hoffman's/control group, 27% were found to have severe cord compression and/or myelomalacia. Twenty-three control patients had brain imaging, of which 8% had positive findings. Grijalva and coworkers[50] reported 59% sensitivity, 49% specificity, 35% positive predictive value, and 72% negative predictive value for cervical cord compression. For brain pathology, there was 71% sensitivity, 33% specificity, 10% positive predictive value, and 95% negative predictive value. The authors similarly concluded that Hoffmann's sign should not be solely relied on as a screen tool for predicting presence of cervical spinal cord or brain pathology.

In summary, the significance of Hoffman's sign remains disputed in the literature. The validity has not been well studied although poor to fair sensitivity, fair to good specificity, and poor positive predictive values are reported. There are no known studies assessing the interexaminer reliability of Hoffman's sign.

THORACIC OUTLET SYNDROME

Although not a true cervical spine condition, examination for thoracic outlet syndrome (TOS) is appropriately discussed here because it is ascribed to a constellation of symptoms into the upper extremities including pain, weakness, numbness, or paresthesias, which are similar to those in patients suffering from cervical radicular pain. Symptoms are caused by compression of the vascular structures (subclavian artery and vein, axillary artery and vein), and/or neurologic structures (lower trunk or cords of the brachial

plexus). Anatomically, the outlet can be defined by its bony borders including the first rib, first thoracic vertebra, clavicle, and manubrium of the sternum or within the muscular space between the anterior and middle scalenes. The four main sites of compression described are (Fig. 3.7):

- within the scalene musculature (scalenus anticus syndrome)
- under a congenital band or bony extension of the seventh cervical transverse process (cervical rib)
- between the clavicle and the first rib (costoclavicular syndrome)
- under the pectoralis minor (pectoralis minor syndrome)

The syndrome is controversial, and the diagnostic tests used to assess this condition are of questionable value. Warren and Heaton[51] found that 58% of 62 randomly chosen individuals had at least one diagnostic test result positive including the Adson's, costoclavicular, and hyperabduction tests. Only 2% had more than one test result positive, bringing into question the specificity of the various tests. Rayan and Jensen[52] found that 91% of normal individuals developed symptoms from at least one of the tests for TOS.

ADSON TEST

In 1927, Adson and Coffey[53] described a physical exam maneuver that could be used to assess compression of the subclavian artery between a cervical rib and the scalenus anticus muscle; this maneuver later became known as the Adson maneuver (Fig. 3.8). Simply stated:

> sitting upright, with arms resting on knees [the patient] takes a deep breath, extends the neck, and turns the head toward the affected side. An alteration of the radial pulse or blood pressure in the affected arm was considered "a pathognomonic sign of the presence of a cervical rib or scalenus anticus syndrome (Video 3-5).
>
> However, the efficacy of this test remains controversial. Based on the biomechanics of the Adson test, one would expect that the scalene angle should increase, not decrease, thus causing the aforementioned compression. Instead, the scalene angle actually increases and, in fact, this would allow more room for the brachial plexus to exit the neck and reduce the likelihood of compression.[54-57] Moreover, to date, no studies have been performed to document the reliability of this test. The specificity has been noted to range from 18% to 87%, but the sensitivity has been documented to approach 94%.[58]

WRIGHT'S HYPERABDUCTION TEST

In 1945, Wright[59] originally described the obliteration of the radial pulse in at least one upper extremity in 93% of 150 asymptomatic subjects with the arm held overhead at a 90-degree angle with the elbow flexed. He attributed the neurovascular symptom to entrapment by pectoralis minor tendon (Fig. 3.9). Gilroy and Meyer[60] and Raaf[61] found that arm elevation induced radial pulse obliteration or bruit in the former, in 60% to 69% of normal subjects. The existing research clearly demonstrates that pulse diminution is a

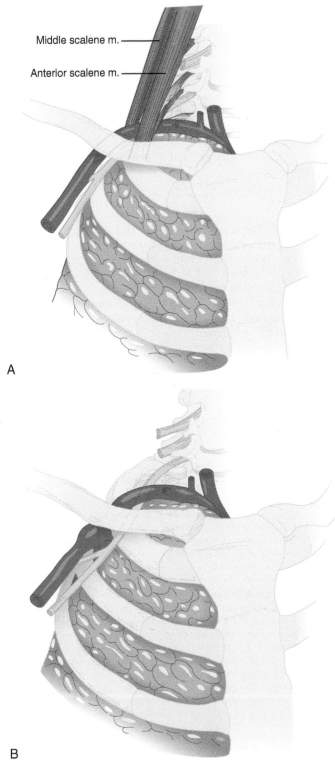

Middle scalene m.

Anterior scalene m.

A

B

Figure 3.7   Thoracic outlet anatomy. Compression of neurovascular structures may occur, (A) within the scalene musculature, or (B) between the clavicle and the first rib. (Reproduced with permission from Bennett JB, Mehlhoff TL: Thoracic outlet syndrome. In Delee JC, Drez D, eds. *Orthopedic Sports Medicine: Principles and Practices.* Philadelphia: WB Saunders; 1994:795.)

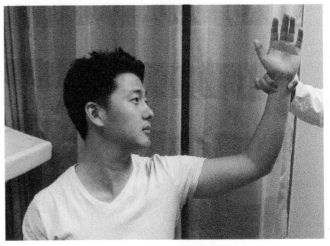

Figure 3.8   Adson test.

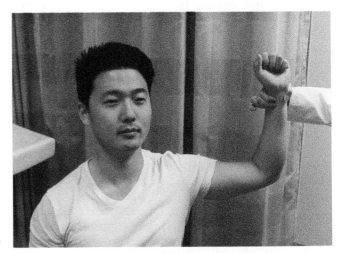

Figure 3.9   Wright hyperabduction test.

normal phenomenon in the general population with overhead activity. According to Roos, "these studies clearly indicate that pulse obliteration with the arms and head in various positions is a normal finding in the majority of asymptomatic people and therefore has no relation to the etiology or presence of symptoms."[62] Rayan and Jensen[52] suggested modification of the hyperabduction test with the elbow maintained in extension to avoid inducing ulnar nerve symptoms with elbow flexion. No studies have described the reliability, sensitivity, or specificity of this test.

ROOS TEST

In 1976, Roos described this elevated arm stress test as follows:

> [The patient holds the] brachium at right angles to the thorax and the forearm flexed to 90 degrees. The patient is instructed to open and close his fist at moderate speed for 3 minutes, with the elbows braced somewhat posteriorly. It reproduces the patient's usual symptoms within 3 minutes [Fig. 3.10] (Video 3-6).[62]

Symptoms produced with this test include early fatigue and heaviness of the involved arm, gradual onset of

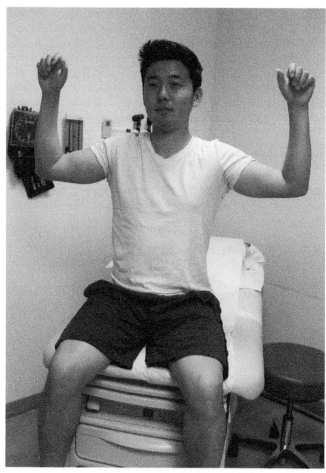

Figure 3.10 Roos test.

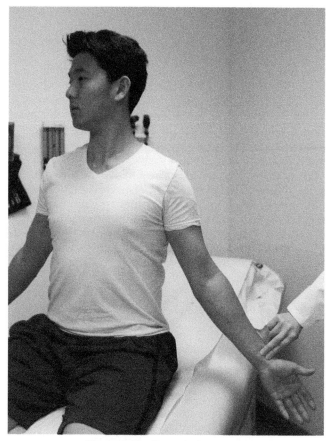

Figure 3.11 Costoclavicular test.

numbness and tingling of the hand, increasing vocal complaints, sudden dropping of the limb into the lap, involved limb slow to recover to normal, and totally abnormal response commonly seen while radial pulses are strong.[62] Roos indicated that his elevated arm test was perhaps the most reliable of all and will delineate TOS from other problems with similar symptoms. Unfortunately, no specific data are presented to support these claims.

Plewa and Delinger[63] demonstrated in a study of four of the common tests for TOS in normal subjects that the elevated arm stress test resulted in diminution of pulse in 62% compared with 11% for Adson's or costoclavicular tests. This points to the high false-positive rate among these tests and brings into question the sensitivity and specificity of this maneuver.

COSTOCLAVICULAR TEST

The original description of the costoclavicular maneuver may be ascribed to Falconer and Wedell who, in 1943, reported in a case series of three subjects with subclavian artery and vein compression that:

> costoclavicular compression of the subclavian vessels can be recognized by observing the effect of postural maneuvers of the shoulder girdle on the arterial pulse of the limb. Backward and downward bracing of the shoulders is the movement which obliterates the pulses most readily.[64]

The test is performed with the patient asked to retract and then depress the shoulders. This is followed by protrusion of the chest and a request to hold the position for 1 minute (Fig. 3.11). The examiner identifying the radial pulse on the involved extremity monitors the pulse for reduction. Telford and Modershead[56] found an alteration of the radial pulse in 64% of normal individuals with shoulder depression and 68% after shoulder retraction. No studies are available that identify the sensitivity or specificity of this maneuver.

AUTHOR'S PREFERRED APPROACH

As with all aspects of a patient's clinical exam, it is important to start with a detailed history because this can aid in narrowing the focus of the physical examination. The cervical spine physical examination should start with overall inspection of the patient, paying particular attention to spinal alignment, including head forward posture or loss of normal lordosis. Palpatory exam can be helpful for assessing tender points and establishing rapport. Segmental evaluation of the cervical z-joints may be limited in determining exact levels of pathology especially in patients with significant soft tissue/musculature; however, relative levels (high cervical, mid cervical, lower cervical) may still be determined. Range of motion is typically performed actively with the patient standing or sitting. Passive range of motion is reserved for those with identified deficits and is done with the patient supine. Range of motion may also be useful to narrow suspected areas of pathology; that is, limited rotation due to atlantoaxial joint dysfunction vs limited flexion/extension due to atlanto-occipital joint dysfunction.

A neurologic exam is imperative to assess potential deficits and the need for additional imaging studies. This should include manual muscle testing, deep tendon reflexes, and sensory exam. If there is concern for cervical myelopathy, balance testing including Romberg's should be included. Hoffman's may be useful, especially in the setting of asymmetric positive Hoffman's or hyperreflexia.

Provocative exam maneuvers in general have low sensitivity, but relatively higher specificity. Therefore, they are used based on the history and examination to help confirm a diagnosis. Typical exam maneuvers used include the Spurling test and shoulder abduction test to assess for cervical radiculopathy. In performing the Spurling test, we rarely perform axial compression because this may severely exacerbate pain, much to the patient's dismay. Instead, we may place an index finger on the patient's chin and gently guide them into a hyperextended and lateral flexed position.

Other considerations should include performing a shoulder exam or upper extremity exam to assess for concordant peripheral joint pathology or peripheral mononeuropathies. Thoracic outlet syndrome maneuvers are not regularly performed as part of our cervical spine exam although they certainly should be considered when there is clinical suspicion based on history including predominant upper extremity symptoms as opposed to associated neck pain.

CONCLUSION

The majority of the specialized provocative tests commonly used in examination of the cervical spine and related neck structures are purported to assist in identification of radiculopathy, spinal cord pathology, or brachial plexus pathology. Each of the tests described originated from the anecdotal observations of experienced, well-respected clinicians. They are summarized in Table 3.4.

Few studies have been performed addressing the interexaminer reliability or validity of these tests. Of the studies

Table 3.4   Cervical Spine and Thoracic Outlet Tests

Test	Original Description	Reliability Studies	Validity Studies
Spurling/neck compression test	Passive lateral flexion and compression of head. Positive test is reproduction of radicular symptoms distant from neck.	Viikari-Juntura 1987[26] Seated position. Kappa = 0.40–0.77 Proportion specific agreement = 0.47–0.80	Viikari-Juntura (1989)[27] Seated position. Sensitivity: 40–60% Specificity: 92–100%
Shoulder abduction(relief) sign	Active abduction of symptomatic arm, placing patient's hand on head. Positive test is relief or reduction of ipsilateral cervical radicular symptoms.	Viikari-Juntura 1987[26] Seated position. Kappa = 0.21–0.40 Proportion specific agreement = 0.57–0.67	Viikari-Juntura (1989)[27] Seated position. Sensitivity: 43–50% Specificity: 80–100%
Neck distraction test	Examiner grasps patient's head under occiput and chin and applies axial traction force. Positive test is relief or reduction of cervical radicular symptoms.	Viikari-Juntura 1987[26] Supine position. 10–15 kg traction force applied. Kappa = 0.50 Proportion specific agreement = 0.71	Viikari-Juntura (1989)[27] Supine position. 10–15 kg traction force applied. Sensitivity: 40–43% Specificity: 100%
Lhermitte sign	Passive anterior cervical flexion. Positive test is presence of "electric-like" sensations down spine or extremities.	Not reported.	Uchihara 1994[29] Sensitivity: <28% Specificity: "High"
Hoffmann's sign	Passive snapping flexion of middle finger distal phalanx. Positive test is flexion-adduction of ipsilateral thumb and index finger.	Not reported	Glaser (2000)[49] Sensitivity: 58% Specificity: 78% Positive predictive value: 62% Negative predictive value: 75%
Adson test	Inspiration, chin elevation, and head rotation to affected side. Positive test is alteration or obliteration of radial pulse.	Not reported	Marx (1999)[58] Specificity: 18–87% Sensitivity: 94%
Wright hyperabduction test	Arms elevated to 90 degrees, pulse palpated at wrist. Positive test is obliteration of radial pulse.	Not reported	Not reported
Roos test	Arms and elbows flexed to 90 degrees. The patient is instructed to open and close his fist at moderate speed for 3 minutes. Positive test reproduces the patient's usual symptoms within 3 minutes.	Not reported	Not reported
Costoclavicular test	Patient asked to retract and then depress the shoulders, followed by protrusion of the chest. Positive test indicated by reduction in radial pulse.	Not reported	Not reported

performed, most were not methodologically sound or had other limitations. The existing literature appears to indicate high specificity, low sensitivity, and good to fair interexaminer reliability for Spurling's neck compression test, the neck distraction test, and the shoulder abduction (relief) test when performed as described. For Hoffmann's sign, the existing literature does not address interexaminer reliability but appears to indicate fair sensitivity and specificity. For the Lhermitte sign and Adson test, not even tentative statements can be made with regard to interexaminer reliability, sensitivity, and specificity, based on the existing literature. It should be emphasized that more research is indicated to understand the clinical utility of all these tests.

REFERENCES

1. Hogg-Johnson S, van der Velde G, Carroll LJ, et al. The burden and determinants of neck pain in the general population: results of the Bone and Joint Decade 2000-2010 Task Force on Neck Pain and Its Associated Disorders. *Spine.* 2008;33:S39-S51.
2. Fejer R, Kyvik KO, Hartvigsen J. The prevalence of neck pain in the world population: a systematic critical review of the literature. *Eur Spine J.* 2006;15(6):834-848.
3. Caillet R. *Neck and Arm Pain.* Philadelphia: FA Davis; 1991:81-123.
4. Shin S, Yoon DM, Yoon KB. Identification of the correct cervical level by palpation of spinous processes. *Anesth Analg.* 2011;112:1232-1235.
5. Seffinger MA, Najm WI, Mishra SI, et al. Reliability of spinal palpation for diagnosis of back and neck pain: a systematic review of the literature. *Spine.* 2004;29:E413-E425.
6. Myburgh C, Larsen AH, Hartvigsen J. A systematic, critical review of manual palpation for identifying myofascial trigger points: evidence and clinical significance. *Arch Phys Med Rehabil.* 2008;89:1169-1176.
7. Sandmark H, Nisell R. Validity of five common manual neck pain provoking tests. *Scand J Rehabil Med.* 1995;27:131-136.
8. Sobel JB, Sollenberger P, Robinson R, et al. Cervical nonorganic signs: a new clinical tool to assess abnormal illness behavior in neck pain patients: a pilot study. *Arch Phys Med Rehabil.* 2000;81:170-175.
9. White AA, Panjabi MM. *Clinical Biomechanics of the Cervical Spine.* Philadelphia: JB Lippincott; 1978.
10. April C, Bogduk N. The prevalence of cervical zygapophysial joint pain: a first approximation. *Spine.* 1992;17:744-747.
11. Mooney V, Robertson J. Facet joint syndrome. *Clin Orthop.* 1976;115:149-156.
12. Bennett JG, Bergmanis LE, Carpenter JK, et al. Range of motion of the neck. *J Am Phys Ther Assoc.* 1963;43:45-47.
13. Defibaugh JJ. Measurement of head motion. II: An experimental study of head motion in adult males. *Phys Ther.* 1964;44:163-168.
14. Kottke FJ, Blanchard RS. A study of degenerative changes of the cervical spine in relation to age. *Bull Univ Minn Hosp.* 1953;24:470-479.
15. Youdas JW, Garrett TR, Suman VJ, et al. Normal range of motion of the cervical spine: an initial goniometric study. *Phys Ther.* 1992;72:770-780.
16. Youdas JW, Carey JR, Garrett TR. Reliability of measurements of cervical range of motion comparison of three methods. *Phys Ther.* 1991;71:98-104.
17. Dall'Alba PT, Sterling MM, Treleaven JM, et al. Cervical range of motion discriminates between asymptomatic persons and those with whiplash. *Spine.* 2001;26:2090-2294.
18. Dvorak J, Antinnes JA, Panjabi M, et al. Age and gender related normal motion of the cervical spine. *Spine.* 1992;17:S393-S398.
19. Gore DR, Sepic SB, Gardner GM. Roentgenographic findings of the cervical spine in asymptomatic people. *Spine.* 1986;11:521-524.
20. Spurling RG, Scoville WB. Lateral rupture of the cervical intervertebral discs: a common cause of shoulder and arm pain. *Surg Gynecol Obstet.* 1944;78:350-358.
21. Anekstein Y, Blecher R, Smorgick Y, et al. What is the best way to apply the Spurling test for cervical radiculopathy? *Clin Orthop Relat Res.* 2002;470:2566-2572.
22. Bradley JP, Tibone JE, Watkins RG. History, physical examination, and diagnostic tests for neck and upper-extremity problems. In: Watkins RG, ed. *The Spine in Sports.* St Louis: Mosby–Year Book; 1996.
23. Ellenberg M, Honet JC. Clinical pearls in cervical radiculopathy. *Phys Med Rehabil Clin N Am.* 1996;7:487-508.
24. Magee DJ. Cervical spine. In: *Orthopedic Physical Assessment.* 3rd ed. Philadelphia: WB Saunders; 1997.
25. Malanga GA. The diagnosis and treatment of cervical radiculopathy. *Med Sci Sports Exerc.* 1997;29(suppl):S236-S245.
26. Viikari-Juntura E. Interexaminer reliability of observations in physical examinations of the neck. *Phys Ther.* 1987;67:1526-1532.
27. Viikari-Juntura E, Porras M, Laasonen EM. Validity of clinical tests in the diagnosis of root compression in cervical disease. *Spine.* 1989;14:253-257.
28. Tong HC, Haig AJ. Spurling's test and cervical radiculopathy. *Presented at the American Academy of Physical Medicine and Rehabilitation Annual Assembly,* San Francisco, 2000.
29. Uchihara T, Furukawa T, Tsukagoshi H. Compression of brachial plexus as a diagnostic test of cervical cord lesion. *Spine.* 1994;19:2170-2173.
30. Davidson RI, Dunn EJ, Metzmaker JN. The shoulder abduction relief test in the diagnosis of radicular pain in cervical extradural compressive monoradiculopathies. *Spine.* 1981;6:441-446.
31. Beatty RM, Fowler FD, Hanson EJ. The abducted arm as a sign of ruptured cervical disc. *Neurosurgery.* 1987;21:731-732.
32. Fast A, Parikh S, Marin EL. The shoulder abduction relief sign in cervical radiculopathy. *Arch Phys Med Rehabil.* 1989;70:402-403.
33. Ellenberg MR, Honet JC, Treanor WJ. Cervical radiculopathy. *Arch Phys Med Rehabil.* 1994;75:342-352.
34. Gutrecht JA. Lhermitte's sign: from observation to eponym. *Arch Neurol.* 1989;46:557-558.
35. Marie P, Chatelin C. Sur certains symtomes vraisemblablement d'orogine radiculaire chez les blesses du crane. *Rev Neurol.* 1917;31:336.
36. Babinski J, Dubois R. Douleurs a forme de decharge electrique, consecutives aux traumatismes de la nuque. *Presse Med.* 1918;26:64.
37. L'hermitte J. Les formes douloureuses de commotion de la moelle epiniere. *Rev Neurol.* 1920;36:257-262.
38. Bendheim OL. On the history of Hoffmann's sign. *Bull Inst Hist Med.* 1937;5:684-685.
39. Keyser TS. Hoffman's sign or the "digital reflex." *J Nerv Ment Dis.* 1916;44:51-62.
40. Curschmann H. Uber die diagnostiche bedeutung des Babinskischen phanomens im prauramischen zustand. *Munch Med Wchnschr.* 1911;58:2054-2057.
41. Echols DH. The Hoffmann sign: its incidence in university students. *J Nerv Ment Dis.* 1936;84:427-431.
42. Cooper MJ. Mechanical factors governing the Tromner reflex. *Arch Neurol Psychiat.* 1933;30:166-169.
43. Tromner E. Ueber sehnen-respective muskelreflexe und die merkmale ihrer schwachung und steigerung. *Berl Klin Wchnschr.* 1913;50:1712-1715.
44. Madonick MJ. Statistical control studies in neurology. III: The Hoffmann sign. *Arch Neurol Psychiat.* 1952;68:109-115.
45. Schneck JM. The unilateral Hoffmann reflex. *J Nerv Ment Dis.* 1946;104:597-598.
46. Pitfield RL. The Hoffmann reflex: a simple way of reinforcing it and other reflexes. *J Nerv Ment Dis.* 1929;69:252-258.
47. Denno JJ, Meadows GR. Early diagnosis of cervical spondylotic myelopathy: a useful clinical sign. *Spine.* 1991;16:1353-1355.
48. Sung RD, Wang JC. Correlation between a positive Hoffman's reflex and cervical pathology in asymptomatic individuals. *Spine.* 2001;26:67-70.
49. Glaser JA, et al. Cervical cord compression and the Hoffman's sign. *Presented at the 14th Annual Meeting of the North American Spine Society,* October 21, 1999.
50. Grijalva RA, Hsu FPK, Wycliffe ND, et al. Hoffmann's sign: clinical correlation of neurological imaging findings in the cervical spine and brain. *Spine.* 2015;40:475-479.

51. Warren AN, Heaton JM. Thoracic outlet compression syndrome: the lack of reliability of its clinical assessment. *Ann R Coll Surg Engl.* 1987;69:203-204.

52. Rayan GM, Jensen C. Thoracic outlet syndrome: provocative examination maneuvers in a typical population. *J Shoulder Elbow Surg.* 1995;4:113-117.

53. Adson AW, Coffey JR. Cervical rib: a method of anterior approach for relief of symptoms by division of the scalenus anticus. *Ann Surg.* 1927;85:839-857.

54. Adson AW. Cervical ribs: symptoms, differential diagnosis, and indications for section of the insertion of the scalenus anticus muscle. *J Int Coll Surg.* 1951;16:546-559.

55. Nachlus IW. Scalenus anticus syndrome or cervical foraminal compression? *South Med J.* 1942;35:663-667.

56. Telford E, Modershead S. Pressure of the cervical brachial junction: an operative and anatomical study. *J Bone Joint Surg Br.* 1948;308:249-265.

57. Walshe FMR, Jackson H, Wyburn-Mason R. On some pressure effects associated with rudimentary and "normal" first ribs, and the factors entering into their causation. *Brain.* 1944;67:141-177.

58. Marx RG, Bombardier C, Wright JG. What we know about the reliability and validity of physical examination tests used to examine the upper extremity. *J Hand Surg Am.* 1999;24A:185-192.

59. Wright IS. The neurovascular syndrome produced by abduction of the arms: the immediate changes produced in 150 normal controls and the effects on some persons of prolonged hyperabduction of the arms as in sleeping and some occupations. *Am Heart J.* 1945;29:1-19.

60. Gilroy J, Meyer JS. Compression of the subclavian artery, a cause of ischemic brachial neuropathy. *Brain.* 1963;86:733-746.

61. Raaf J. Surgery for cervical rib and scalenus anticus syndrome. *J Am Med Assoc.* 1965;157:219.

62. Roos DB. Congenital anomalies associated with thoracic outlet syndrome: anatomy, symptoms, diagnosis, and treatment. *Am J Surg.* 1976;132:771-778.

63. Plewa MC, Delinger M. The false positive rate of thoracic outlet syndrome shoulder maneuvers in healthy subjects. *Acad Emerg Med.* 1998;5:337-342.

64. Falconer MA, Weddell G. Costoclavicular compression of the subclavian artery and vein. *Lancet.* 1943;2:539-543.

Physical Examination of the Shoulder

Edward G. McFarland, MD | Jay E. Bowen, DO | Amrut Borade, MD |
Gerard A. Malanga, MD | Tutankhamen Pappoe, MD

INTRODUCTION

The shoulder girdle allows for a large degree of motion in multiple planes, with the glenohumeral joint being the most mobile joint in the body. The tradeoff for this freedom of motion is a relative lack of stability, which makes the shoulder girdle susceptible to an array of injuries. A number of physical examination maneuvers have been developed to assist examiners in diagnosing shoulder problems. Performing these maneuvers accurately and understanding their reliability and validity are paramount to a proper shoulder examination. In this chapter, we review common shoulder examination maneuvers, identifying the original descriptions and presenting research examining the sensitivity, specificity, positive predictive value (PPV), and negative predictive value (NPV) of the various tests.

EXAMINATION OF THE SHOULDER

A thorough examination of shoulder symptoms should include the cervical spine, contralateral shoulder, elbow, trunk, and upper-limb neurovascular structures. We limit our focus to the shoulder girdle, which includes the sternoclavicular, acromioclavicular (AC), glenohumeral, and scapulothoracic (ST) joints. Doing the basic aspects of a musculoskeletal examination is especially important in the shoulder: The key to performing a good shoulder examination is to develop a system in which the patient is prepped so you can (1) see the shoulders; (2) compare both sides; (3) do a neurovascular examination; and (4) consider the joint above, which in this case is the cervical spine.

INSPECTION

The first step of shoulder examination is to have the patient undress so that both shoulders can be examined and compared. For men, this is accomplished by taking off the shirt, and for women a sports bra or a gown worn around the thorax can suffice (Fig. 4.1). The patient should be examined from the front and the back, where elements such as muscle bulk and scapular positioning can be easily observed. Posture should be observed in both the seated and standing positions and from different angles. Scars, atrophy, swelling, ecchymosis, erythema, rashes, deformities, shoulder heights, and scapular positioning should be evaluated. Posture in the standing and seated positions should be observed for a forward set, protracted head, and rounded shoulders (humeral internal rotation and scapular protraction), which will cause functional narrowing of the subacromial space. Scapular winging may be seen and can be accentuated by muscle activation (Fig. 4.2). Observing the shoulder girdle from the back of the patient during arm flexion and abduction may reveal altered movement of the scapula secondary to muscle weakness or imbalances in flexibilities.

PALPATION

The superficial structures that should be evaluated are the sternal notch, sternoclavicular joint, clavicle, AC joint, long head of the biceps tendon, subacromial bursae, greater and lesser tuberosities of the humerus, coracoid process, supraclavicular fossa, and spine of the scapula with its borders (Fig. 4.3). The AC joint is superficial and is identified with palpation of the clavicle and spine of the scapula until they meet laterally. The long head of the biceps is anterior, between the lesser and greater humeral tuberosities, and is difficult to palpate because of the large deltoid muscle. By externally rotating the arm and flexing and extending the elbow, the examiner may be able to feel the tendon moving in the anterior shoulder. The cervical spine and trapezius should be palpated if the patient has neck pain.

The attachments of the muscles to the scapula are noted in Figure 4.4. When indicated, the axilla should be evaluated for masses, lymph nodes, and palpation of the muscles. The pectoralis major lies anterior and covers the pectoralis minor, which is difficult to palpate. The pectoralis minor muscle, when tight, has been implicated in an internally rotated and protracted scapula. The latissimus dorsi forms the posterior border and may occasionally be torn, especially in baseball pitchers.

RANGE OF MOTION TESTING

Active range of motion testing is usually performed first to allow the patient to feel comfortable and avoid painful positions. Passive motion testing can then be performed to isolate motions for accurate evaluation. The active and passive range of motion of both sides should be compared. The planes of shoulder girdle motion include forward

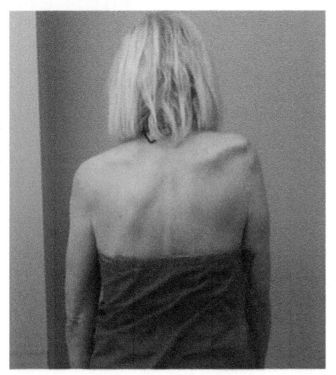

Figure 4.1 It is helpful to dress the patient so that both shoulders can be seen completely, allowing side-to-side comparison.

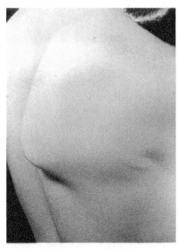

Figure 4.2 Winging of the scapula. (Reproduced with permission from Hawkins RJ, Bokor DJ: Clinical evaluation of shoulder problems. In Rockwood CA, Matsen FA (eds), *The Shoulder*, 2nd edn. Philadelphia: WB Saunders, 1998, p. 172.)

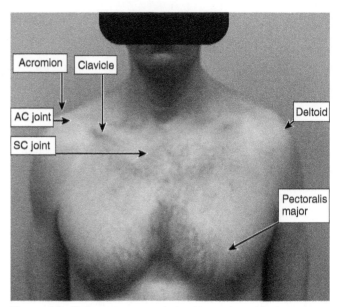

Figure 4.3 Surface anatomy of shoulder region. *AC*, Acromioclavicular; *SC*, sternoclavicular.

flexion, extension, internal/external rotation, abduction/adduction, and a combination called *circumduction*. Range of motion is noted by degrees from a reference position; usually the anatomic position is used without scapular fixation unless otherwise specified.

The first measure of shoulder motion should be elevation of the arm. Elevation can be performed with the arm in abduction or flexion. Abduction of the arm can be performed in the plane of the body but is best performed in the "scapular plane," which is approximately 30 degrees in front of the plane of the body (Fig. 4.5). Both forward flexion and abduction are typically at least 160 degrees but

may exceed this in flexible athletes. The next motions to evaluate are shoulder rotations. The neutral position is with the arm and forearm in the horizontal plane (Fig. 4.6A). The first is done with the arm abducted 90 degrees and typically supported by the examiner holding the elbow. External rotation (Fig. 4.6B) and internal rotation (Fig. 4.6C) at this elevation typically include not only motion of the ST articulation but also the glenohumeral joint. Next, external rotation with the arm at the side should be compared with that of the opposite extremity.

Internal rotation cannot be accurately measured with the arm at the side in this position because the trunk impedes the motion. Internal rotation of the shoulder can be performed by asking the patient to place the arms up the back with the thumbs up (Fig. 4.7). The landmarks typically used for this measure are the hip, buttock, sacrum, L1 body, lower border of the scapula around T8, and prominent C4 vertebral spinous process. This method of measurement can be reproducible for one individual, but the relationship of the thumb tip to various vertebral levels has not been shown to be accurate or reproducible.[1] One functional measure of internal rotation is the Apley scratch test, but it is not practical because most people cannot perform the maneuver (Fig. 4.8).

Normal values of active range of motion for the shoulder joint are shown in Table 4.1. When evaluating shoulder motion, it is sometimes important to measure glenohumeral motion while preventing ST motion. Isolating glenohumeral motion with the arm abducted 90 degrees involves externally or internally rotating the arm until scapular motion is perceived manually and visually. Internal and external rotation from this position can vary greatly, particularly in overhead athletes. Generally, glenohumeral external rotation is 90 degrees or more, and internal rotation is 0 to 30 degrees with the arm abducted 90 degrees. External rotation with the arm at the side can be measured either as glenohumeral motion alone or combined with ST motion.

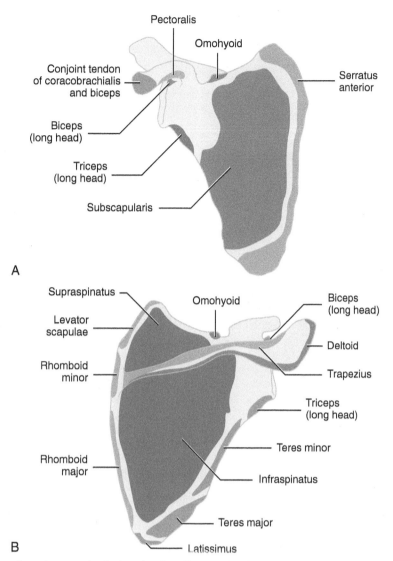

Figure 4.4   Muscular anatomy about the scapula. **A,** Anterior view. **B,** Posterior view. (Adapted from Jobe CM. Gross anatomy of the shoulder. In: Rockwood CA, Matsen FA, eds. *The Shoulder.* 2nd ed. Philadelphia: W.B. Saunders; 1998.44.)

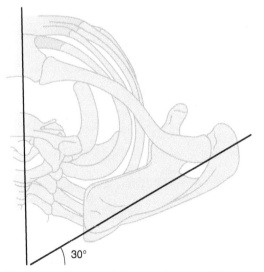

Figure 4.5   Plane of the scapula is approximately 30 degrees in front of the plane of the body. (Redrawn from McFarland EG: TK Kim, HB Park, G El Rassi, H Gill, E Keyurapan: Examination of the Shoulder: The Complete Guide, New York, Thieme, 2006, pp 162-212 Fig 2.4.)

Table 4.1   Normal Active Shoulder Range of Motion

Position	Degrees
Forward flexion/elevation[a]	0–180
Extension[a]	0–60
Abduction[a]	0–180
Glenohumeral internal rotation[b]	0–70
Glenohumeral external rotation[b]	0–90

[a]Zero begins at the anatomic position.
[b]Zero begins with the humerus abducted to 90 degrees.
Reproduced with permission from Moore KL. The upper limb. In: Clinically Oriented Anatomy. *2nd ed. Baltimore: Williams & Wilkins; 1985.*

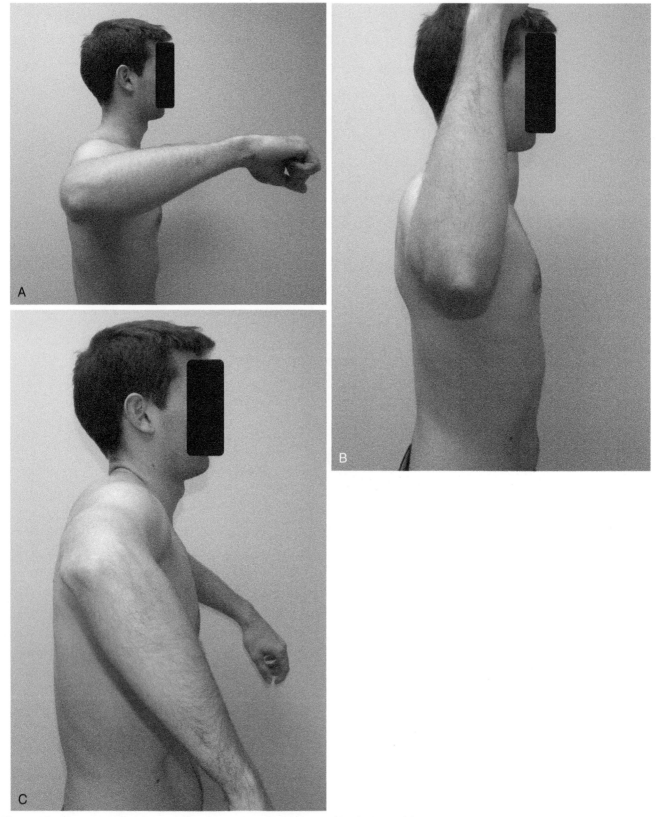

Figure 4.8   When examining the shoulders for rotation, the starting position is shown (**A**) with the arms in a neutral position, **B,** External rotation and (**C**) internal rotation can be measured from the side.

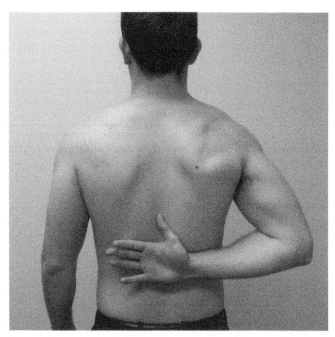

Figure 4.7   Internal rotation of the arm up the back is performed as pictured here.

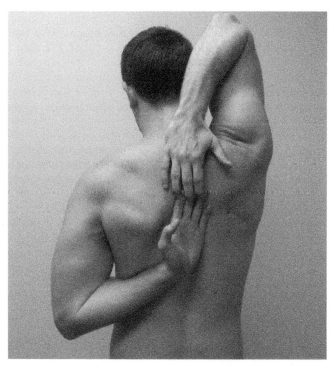

Figure 4.8   The Apley scratch test is a measure of several joint ranges of motion and not just the shoulder.

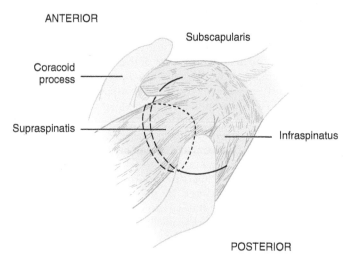

Figure 4.9   The rotator cuff muscles function to compress the humeral head into the glenoid and to rotate the arm. (Reproduced with permission from Perry J. Anatomy and biomechanics of the shoulder in throwing, swimming, gymnastics, and tennis. *Clin Sports Med.* 1983;2(2):252.)

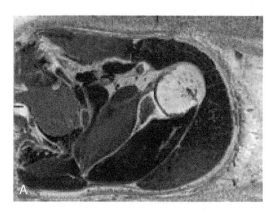

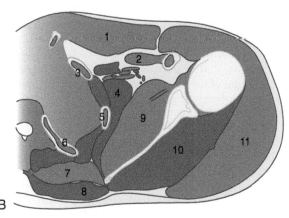

Figure 4.10   Prime movers about the shoulder girdle shown on magnetic resonance imaging (**A**) and illustrated (**B**): *1,* pectoralis major; *2,* pectoralis minor; *3,* first rib; *4,* serratus anterior; *5,* second rib; *6,* third rib; *7,* rhomboid; *8,* trapezius; *9,* subscapularis; *10,* infraspinatus; *11,* deltoid. (Adapted from Jobe CM. Gross anatomy of the shoulder. In: Rockwood CA, Matsen FA, eds. *The Shoulder.* 2nd ed. Philadelphia: W.B. Saunders; 1998:43.)

MUSCLES, INNERVATIONS, AND BIOMECHANICS

The muscles of the shoulder consist of the stabilizing rotator cuff (supraspinatus, infraspinatus, teres minor, and subscapularis; Fig. 4.9), trapezius, serratus anterior, rhomboids, and the prime movers (pectoralis major/minor, latissimus dorsi, teres major, triceps, biceps, and deltoid; Fig. 4.10). Most of the shoulder girdle is supplied by the fifth and sixth cervical roots through the upper trunk of the brachial plexus.

The suprascapular nerve (C5–C6) innervates the supraspinatus and infraspinatus, which originate from the supraspinatus and infraspinatus fossa, respectively. The supraspinatus inserts onto the superior facet of the greater tuberosity, whereas the infraspinatus inserts on the middle facet. The axillary nerve (C5–C6) innervates the deltoid and teres minor. The deltoid originates from the lateral third of the clavicle and scapular spine and includes the AC joint; it inserts onto the deltoid tuberosity of the humerus. The teres minor originates from the superior lateral portion of the scapula and inserts onto the inferior aspect of the greater tuberosity. The subscapularis is innervated by the nerve to the subscapularis (upper and lower), composed of the cervical 5, 6, and 7 roots. It originates from the anterior portion of the scapula (subscapularis fossa) and inserts onto the lesser tuberosity of the humerus.

The trapezius contains three portions—upper, middle, and lower. It is innervated by the spinal accessory, 11th cranial nerve (C3–C4). It has a vast origin from the occipital protuberance and superior nuchal line superiorly to the 12th thoracic vertebra inferiorly. It inserts onto the lateral third of the clavicle, acromion, and spine of the scapula. The long thoracic nerve (C5–C7) innervates the serratus anterior. It originates from the lateral portions of the first eight ribs and inserts onto the anterior surface of the medial border of the scapula. The rhomboids include the major and minor divisions and are innervated by the dorsal scapular nerve (C5). They originate from the ligamentum nuchae and spinous processes from C7 to T5 and insert onto the medial border of the scapula from the scapular spine to the inferior angle.

The pectoralis major has two components, the clavicular and sternocostal divisions, which are innervated by the lateral and medial pectoral nerves (clavicular, C5–C6 and sternocostal, C7–T1). The pectoralis minor is also innervated by these nerves (C6–C8). The major originates from the medial portion of the clavicle, sternum, and second to sixth ribs and inserts onto the humeral lateral lip of the intertubercular groove. The minor originates from ribs 3 to 5 and inserts onto the medial coracoid. The latissimus dorsi is supplied by the thoracodorsal nerve (C6–C8) and has a large origin of the spinous processes of T6 to the sacrum, the thoracolumbar fascia, iliac crest, and the caudal three ribs while inserting onto the floor of the intertubercular groove. The teres major is supplied by the lower subscapular nerve (C6–C7). It originates on the dorsal surface of the inferior angle of the scapula and inserts onto the medial lip of the intertubercular groove. The triceps has three heads, the long, lateral, and medial, which are supplied by the radial nerve (C6–C8). The long head originates from the infraglenoid tubercle of the scapula, and the lateral and medial heads originate from the posterior surface of the humerus superior and inferior to the spiral groove, respectively. They insert onto the proximal ulna (olecranon). The biceps comprises the long and short heads innervated by the musculocutaneous nerve (C5–C6). The long head originates from the supraglenoid tubercle of the scapula and the short head from the coracoid process of the scapula, and both insert onto the radial tuberosity and flow into the bicipital aponeurosis.

SCAPULAR BIOMECHANICS

Saha[2] has discussed three layers of muscles that stabilize the scapula and assist in force production from the musculature. The rotator cuff muscles (supraspinatus, infraspinatus, subscapularis, and teres minor) are the inner layer; these muscles serve first to provide compressive force of the humeral head into the glenoid and secondly to provide rotation of the arm. The middle layer comprises the teres major, pectoralis major, the latissimus dorsi, and the short fibers of the anterior and posterior deltoid. The superficial layer is the triceps, long head of the biceps, coracobrachialis, and superficial fibers of the anterior and posterior deltoid. The trapezius, rhomboids, and serratus anterior provide stabilizing forces because the scapula lacks rigid, bony fixation.

The upper trapezius, levator scapula, and superior serratus anterior elevate the scapula; the pectoralis minor and major and latissimus dorsi depress the scapula; the serratus anterior, pectoralis minor, and levator scapula protract the scapula; the trapezius, rhomboids, and latissimus dorsi retract the scapula; the superior and inferior portions of the trapezius and inferior portion of the serratus anterior cause lateral scapular rotation; and the levator scapula, rhomboids, pectoralis minor, and major and latissimus dorsi cause medial scapular rotation. These muscles fire in a coordinated fashion to perform the resultant actions in a smooth and effective manner, known as *force couples.*

Proper positioning of the scapula throughout motion allows the muscles associated with the scapula to have the appropriate length–tension relationships for the greatest efficiency of limb positioning. With the scapula stabilized, the glenoid can be maintained for humeral motion upon it. As the humerus is abducted, the glenohumeral to ST range of motion occurs at approximately a 2:1 ratio. This ratio changes through the arc of motion; that is, the 2:1 ratio is not constant throughout the entire range of motion. In the initial portion of abduction, glenohumeral motion predominates, and the ratio has been found to be 4.4 degrees of glenohumeral motion for every degree of ST motion. As the shoulder moves above 90 degrees of abduction, this ratio becomes 1.1 degrees of glenohumeral to 1 degree of ST motion. This scapular rotation during abduction also elevates the acromion, which has been postulated to help prevent impingement of the rotator cuff upon the acromion.[3,4]

Although the muscles are the dynamic stabilizers, the static stabilizers of the ligaments and joint capsule should not be forgotten (Fig. 4.11).[5,6] The primary stabilizer of anterior translation with the arm abducted to 90 degrees is the anterior band of the inferior glenohumeral ligament complex (IGHLC). With the arm in lesser degrees of abduction, the middle glenohumeral ligament restricts external rotation. Limitation of posterior translation is by the posterior band of the IGHLC, whereas inferior translation is limited by the inferior capsule and, at the top of the shoulder, the superior glenohumeral ligament (Fig. 4.12).[7] Recently, it has been noted that the inferior glenohumeral ligament also contributes to limitation of inferior motion with the arm abducted.[8]

TESTS OF ROTATOR CUFF STRENGTH AND INTEGRITY

See Table 4.2.

Dynamic stability of the glenohumeral joint is provided by contraction of the rotator cuff and, to a lesser degree, the long head of the biceps. These tendons increase compression across the glenohumeral joint and dynamically

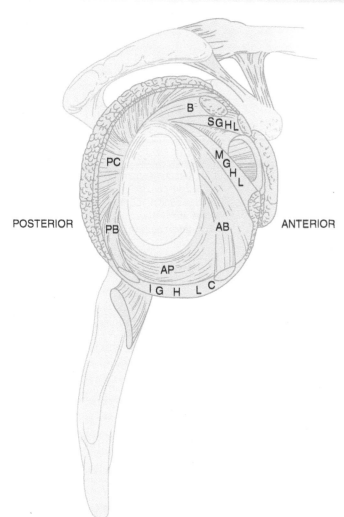

Figure 4.11 Anatomy of the glenohumeral ligaments. *AB,* anterior band; *B,* long head of biceps; *IGHLC,* inferior glenohumeral ligament complex; *MGHL,* middle glenohumeral ligament; *PB,* posterior band; *PC,* posterior capsule; *SGHL,* superior glenohumeral ligament. (From Bowen, MK, Warren RF; Ligamentous control of shoulder stability based on selective cutting and static translation experiments. *Clin Sports Med.* 1991;10:763.)

Figure 4.12 The superior glenohumeral ligament (SGHL) is the primary restraint to inferior translation. *AB,* Anterior band; *MGHL,* middle glenohumeral ligament; *PB,* posterior band. (Reproduced with permission from Bowen MK, Warren, RF. Ligamentous control of shoulder stability based on selective cutting and static translation experiments. *Clin Sport Med.* 1991;10:769.)

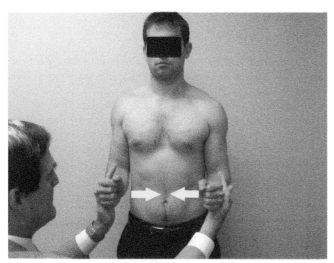

Figure 4.13 The infraspinatus is best assessed by testing external rotation with the arms at the side. *Arrows* show direction of examiner's force.

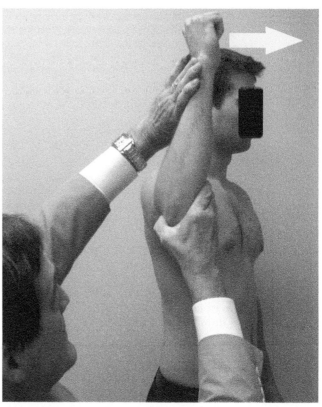

Figure 4.14 Patte test for testing teres minor and infraspinatus. *Arrow* shows direction of examiner's force.

Table 4.2   Tests of Rotator Cuff Strength and Integrity

Test	Description	Clinical Utility
Empty can test	The supraspinatus test is first performed by assessing the deltoid with the arm at 90 degrees of abduction and neutral rotation. The shoulder is then internally rotated and angled forward 30 degrees: the thumb should be pointing toward the floor. Muscle testing against resistance is then performed.	Naredo et al.[9] For detecting supraspinatus lesion: Sensitivity: 79.3% Specificity: 50% For detecting supraspinatus tendonitis: Sensitivity: 77.2% Specificity: 38.4% For detecting supraspinatus tears: Sensitivity: 18.7% Specificity: 100% Park et al.[10] For detecting partial-thickness RC tear: Sensitivity: 32.1% Specificity: 67.8% For detecting full-thickness RC tear: Sensitivity: 52.6% Specificity: 82.4%
Full can test	The examiner abducts the arm at 90 degrees of abduction and neutral rotation. The shoulder is then externally rotated with thumb pointing toward the roof. Muscle testing against the resistance is then performed.	Itoi et al.[11] For detecting partial-thickness RC tear: Sensitivity: 83% Specificity: 53% Accuracy: 78%
Drop arm test	The examiner abducts the patient's shoulder to 90 degrees and then asks the patient to slowly lower the arm to the side in the same arc of movement. A positive test result is indicated if the patient is unable to return the arm to the side slowly or has severe pain when attempting to do so.	Bryant et al.[12] For detecting RC tear: Positive predictive value: 100% Sensitivity: 10%
Patte test	The examiner supports the patient's elbow in 90 degrees of forward elevation in the plane of the scapula while the patient is asked to rotate the arm laterally to compare the strength of lateral rotation. Jobe and Patte maneuvers can produce three types of responses: (1) absence of pain, indicating that the tested tendon is normal; (2) the ability to resist despite pain, denoting tendonitis; or (3) the inability to resist with gradual lowering of the arm or forearm, indicating tendon rupture.	Naredo et al.[9] For detecting infraspinatus lesions: Sensitivity: 70.5% Specificity: 90% For detecting infraspinatus tendonitis: Sensitivity: 57.1% Specificity: 70.8% For detecting infraspinatus tears: Sensitivity: 36.3% Specificity: 95%

RC, rotator cuff.

maintain the position of the humeral head within the glenoid.[13-17] As the load on the arm increases, these muscles increase the contraction necessary to keep the humeral head in the socket.

Jenp and coworkers[18] used electromyography to detect the most specific positions for activating particular rotator cuff muscles. The supraspinatus could not be effectively isolated from the deltoid muscle when resisting abduction of the arm, but it is typically tested with the arm elevated 90 degrees with the thumb in internal, neutral, or external rotation.[18] With the arm in this position and the thumb in internal rotation, this test is known as the "Jobe test."[19] However, subsequent study has found that the test has equal validity whether the thumb is pointing down, neutral, or up.[20,21] The subscapularis' greatest activation was with the arm in the scapular plane at 90 degrees of elevation and neutral humeral rotation. The infraspinatus is best tested with the arms at the side (Fig. 4.13). The teres minor is best tested with the arm abducted 90 degrees and externally rotated 90 degrees (Fig. 4.14).

Author comment: You can have a complete tear of the rotator cuff but have complete range of motion. The difference between a shoulder with an intact rotator cuff and a torn rotator cuff is that the latter will be weak with abduction and external rotation.

EMPTY CAN TEST

Jobe[19] described the empty can test—also known as the supraspinatus test—to help in evaluating the strength of the supraspinatus muscle (Fig. 4.15). Jobe originally described the test as follows:

The supraspinatus test is first performed by assessing the deltoid with the arm at 90 degrees of abduction and neutral

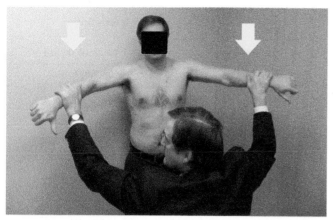

Figure 4.15 The Jobe (empty can) test is a test of the supraspinatus and deltoid muscles. The arms are abducted 90 degrees in the scapular plane with the elbows extended and the thumbs pointing down. The examiner pushes down, and a positive test result is pain or weakness. *Arrows* show the direction of the examiner's force.

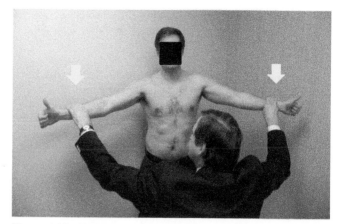

Figure 4.16 Electromyographic studies have shown that the Jobe test can test the supraspinatus and deltoid equally to the empty can test. This position is the "full can test" and is often less painful for patients than the empty can test. *Arrows* show direction of examiner's force.

rotation. The shoulder is then internally rotated and angled forward 30 degrees: the thumb should be pointing toward the floor. Muscle testing against resistance is then performed (Video 4-1).

The test result was positive when the patient reported pain or demonstrated weakness with the arm in this position. Unfortunately, the empty can test can be painful for many patients with shoulder conditions. We recommend performing this test first with the elbows bent to avoid injuring or aggravating the shoulder. Electromyographic study has shown that, in this position, the downward force is resisted by the deltoid and the supraspinatus muscles, so this test does not isolate the supraspinatus.[22] Malanga and associates[22] examined the rotator cuff muscles via electromyography using two testing positions on the basis of recommendations by Jobe and Moynes[23] and Blackburn and coworkers.[24] They noted the supraspinatus was sufficiently activated in both positions (Figs. 4.15 and 4.16).

The sensitivity and specificity of the Jobe test depend on the methods used for each study but also vary according to the type of rotator cuff lesion. The literature suggests that a positive Jobe test is sensitive and moderately specific for a tear of the supraspinatus tendon.[11,25]

FULL CAN TEST

The Jobe test for strength testing of the supraspinatus can be performed in the thumb-up position (see Fig. 4.16).

The examiner abducts the arm at 90 degrees of abduction and neutral rotation.[26] The shoulder is then externally rotated with the thumb pointing toward the roof. Muscle testing against the resistance is then performed. A positive test result is indicated by pain, weakness, or both.

Itoi and others[11] reported a sensitivity of 83%, specificity of 53%, and accuracy of 78% for the full can in detecting partial-thickness rotator cuff tears.

DROP ARM TEST

The drop arm test has been used to assess for rotator cuff tears, particularly of the supraspinatus. Although the original description of the drop arm test remains obscure, it has been ascribed to Codman and described by Magee[27] as follows:

> The examiner abducts the patient's shoulder to 90 degrees and then asks the patient to slowly lower the arm to the side in the same arc of movement. A positive test is indicated if the patient is unable to return the arm to the side slowly or has severe pain when attempting to do so (Video 4-2).

Bryant and coworkers[12] studied 53 patients with a suspicion for rotator cuff tear and compared physical examination tests to the results of MRI and ultrasonography of the shoulder. They found the drop arm test to have a 100% PPV (ie, if present, the patient has a tear) and 10% sensitivity (ie, if negative, the patient could still have a tear). It is important to realize that a positive drop arm test result can be caused by weakness of any cause, including cervical disc disease, brachial plexopathy, brachial neuritis, stroke, amyotrophic sclerosis, and many other neurologic factors.

TEST OF INFRASPINATUS AND TERES MINOR INTEGRITY

See Table 4.2.

As noted, previous electromyographic data have failed to differentiate the function of the infraspinatus and teres minor.[18,28] However, the strength of the infraspinatus can best be tested with resisted external rotation with the arm at the side (see Fig. 4.13).

PATTE TEST (Video 4-3)

Naredo and coworkers[9] reported a test described by Patte in 1995 for assessing tears of the infraspinatus and teres minor (see Fig. 4.14). They write:

> ... the examiner supports the patient's elbow in 90 degrees of forward elevation in the plane of the scapula while the patient is asked to rotate the arm laterally in order to compare the strength of lateral rotation. Jobe's and Patte's manoeuvres can produce three types of response: (a) absence of pain, indicating that the tested tendon is normal; (b) the ability to resist

despite pain, denoting tendinitis; or (c) the inability to resist with gradual lowering of the arm or forearm, indicating tendon rupture.

Naredo and associates[9] compared the Patte test with findings on ultrasonography and showed the test to have a sensitivity of 70.5%, specificity of 90%, PPV of 85.7%, and NPV of 70.5% for detecting infraspinatus lesions; a sensitivity of 57.1%, specificity of 70.8%, PPV of 36.3%, and NPV of 85% for detecting infraspinatus tendonitis; and a sensitivity of 36.3%, specificity of 95%, PPV of 80%, and NPV of 73% for detecting infraspinatus tears.

TESTS OF SUBSCAPULARIS STRENGTH

See Table 4.3.

LIFT-OFF TEST

Muscle strength of the subscapularis can be tested with the lift-off maneuver. The test was first described by Gerber and Krushell[32] in 1991 and was originally performed with the hand up the back (Fig. 4.17). The patient was asked to lift the hand off the buttocks, and if this was not possible, then a subscapularis tendon tear was considered present. Electromyographic study has demonstrated the validity of this test for specificity of the subscapularis (Video 4-4).[33]

LIFT-OFF LAG SIGN

A variation of the lift-off test is the lift-off lag sign. In this test, the examiner holds the elbow of the patient and lifts the hand off the midsacrum level (Fig. 4.18A). The patient is asked not to let the arm or forearm fall to the buttocks; a test result is considered positive if the arm falls to the buttocks or toward the floor (Fig. 4.18B).[34]

BEAR HUG TEST (Video 4-5)

The bear hug test was described by Barth and associates[31] and is performed by asking the patient to place the hand on the side of the shoulder to be tested on the opposite shoulder (Fig. 4.19). The examiner then asks the patient to try to keep the hand on the shoulder while the examiner attempts to pull it off the opposite shoulder. A test result is considered positive when the patient cannot keep the hand on the shoulder and it pulls away.

TESTS OF SCAPULAR PATHOLOGY

See Table 4.4.

The role of the scapula in normal and abnormal shoulder conditions has been controversial. Kibler and coworkers[38] suggested that changes in scapular position contribute to rotator cuff symptoms, labral tears, and shoulder pain. These conclusions are based on observations that patients with shoulder pathologies often have what appear to be malpositioning of the scapula at rest and abnormal motion of the scapula upon the chest wall with activity. This abnormal scapular motion on the thorax with activity has been called "scapular dyskinesis."[38] Although there is little doubt that there are scapular dyskinesia patterns, it is unknown whether the patterns are a cause of shoulder pathologies or the result of shoulder pathologies. Therefore, scapular movement issues are typically addressed simultaneously with the painful conditions associated with the scapular motions.[39]

Although measurement of scapular position and movement had become very popular, these concepts have undergone increasing scrutiny. The tests are described below in detail, but the relationships between these findings and the pathophysiology of the clinical findings is being questioned. For example, Kibler and associates[40] proposed that there were four patterns of scapular dyskinesia. Subsequent study

Table 4.3   Tests of Subscapularis Strength

Test	Description	Clinical Utility
Lift-off test	The hand of the affected arm is placed on the back at the mid-lumbar region, and the patient is asked to rotate the arm internally and lift the hand posteriorly off the back. A positive test result is when the patient cannot lift the hand off the back.	Bartsch et al.[29]: Sensitivity: 40% Specificity: 79% PPV: 50% NPV: 71% Accuracy: 66% Salaffi et al.[5]: Sensitivity: 35% Specificity: 75% PPV: 85% NPV: 21% Accuracy: 64%
Lift-off lag sign	In sitting position, the hand on the side of the painful shoulder is placed at the lumbar region (hand behind back). The hand is passively lifted from the lumbar spine until almost full internal rotation is reached, and the patient is asked to maintain the position actively. The test result is positive if the patient cannot maintain the position.	Miller et al.[30]: Sensitivity: 100% Specificity: 84% PPV: 28% NPV: 100% Bartsch et al.[29]: Sensitivity: 71% Specificity: 60% PPV: 45% NPV: 81% Accuracy: 63%
Bear hug test	The bear hug test was described by Barth et al.[31] and is performed by asking the patient to place the hand on the side of the shoulder to be tested on the opposite shoulder. The examiner then asks the patient to try to keep the hand on the shoulder while the examiner attempts to pull it off the opposite shoulder. A test result is considered positive when the patient cannot keep the hand on the shoulder and it pulls away.	Barth et al.[31]: Sensitivity: 60% Specificity: 92% PPV: 75% NPV: 85% Accuracy: 82%

NPV, Negative predictive value; *PPV*, positive predictive value.

found that independent observers could not agree when trying to classify dyskinesia patterns, and the study concluded that agreement was best when the observers merely made a "yes" or "no" assessment of the presence of dyskinesia.[41] Similarly, it was originally suggested that dyskinesia patterns could be associated with specific disease states.[39] This has since been disproven,[42] and although scapular dyskinesia can be associated with a variety of shoulder conditions, it cannot be used reliably as a diagnostic tool for specific shoulder conditions. Consequently, these tests

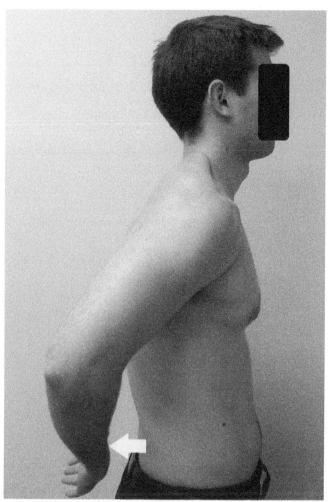

Figure 4.17 The lift-off test is performed by having the patient lift the hand off the lower back as shown *(arrow)*. If the patient cannot do this, then the test result is positive for a subscapularis tendon tear.

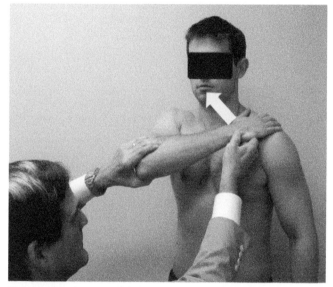

Figure 4.19 The bear hug test is performed by having the patient place the hand of the affected shoulder on the opposite shoulder. The examiner then tries to pull the hand off the shoulder. The *arrow* shows direction of examiner's force. A positive test result is when the wrist flexes or the hand can be pulled away from the shoulder.

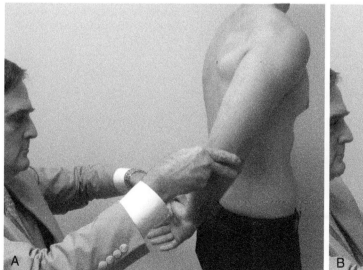
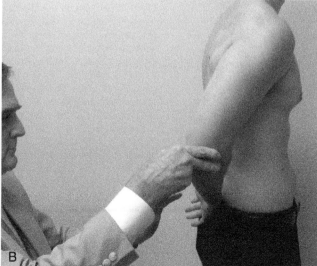

Figure 4.18 **A,** The lift-off lag sign is performed by holding the patient's hand away from the lower back while stabilizing the elbow. **B,** A positive test result is when the hand falls back to the torso and cannot stay in the starting position.

Table 4.4   Tests of Scapular Pathology

Test	Description	Reliability/Validity
Lateral scapular slide test	The first position of the test is with the arm relaxed at the side. The second is with the hands on the hips with the fingers anterior and the thumb posterior with approximately 10 degrees of shoulder extension. The third position is with the arms at or below 90 degrees of arm elevation with maximal internal rotation at the glenohumeral joint. These positions offer a graded challenge to the functioning of the shoulder muscles to stabilize the scapula. The final position presents a challenge to the muscles in the position of most common function at 90 degrees of shoulder elevation.	Odom et al.[35] With 1.5-cm difference as positive: In first position: Sensitivity: 28% Specificity: 53% In second position: Sensitivity: 50% Specificity: 58% In third position: Sensitivity: 34% Specificity: 52% With 1-cm difference as positive: In first position: Sensitivity: 35% Specificity: 48% In second position: Sensitivity: 41% Specificity: 54% In third position: Sensitivity: 43% Specificity: 56%
Isometric pinch test	The test is performed by having the patient pinch the scapulas together posteriorly in retraction. A positive test for scapular muscle weakness is if the patient has burning pain prior to holding this position for 15 to 20 seconds.	Unable to find any tests of sensitivity or specificity
Scapular assistance test	The scapular assistance test involves assisting the lower trapezius by stabilizing the upper medial border of the scapula and rotating the inferomedial border as the arm is abducted or adducted. The test result is positive, indicating lower trapezius weakness as part of the injury, when it gives relief of symptoms of impingement, clicking, or rotator cuff weakness.	Wright et al.[36] Sensitivity: 100 Specificity: 33 Likelihood ratio: 1.49 Intertester reliability has been studied. In the scapular plane, there was 77% agreement between two examiners, and the kappa coefficient was 0.53. In the sagittal plane, there was 91% agreement between two examiners, and the kappa coefficient was 0.62. The authors concluded that it has acceptable interrater reliability.[37]
Scapular retraction test	The test involves manually positioning and stabilizing the entire medial border of the scapula. This test is helpful in two groups of patients. The first group has decreased retraction and apparent muscle weakness. The test result is positive when retesting reveals increased muscle strength with the scapula in the stabilized position. The second group has a positive Jobe relocation test. The test result is positive when scapular retraction decreases the pain or impingement associated with the Jobe relocation test. This indicates that decreased scapular retraction is a component of the overall injury and must be addressed in rehabilitation. A positive scapular retraction test indicates trapezius and rhomboid weakness.	We have found no tests assessing the validity, reliability, sensitivity, specificity, positive predictive value, or negative predictive value of this test.

should be used with an understanding of their limitations and clinical applications.

LATERAL SCAPULAR SLIDE TEST (Video 4-6)

Kibler[43] described the lateral scapular slide test (LSST) in identification of subtle ST motion abnormalities as follows Fig. 4.20:

> The first position is with the arms relaxed at the sides. The second is with the hands on the hips with the fingers anterior and the thumb posterior with about 10 degrees of shoulder extension. The third position is with the arms at or below 90 degrees of arm elevation with maximal internal rotation at the glenohumeral joint.
>
> These positions offer a graded challenge to the functioning of the shoulder muscles to stabilize the scapula. The final position presents a challenge to the muscles in the position of most common function at 90 degrees of shoulder elevation ...
>
> The reference point on the spine is the nearest spinous process, which is then marked with an X. The measurements from the reference point on the spine to the medial border of the scapula are measured on both sides. In the second position, the new position of the inferomedial border of the scapula is marked, and the reference point on the spine is maintained. The distances once again are calculated on both sides. The same protocol is done for the third position.

The exact amount of asymmetry that should be considered pathologic is controversial. Kibler[43] defined 1.5 cm of asymmetry as positive for ST motion abnormality. Odom and coworkers[35] reported 1 cm of asymmetry as being positive when correlated with patients who did or did not have shoulder pathologies. The sensitivities and specificities of this test for pathologic conditions were low regardless of the position measured. Odom and coworkers[35] concluded that "the LSST should not be used to identify people with [or] without shoulder dysfunction."

ISOMETRIC PINCH TEST

In Kibler's 1998 paper, "the role of the scapula in athletic shoulder function" is described by a provocative maneuver for evaluating scapular muscular strength.[43] Kibler writes:

> A good provocative maneuver to evaluate scapular muscle strength is to do an isometric pinch of the scapulae in retraction. Scapular muscle weakness can be noted as a burning pain in less than 15 seconds. Normally, the scapula can be held in this position for 15 to 20 seconds with the patient having no burning pain or muscle weakness.

No independent studies have validated this test or examined its clinical utility. A similar test is the costoclavicular maneuver for making the diagnosis of thoracic outlet syndrome.[44,45]

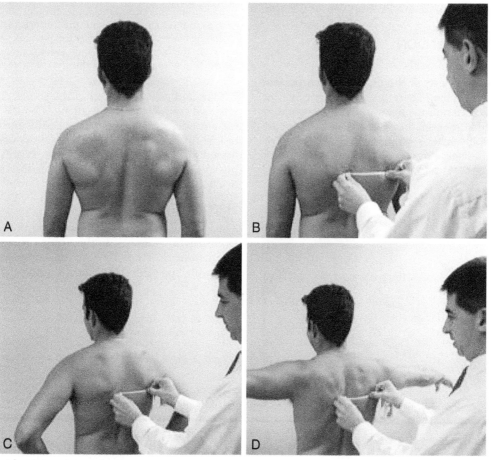

Figure 4.20 Lateral scapular slide test. Measurements are made from a reference point (eg, nearest spinous process) to the inferomedial border of the scapula. **A,** Initial position for examination of the scapula. **B,** Measurement in the first position with arm relaxed at the side. **C,** Second position with hands on hips, fingers anterior, and thumb posterior with approximately 10 degrees of shoulder extension. **D,** Third position with arms at or below 90 degrees of elevation with maximal internal rotation at the glenohumeral joint.

SCAPULAR ASSISTANCE TEST (Video 4-7)

Another test for the strength of the scapular stabilizers is the scapular assistance test (Fig. 4.21) described by Kibler and McMullen[42] in 2003. They described the test as follows:

> The scapular assistance test evaluates scapular and acromial involvement in subacromial impingement. In a patient with impingement symptoms with forward elevation or abduction, assistance for scapular elevation is provided by manually stabilizing the scapula and rotating the inferior border of the scapula as the arm moves. This procedure simulates the force-couple activity of the serratus anterior and lower trapezius muscles. Elimination or modification of the impingement symptoms indicates that these muscles should be a major focus in rehabilitation.

There has been no independent verification of this study, and its clinical usefulness has not been adequately studied.

SCAPULAR RETRACTION TEST

The scapular retraction test was described by Kibler and associates[46] to distinguish a scapular cause of weakness of the supraspinatus. After initial standard supraspinatus testing (Jobe test), the medial border of the scapula is stabilized by the examiner, and muscle testing is repeated. The test is considered positive if supraspinatus strength increases after stabilization of the scapula.[46] We have found no reports assessing the sensitivity, specificity, PPV, or NPV of this test.

TESTS OF THE BICEPS TENDON

See Table 4.5.

Physical examination tests of the biceps tendon present challenges to the clinician. There are several reasons for this. First, the biceps tendon is deep in the joint where it cannot be palpated. Also, even the extra-articular part of the tendon in the bicipital groove is difficult to palpate because other structures (namely the rotator cuff tendons) attach near the bicipital groove. Second, a click or a catch in the

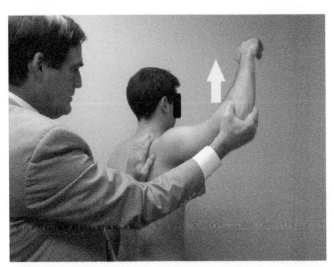

Figure 4.21 The scapular assistance test is designed to determine if stabilizing the scapula improves shoulder pain. The examiner stabilizes the scapula and elevates the arm. The *arrow* shows the direction of the examiner's force.

shoulder cannot be assumed to be caused by the biceps tendon. One study found that only 5% of patients with superior labral tears have a click, but 5% of a control group also had a click.[50]

LUDINGTON TEST

In 1923, Nelson Ludington described a test for diagnosing rupture of the long head of the biceps.[51] Ludington asked the patient to put his or her hands on the head with the palm down and to contract the biceps muscle (Fig. 4.22). The test result was positive if there was a visible deformity of the biceps (Popeye deformity) or if the biceps tendon could not be felt proximally in the arm. This test has never been studied clinically, but palpation of the long head of the biceps tendon is not typically reliable in the proximal arm. Also, in most patients with a torn biceps tendon, a bulge is seen simply by asking the patient to contract the biceps muscle with the arm at the side.

There are no reported studies assessing the sensitivity, specificity, PPV, or NPV of this maneuver.

YERGASON'S TEST

Robert Yergason originally described his "supination sign" for evaluating tendonitis of the biceps tendon in 1931.[52] He described the test as follows (Fig. 4.23):

> If the elbow is flexed to 90 degrees, the forearm being pronated; and the examining surgeon holds the patient's wrist so as to resist supination, and then directs that active supination be made against his resistance; pain, very definitely localized in the bicipital groove, indicates a condition of wear and tear of the long head of the biceps... (Video 4-8)

Calis and associates[47] found the Yergason's test to have a sensitivity of 37% and a specificity of 86.1% for diagnosis of subacromial impingement using MRI and Neer injection test as the gold standards. The authors described the test for a disorder of the long head of the biceps tendon but did not specify how this related to the diagnosis of biceps disease or conditions.

SPEED'S TEST

The earliest reference to this study in the literature was by Crenshaw and Kilgore on "the surgical treatment of bicipital tenosynovitis" in 1996.[53] They cite a personal communication with Speed in 1952 and describe the test as follows (Fig. 4.24):

> [Have] the patient flex his shoulder [elevate it anteriorly] against resistance while the elbow is extended and the forearm supinated. The test is considered positive when pain is localized to the bicipital groove (Video 4-9).

Several studies have shown that Speed's test does not actually help the clinician in making the diagnosis of biceps tendon disorders. Bennett[48] found Speed's test to have a specificity of 13.8% and a sensitivity of 90% for biceps tendon disorders. Gill and coworkers[49] found that Speed's test had a sensitivity of 50%, specificity of 67%, PPV of 8%, NPV of 96%, and likelihood ratio of 1.51 for detecting partial tears of the biceps tendon. Calis and associates[47] noted the Speed's test to have a sensitivity of 68.5% and a

Table 4.5 Tests of the Biceps Tendon

Test	Description	Reliability/Validity
Yergason's test	The elbow is flexed to 90 degrees with the forearm pronated, and the examiner holds the patient's wrist to resist supination and then directs that active supination be made against the resistance; pain, very definitely localized in the bicipital groove, indicates a condition of wear and tear of the long head of the biceps.	Calis et al.[47] For diagnosis of subacromial impingement (not evaluating the biceps tendon) using MRI and Neer injection test as the gold standards: Sensitivity: 37% Specificity: 86%
Speed's test	Have the patient flex the shoulder (elevate it anteriorly) against resistance while the elbow is extended and the forearm supinated. The test result is considered positive when pain is localized to the bicipital groove.	Bennett[48] Sensitivity: 90% Specificity: 13.8% Calis et al.[47] For subacromial impingement: Sensitivity: 68.5% Specificity: 55.5%
Lift-off test for partial tears of the biceps tendon	The hand of the affected arm is placed on the back at the midlumbar region, and the patient is asked to rotate the arm internally and lift the hand posteriorly off the back. A positive test result is when the patient cannot lift the hand off of the back.	Gill et al.[49] Sensitivity: 28% Specificity: 89% PPV: 15% NPV: 95% Likelihood ratio: 2.61 Accuracy: 85%
Ludington test	The patient is asked to put hands on the head with palms down and to contract the biceps muscle. The test result is positive if there is a visible deformity or if the biceps tendon cannot be felt proximally in the arm.	There are no reported studies assessing the sensitivity, specificity, PPV, or NPV of this maneuver.

MRI, magnetic resonance imaging; *NPV,* negative predictive value; *PPV,* positive predictive value.

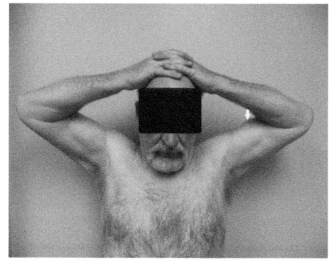

Figure 4.22 The Ludington test was designed to compare the biceps muscle shape side to side. The *arrow* shows the Popeye deformity.

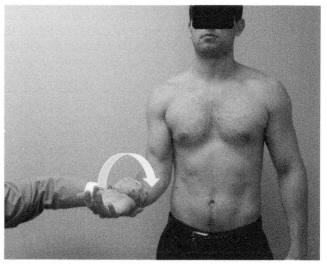

Figure 4.23 Yergason's test is performed by the examiner resisting forearm supination by the patient with the elbow bent. The *arrow* shows the direction of the examiner's force.

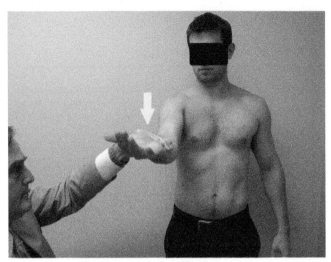

Figure 4.24 Speed's test is performed by the patient resisting a downward force by the examiner *(arrow)*. A positive test result is pain in the biceps area of the shoulder.

specificity of 55.5%. Burkhart and others[15] evaluated Speed's test for labral pathology. They found that it had a sensitivity of 100% and a specificity of 70% for anterior labral lesions and a sensitivity of 29% and a specificity of 11% for posterior labral lesions. The combined sensitivity and specificity for both lesions were 78% and 37%, respectively.

TESTS OF ROTATOR CUFF DISEASE

See Table 4.6.

Over the past 15 years, it has become increasingly appreciated that rotator cuff tendon disease is a complex condition characterized by aging of the tendons with subsequent tendinopathy, partial tears of the tendons, and eventually full-thickness tears of the tendons. It is now recognized that rotator cuff tears are attributable to intrinsic causes (ie, the tendons wear out over time). It cannot be totally ruled out that contact of the rotator cuff with the acromion or other structures might contribute to the pain seen with some rotator cuff tears, so it is thought that the disease spectrum should be called "rotator cuff disease" and not "impingement."[55,56]

There is also increasing appreciation that there is no consistent relationship between rotator cuff disease and pain. Some patients have complete tears of three of the four rotator cuff tendons and have full range of motion of the shoulder. Other patients have only a partial tear and have symptoms that awaken them at night or keep them from sports participation. Many factors seem to influence which rotator cuff pathologies cause pain in certain individuals but not others.

As a result of this shift in how we think of rotator cuff disease, tests for "impingement" are known not to be diagnostic for any one type of rotator cuff disorder. Typically, rotator cuff pain is present on the lateral side of the shoulder into the deltoid and midarm. It is typically made worse with lifting overhead or lifting weights away from the body. Patients with full tears can have a spectrum of findings but typically have weakness when lifting overhead and lifting away from the body with the elbows extended.

Studies have shown that results of "impingement tests" such as the Neer sign and the Hawkins sign can be positive with a myriad of shoulder disorders and not just with rotator cuff disease. The most reliable tests for rotator cuff tears are weakness to resisted abduction, weakness to resisted external rotation with the arm at the side, and a "painful arc." A study by Murrell and Walton[57] found that if a patient was older than 65 years of age, had a positive Neer or Hawkins sign, and had weakness in external rotation, then there was a 98% chance the patient had a full-thickness rotator cuff tear. A study by Park and others[10] similarly found that a patient older than 65 years of age with a painful arc and weakness in abduction had a 91% chance of a full-thickness rotator cuff tear. It should be noted that if a patient has only pain and not weakness with resisted abduction or external rotation, this is not diagnostic for rotator cuff disease.[11]

NEER SIGN

In 1972, Neer[58] hypothesized that with forward flexion of the arm, the damaged rotator cuff would create pain into the deltoid region or into the anterior shoulder (Fig. 4.25). Neer also noted that at approximately 80 degrees of flexion, the rotator cuff was flexed past the acromial edge. However, the Neer sign is positive typically around 120 degrees of flexion, where the rotator cuff hits the superior glenoid (Video 4-10).[59] The Neer test also can be positive with a wide variety of shoulder conditions, including stiff shoulders, superior labral lesions, arthritis, and fractures.

THE PAINFUL ARC

The painful arc was first described by Neer,[58] who noted that patients with an inflamed rotator cuff would often have pain from approximately 70 to 120 degrees, and the pain would diminish at about that level of elevation (Fig. 4.26). The pain is typically into the deltoid area and sometimes worsens when bringing the arm down from an elevated position. Neer also noted that in terminal flexion there may be pain at the top of the arc of motion; he suggested this pain was caused by arthritic AC joints. This test alone does not make the diagnosis of rotator cuff disorders, but in combination with other tests, it has a role in the shoulder evaluation.

NEER SUBACROMIAL INJECTION TEST

In 1977, Neer reported a "test" (called a "test" to distinguish it from the Neer "sign") to evaluate impingement of the rotator cuff tendons against the acromion and coracoacromial ligament, which involved injecting the subacromial space with local anesthetic.[58] Neer suggested that if injection of local anesthetic into the subacromial space did not relieve the pain, then the pain was most likely coming from another location than bursa and rotator cuff.

In 1980, Hawkins also suggested that in patients with painful rotator cuff disease, the diagnosis could be confirmed with an injection into the subacromial space. This test is known as the Neer test or the subacromial injection test.[60] There are no studies that validate this test.

Kirkley and associates[61] used the Neer test unsuccessfully to predict outcomes from subacromial decompression for rotator cuff tendinosis. There was no correlation between postoperative Western Ontario Rotator Cuff Index scores and the result of the injections, suggesting that there were

Table 4.6   Tests of Rotator Cuff Disease

Test	Description	Reliability/Validity

Neer sign	Passive elevation of the arm in flexion with the arm in internal rotation while stabilizing the scapula from the back should result in pain into the deltoid region. Typically, pain occurs around 120 degrees of flexion.	Calis et al.[47]
		  Sensitivity: 88.7%
		  Specificity: 30.5%
		MacDonald et al.[54]
		  For assessing subacromial bursitis:
		    Sensitivity: 75%
		    Specificity: 47.5%
		  For detecting RC pathology:
		    Sensitivity: 83.3%
		    Specificity: 50.8%
		Park et al.[10]
		  For assessing subacromial bursitis:
		    Sensitivity: 85.7%
		    Specificity: 49.2%
		    PPV: 20.9%
		    NPV: 95.7%
		    +LR: 1.69
		    Accuracy: 54.2
		  For partial RC tears:
		    Sensitivity: 75.4%
		    Specificity: 47.5%
		    PPV: 18.1%
		    NPV: 92.6%
		    +LR: 1.44
		    Accuracy: 51.3
		  For full-thickness RC tears:
		    Sensitivity: 59.3%
		    Specificity: 47.2%
		    PPV: 41.3%
		    NPV: 64.9%
		    +LR: 1.12
		    Accuracy: 51.8%

Neer subacromial injection test	Neer sign pain may be temporarily stopped by instilling 1% lidocaine into the bursa.	There are no studies that validate the Neer test.

Hawkins test	This involves forward flexing the humerus to 90 degrees and internally rotating. Pain should radiate into the deltoid region.	MacDonald et al.[54]
		  For assessing subacromial bursitis:
		    Sensitivity: 91.7%
		    Specificity: 44.3%
		  For RC pathology:
		    Sensitivity: 87.5%
		    Specificity: 42.6%
		Calis et al.[47]
		  Sensitivity: 92.1%
		  Specificity: 25%
		MacDonald et al.[54]
		  When Neer and Hawkins tests were both positive for detecting bursitis:
		    Sensitivity: 70.8%
		    Specificity: 50.8%
		  For detecting RC pathology:
		    Sensitivity: 83.3%
		    Specificity: 55.7%
		  If only one of the two tests was positive, for detecting bursitis:
		    Sensitivity: 95.8%
		    Specificity: 41%
		  For detecting RC pathology:
		    Sensitivity: 87.5%
		    Specificity: 37.7%

Continued on following page

Table 4.6   Tests of Rotator Cuff Disease (Continued)

Test	Description	Reliability/Validity

Painful arc sign	The patient is asked to actively abduct the shoulder. In a positive test result, the patient will experience pain from approximately 70 to 120 degrees, and pain will diminish after that level of elevation. The pain is typically into the deltoid area and sometimes worsens when bringing the arm down from an elevated position.	Park et al.[10]
		  For subacromial bursitis:
		    Sensitivity: 70.6%
		    Specificity: 46.9%
		    PPV: 12.3%
		    NPV: 93.8%
		    LR: 1.33
		    Accuracy: 49.2%
		  For partial RC tears:
		    Sensitivity: 67.4%
		    Specificity: 47%
		    PPV: 14.9%
		    NPV: 91.3%
		    LR: 1.27
		    Accuracy: 49.4%
		  For full-thickness RC tears:
		    Sensitivity: 75.8%
		    Specificity: 61.8%
		    PPV: 61%
		    NPV: 76.4%
		    LR: 1.98
		    Accuracy: 68%

Yocum's test	The patient is asked to place the hand on his or her other shoulder and to raise the elbow without elevating the shoulder. This test is positive when it elicits the pain usually experienced by the patient.	Naredo et al.[9]
		  Yocum's test in combination with Hawkins' and Neer's test:
		    Sensitivity: 65%
		    Specificity: 72.7%
		Silva et al.[64]
		    Sensitivity: 79%
		    Specificity: 79%
		    LR: 1.32

LR, likelihood ratio; *NPV,* negative predictive value; *PPV,* positive predictive value; *RC,* rotator cuff.

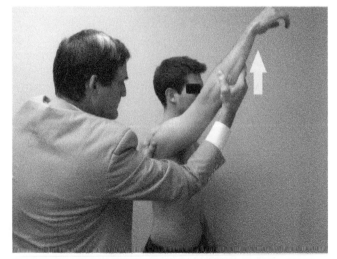

Figure 4.25   The test for the Neer sign is performed by the examiner stabilizing the shoulder blade as the arm is raised in flexion. A positive test is pain in the deltoid or anterior shoulder. The *arrow* shows the direction of the examiner's force.

other factors involved in creating pain other than inflammation of the subacromial space.

HAWKINS TEST (Video 4-11)

Hawkins and Schutte[62] described this test but ascribed it to Dr. John Charles Kennedy. It was performed by forward flexing the arm bent at the elbow (Fig. 4.27). A positive test result is when there is pain into the deltoid or anterior shoulder. Unfortunately, the Hawkins test can be positive in a variety of shoulder conditions and cannot be used alone to make the diagnosis of rotator cuff dysfunction.

Another controversy that is important to understand is that some suggest that looseness of the shoulder joint can lead to shoulder pain and "instability." This type of instability is supposedly experienced by the patient as pain and not typically felt as the pain experienced when the shoulder is coming out of the socket. This is an important distinction for two reasons. First, one theory of shoulder pain in athletes is that their shoulders are unstable, and the treatment is to strengthen the muscles around the shoulder; if that does not work, it is suggested that surgery to tighten the ligaments might be helpful. The second reason that this distinction is important is that physical examination tests for instability are

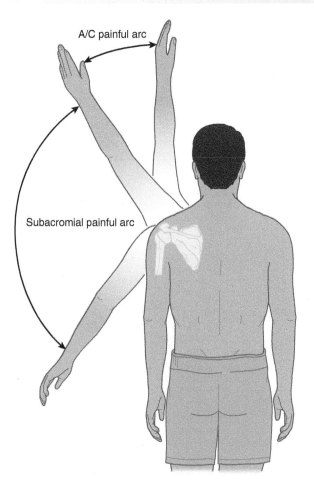

Figure 4.26 Diagrammatic presentation of the painful arc. Patients with inflamed rotator cuffs typically have pain from 70 to 120 degrees.

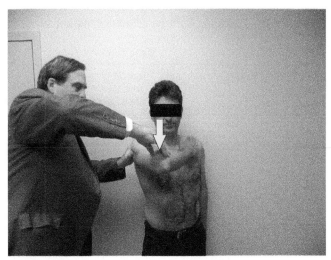

Figure 4.28 In the Yocum test the patient places his hand on the opposite shoulder. The patient is then asked to resist a downward force by the examiner on the elbow. A positive test is pain or weakness with resistance.

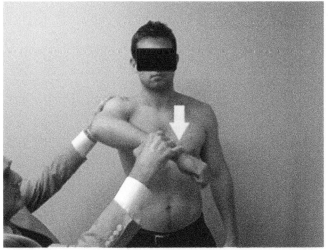

Figure 4.27 The Hawkins test is performed by forward flexing the arm to approximately 90 degrees and then slowly internally rotating the arm. The *arrow* shows the direction of the examiner's force. A positive test result is pain in the anterior or lateral shoulder.

very accurate for traumatic instability but not for patients who have shoulder pain from "too much laxity." A good example is the anterior apprehension test for anterior shoulder instability. If, during the test, the patient feels that the shoulder will come out of the socket, then a diagnosis of

anterior shoulder instability can be made with accuracy. However, if the patient just has pain with an apprehension maneuver, it does not mean the patient has instability and may reflect other conditions in the shoulder.

It also should be noted that the physical examination tests for shoulder instability are among the most clinically helpful and accurate of all shoulder examination tests. Several of these tests accurately diagnose anterior shoulder instability more than 93% of the time and can be used with confidence.

YOCUM'S TEST

Naredo et al.[9] described a test developed by Lewis Yocum[63] for assessing impingement (Figure 4.28). The test is described as follows:

> ... the patient is asked to place the hand on his or her other shoulder and to raise the elbow without elevating the shoulder. These tests are positive when they elicit the pain usually experienced by the patient (Video 4-12).

Naredo et al.[9] showed that Yocum's test in combination with Hawkins' and Neer's test had a sensitivity of 65%, specificity of 72.7%, positive predictive value of 81.2%, and negative predictive value of 53% when compared with findings on ultrasonography. Another study by Silva et al.[64] suggested that the Yocum test had a sensitivity of 79% and a specificity of 70% for rotator cuff pathology found on MRI alone. It should be noted that this latter study used MRI as the gold standard, and the Yocum test had a likelihood ratio of only 1.32.

See also the description of the posterior apprehension test below; this maneuver also assists in assessment of impingement.

TESTS FOR ANTERIOR SHOULDER INSTABILITY

See Table 4.7.

The anterior band of the IGHLC is considered the primary restraint for anterior translation at 90 degrees of

Table 4.7 Tests for Anterior Shoulder Instability

Test	Description	Reliability/Validity
Apprehension test	This test can be carried out with the patient in either a standing or supine position. As the shoulder is moved passively into maximal external rotation in abduction and forward pressure is applied to the posterior aspect of the humeral head, the patient suddenly becomes apprehensive.	Farber et al.[68] With relief of pain: Sensitivity: 30% Specificity: 90% PPV: 19% NPV: 94% Accuracy: 86% +LR: 3 −LR: 0.77 With relief of apprehension: Sensitivity: 81% Specificity: 92% PPV: 53% NPV: 98% Accuracy: 91% +LR: 10.3 −LR: 0.2
Jobe relocation (Fowler) test	The examiner first performs the apprehension test, and at the point where the patient feels pain or apprehension, the examiner applies a posteriorly directed force to the humeral head.	Speer et al.[67] Without the provocative maneuver: Accuracy: 80% With the provocative maneuver: Accuracy: 85% With the provocative maneuver for pain: Sensitivity: 54% Specificity: 44% With the provocative maneuver for apprehension: Sensitivity: 68% Specificity: 100%
Anterior release ("surprise") test	This test is performed with the patient in the supine position, with the affected shoulder over the edge of the examining table. The patient's arm is abducted to 90 degrees while the examiner places a posteriorly directed force on the patient's humeral head with the hand. The posterior force is maintained while the patient's arm is brought into the extreme of external rotation. The humeral head is then released. The test result is considered positive when the patient reports that the shoulder subluxates or dislocates.	Gross and Distefano[70] Sensitivity: 91.9% Specificity: 88.9%
Fulcrum test (Video 4-13)	The patient lies supine at the edge of the examination table with the arm abducted to 90 degrees. The examiner places one hand on the table under the glenohumeral joint to act as a fulcrum. The arm is gently and progressively extended and externally rotated over this fulcrum. Maintenance of gentle passive external rotation for a minute fatigues the subscapularis, challenging the capsular contribution to the anterior stability of the shoulder. A patient with anterior instability will usually become apprehensive as this maneuver is carried out.	There are no studies on the sensitivity or specificity of the fulcrum test for assessing stability.[a]

Table 4.7 Tests for Anterior Shoulder Instability (Continued)

Test	Description	Reliability/Validity
Anterior drawer test	The affected shoulder is held in 80–120 degrees of abduction, 0–20 degrees of forward flexion, and 0–30 degrees of lateral rotation; this position should be quite comfortable. The examiner holds the patient's scapula with the left hand, pressing the scapular spine forward with the index and middle fingers; the thumb exerts counter pressure on the coracoid process. The scapula is now held firmly in the examiner's left hand. With the right hand, the examiner grasps the patient's relaxed upper arm in its resting position and draws anteriorly with a force comparable to that used in the knee Lachman's test.	Farber et al.[68] With pain as criterion: Sensitivity: 28% Specificity: 71% PPV: 13% NPV: 86% Accuracy: 65% +LR: 0.97 −LR: 1.01 With reproduction of instability symptoms as criterion: Sensitivity: 53% Specificity: 85% PPV: 35% NPV: 92% Accuracy: 81% +LR: 0.97 −LR: 1.01 With grade 2 or 3 laxity as criterion: Sensitivity: 60% Specificity: 74% PPV: 26% NPV: 92% Accuracy: 72% +LR: 2.28 −LR: 0.54
Load and shift test	With the patient sitting or supine, the scapula is stabilized by securing the coracoid and the spine process with one hand. The humeral head is then grasped with the other hand to glide it anteriorly and posteriorly. The degree of glide is graded mild, moderate, or severe.	Neer and Foster[71] In diagnosing Bankart lesions: Sensitivity: 90.9% Specificity: 93.3% Liu et al.[72] In predicting labral tears when testing in combination with the apprehension, load and shift, inferior sulcus sign, and crank test: Sensitivity: 90% Specificity: 85%

[a]Holovacs et al.[73] reported the fulcrum test to have sensitivity of 69% and specificity of 50% for detecting labral pathology when compared with findings on arthroscopy.

LR, likelihood ratio; *NPV,* negative predictive value; *PPV,* positive predictive value.

shoulder abduction. At lesser degrees of abduction, the middle glenohumeral ligament and superior glenohumeral ligament are believed to assist in resisting continued translation. The labrum, which is the major site of attachment for these ligaments, plays an important role, as well.[13-17] The primary capsular restraint to posterior translation of the shoulder is the posterior band of the inferior glenohumeral ligament.[65] The primary restraint to inferior translation of the shoulder is the inferior glenohumeral ligament, and the secondary restraints are the superior glenohumeral and coracohumeral ligaments.[65]

APPREHENSION TEST

The apprehension test was first described by Rowe and Zarins in 1981 (Fig. 4.29).[66] They described the test as follows:

This test can be carried out when the patient is either in a standing or in a supine position. As the shoulder is moved passively into maximum external rotation in abduction and forward pressure is applied to the posterior aspect of the humeral head, the patient suddenly becomes apprehensive and complains of pain in the shoulder (Video 4-14).

Speer and coworkers[67] studied 100 patients with a variety of diagnoses, placing the arm in 90 degrees of abduction and 90 degrees of external rotation. They first looked for apprehension or pain in that position and then placed an anterior force on the shoulder and recorded whether the patient became apprehensive or had pain. They found that in patients with anterior instability, the test result was positive in 63% for apprehension and that 46% had pain in that position.

Farber and associates[68] studied 46 patients with shoulder instability for clinical usefulness of three physical examination tests (anterior apprehension, relocation, and anterior drawer test). They found that if apprehension was used as the diagnostic criterion for a positive test result

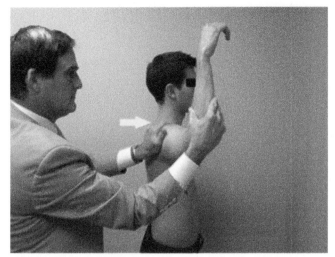

Figure 4.29 The anterior apprehension test is performed with the examiner standing behind the patient. The patient's arm is placed in abduction and slowly externally rotated until the patient becomes apprehensive that the shoulder might subluxate or dislocate. The *arrow* shows the direction of the examiner's force.

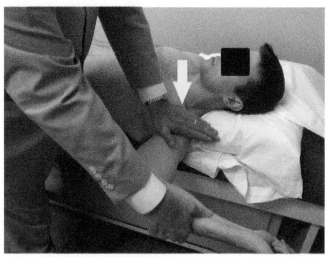

Figure 4.30 The Jobe relocation test is performed with the patient supine. The arm is positioned similarly to the anterior apprehension test. The examiner externally rotates the arm until the patient becomes apprehensive that the shoulder might subluxate. The examiner then places a hand on the humeral head, stabilizing the proximal humerus. A positive test result is when the apprehension is relieved with the stabilizing force. The *arrow* shows the direction of the examiner's force.

for traumatic anterior shoulder instability, the sensitivity, specificity, and likelihood ratio were 72%, 96%, and 20.2, respectively, for the apprehension test and 81%, 92%, and 10.4, respectively, for the relocation test. This means that if the patient is apprehensive with these maneuvers, the diagnosis of anterior instability is practically assured. If pain was used as the diagnostic criterion for a positive test result, the values for the sensitivity, specificity, and likelihood ratio of both tests were lower.

JOBE RELOCATION TEST (FOWLER TEST)

The relocation test initially described by Jobe in 1989 (with credit also given to Fowler in 1982) is complementary to the apprehension test.[67,69] The test is used to help discern whether the pain or discomfort from the apprehension test is attributable to anterior instability or "internal impingement" of the rotator cuff to the superior and posterior glenoid with the arm in this position (Fig. 4.30).

The examiner first performs the apprehension test, and at the point where the patient feels pain or apprehension, the examiner applies a posteriorly directed force to the humeral head. If the pain is related to primary impingement, it will persist despite the posteriorly applied force. If the pain and discomfort is from instability and secondary impingement, this action should "relocate" the humeral head and allow full pain-free external range of motion (Video 4-15).[69]

It is important to note that when the relocation test is applied to patients with traumatic, anterior shoulder instability, a positive Jobe test is when the patient has apprehension that is relieved when the humeral head is stabilized by the examiner. If the patient has pain alone, then the Jobe test is not as helpful in making the diagnosis of traumatic anterior instability. For patients who have pain alone, the source of the pain with this test is not entirely understood. Some suggest that pain alone may indicate problems with the superior labrum or the biceps anchor to the labrum.

The relocation test is not as helpful for creating treatment plans for those who have only pain with this test.

Speer and associates[67] evaluated the relocation test with and without the application of an anterior force to the proximal humerus. They concluded that the test had accuracy of 80% without application of an anterior force (provocative maneuver) and 85% with application of the anterior force. With application of an anterior force and pain as the positive end point, the test had a sensitivity of 54% and specificity of 44%. With application of anterior force and apprehension as the positive end point, the test had a sensitivity of 68% and specificity of 100%.

Farber and coworkers[68] evaluated the anterior drawer test (see section: Anterior Drawer Test) with application of anterior translation force to the humeral head in a position of 60 to 80 degrees of arm abduction. Their conclusions were as follows: (1) with pain as a parameter for a positive anterior drawer test, the sensitivity was 28%, specificity was 71%, PPV was 13%, NPV was 86%, and accuracy was 65%; (2) with reproduction of instability symptoms as a parameter for a positive test, the sensitivity was 53%, specificity was 85%, PPV was 35%, NPV was 92%, and accuracy was 81%; and (3) for grade 2 or 3 laxity, the sensitivity was 60%, specificity was 74%, PPV was 26%, NPV was 92%, and accuracy was 72%.

ANTERIOR RELEASE TEST OR "SURPRISE TEST"

Gross and Distefano[70] describe the anterior release test as a test for assessing traumatic anterior glenohumeral instability (Fig. 4.31). This test is performed with the patient supine and the arm positioned in 90 degrees of abduction and 90 degrees of external rotation, similar to an anterior apprehension test. The arm is externally rotated until the patient feels apprehension that the shoulder might come out of the socket. The examiner then performs a relocation maneuver to stabilize the humeral head but continues to externally

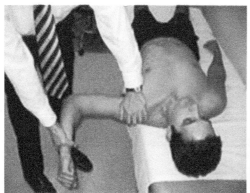

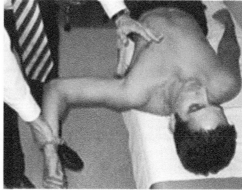

Figure 4.31 In the anterior release test, after the relocation maneuver, the examiner continues the external rotation of the arm and suddenly releases the stabilizing forces on the humeral head. In a positive test result, the patient would resume apprehension or pain or have the shoulder subluxate.

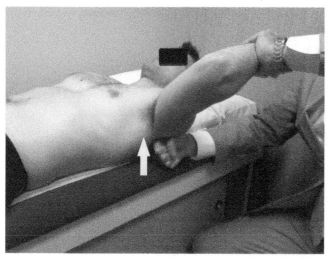

Figure 4.32 The fulcrum test is performed similarly to a supine apprehension sign, but the hand or a bolster is placed behind the shoulder to increase anterior tension on the ligaments. The *arrow* shows the direction of the examiner's force.

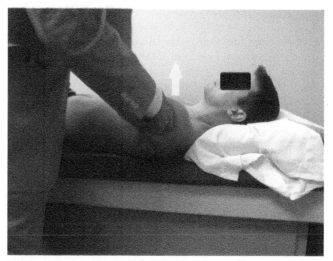

Figure 4.33 The anterior drawer test is performed in 80 to 120 degrees of abduction, 0 to 20 degrees of forward flexion, and 0 to 30 degrees of external rotation of the shoulder. The examiner then grasps the patient's relaxed upper arm and forcibly draws it anteriorly. *Arrow* shows direction of examiner's force.

rotate the arm. The examiner then suddenly releases the stabilizing force on the humeral head, and the patient may resume having apprehension, may have only pain, or may have the shoulder subluxate. One caution with this test is that it can result in dislocation or subluxation of the humeral head. Therefore, this test is not recommended on a routine basis.

FULCRUM TEST

We were unable to find the original description of the fulcrum test (Fig. 4.32). It is classically described by Matsen and Kirby[74] as follows:

> The patient lies supine at the edge of the examination table with the arm abducted to 90 degrees. The examiner places one hand on the table under the glenohumeral joint to act as a fulcrum. The arm is gently and progressively extended and externally rotated over this fulcrum. Maintenance of gentle passive external rotation for a minute fatigues the subscapularis, challenging the capsular contribution to the anterior stability of the shoulder. The patient with anterior

instability will usually become apprehensive as this maneuver is carried out (watch the eyebrows for a clue that the shoulder is getting ready to dislocate).

The only difference between this test and a supine apprehension test is that a bolster or the hand is placed behind the shoulder to increase the anterior stress on the shoulder joint. Holovacs et al.[73] reported the fulcrum test to have sensitivity of 69% and specificity of 50% for detecting labral pathology when compared with findings on arthroscopy. In their study, they did not specify whether the labral tears were in the superior or inferior half of the glenoid.

ANTERIOR DRAWER TEST

The anterior drawer test (Fig. 4.33) is a test of shoulder laxity, which means it is a way to determine how much translation the humeral head has on the glenoid. In this examination, the goal is to judge how much motion there is of the humeral head on the glenoid when pushing the head toward the front of the glenoid. This test was described by Gerber and Ganz[75] as follows:

> The test is performed with the patient supine ... The examiner stands facing the affected shoulder. Assuming the left shoulder is being tested, he fixes the patient's left hand in his own right axilla by adducting his own humerus. The patient should not grasp the surgeon's axilla but should be completely relaxed. To be sure that relaxation is complete, the examining surgeon gently taps the patient's elbow.
>
> The affected shoulder is held in 80 to 120 degrees of abduction, 0 to 20 degrees of forward flexion, and 0 to 30 degrees of lateral rotation; this position should be quite comfortable. The examiner holds the patient's scapula with his left hand, pressing the scapular spine forward with his index and middle fingers; his thumb exerts counter-pressure on the coracoid process. The scapula is now held firmly in the examiner's left hand. With his right hand, he grasps the patient's relaxed upper arm in its resting position and draws it anteriorly with a force comparable to that used at the knee in Lachman's test.

It is important to realize that this examination is a test of laxity of the shoulder and not inherently a test of shoulder instability. The only way that it can be used to make a diagnosis of instability is if the humeral head can be subluxated out the front of the shoulder, and the patient reports that the subluxation is what they feel when they have symptoms. If the patient reports pain alone, then this test is not helpful for making the diagnosis of instability.

The amount of movement or translation of the humeral head on the glenoid has been a subject of confusion because classification systems are myriad.[76] The recommended system is a simplified version of the Hawkins scale (Fig. 4.34). In the original Hawkins scale, grades were defined as follows: grade 0, normal translation; grade 1, the humeral head translates to the glenoid rim but not over it; grade 2, the humeral head moves over the glenoid rim but then reduces; and grade 3, the humeral head translates over the glenoid rim and stays out of the glenoid. This scale was modified by McFarland and others[26] to combine grades 0 and 1 because, in actuality, the humeral head either goes over the rim or it does not; thus, the majority of shoulders are actually type 2, and type 3 laxity is very uncommon, especially in the office, where the patient may be apprehensive or have pain with the test.

The clinical usefulness of the anterior drawer test for traumatic anterior instability was studied by Farber and others.[68] They found that in patients with traumatic anterior instability with use of pain as the criterion, the anterior drawer test had a sensitivity of 28%, specificity of 71%, PPV of 13%, NPV of 86%, accuracy of 65%, and likelihood ratio of 0.97. With reproduction of instability symptoms as the criterion, it had a sensitivity of 53%, specificity of 85%, PPV of 35%, NPV of 92%, accuracy of 81%, and likelihood ratio of 3.57. The anterior drawer test measured grades 2 and 3 laxity with a sensitivity of 60%, specificity of 74%, PPV of 26%, NPV of 92%, accuracy of 72%, and likelihood ratio of 2.28.

LOAD AND SHIFT TEST

The load and shift test is also a test of shoulder laxity that is similar to the anterior drawer test. The load and shift test can be performed with the patient sitting or supine, and it is performed by using one hand to stabilize the scapula

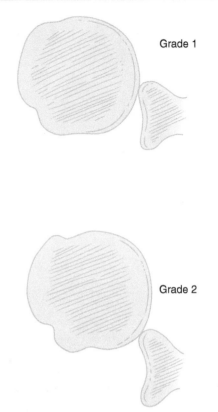

Figure 4.34 The Hawkins scale is based on what the examiner feels when testing laxity of the shoulder. In grade 1 laxity, the humeral head translates to the glenoid rim but not over it. In grade 2 laxity, the humeral head translates over the glenoid rim but reduces on its own. In grade 3 laxity, the humeral head dislocates outside of the glenoid rim and stays out. (Redrawn from McFarland EG, Campbell G, McDowell J. Posterior shoulder laxity in asymptomatic athletes. *Am J Sports Med*. 1996 Jul-Aug;24(4):468-71. Figure 2.)

while the other hand translates the proximal humerus from front to back (Fig. 4.35). The goal of this test is to determine how much laxity the shoulder has in these positions. It can be graded similarly to the anterior and posterior drawer tests with a modified Hawkins system in which the humeral head either subluxates over the rim (grade 2) or does not (grade 1). If it can be subluxated and it stays out of the glenoid, then it is a grade 3. It is helpful as an instability test only if the examiner can subluxate the shoulder over the rim of the glenoid, and the patient says that the subluxation reproduces the symptoms.

TESTS FOR POSTERIOR SHOULDER INSTABILITY

See Table 4.8.

The posterior band of the IGHLC is the primary restraint to posterior translation of the humeral head. The secondary restraints to posterior movement of the shoulder are the superior glenohumeral ligament, coracohumeral ligament, and rotator interval (anterior-superior portion of the capsule).

Similar to the physical examination tests for anterior shoulder instability, there are tests of posterior shoulder laxity that are different from tests that assess posterior shoulder instability. Posterior laxity can be assessed with the posterior drawer test or with a posterior load and shift test.

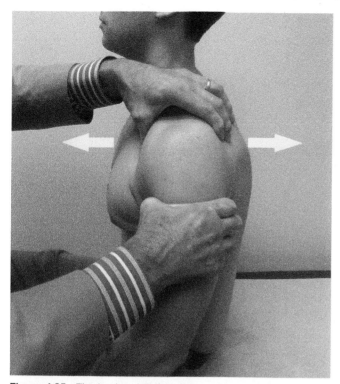

Figure 4.35 The load and shift test is performed with the patient sitting and the scapula stabilized by the examiner's hand. The examiner's other hand grasps the humeral head and translates it anteriorly and posteriorly over the glenoid rim. The *arrows* show the direction of the examiner's force.

Posterior instability can be difficult to establish because the physical examination tests for posterior instability are not as well studied as the anterior instability tests.

POSTERIOR DRAWER TEST

Similar to the anterior drawer test, the posterior drawer test is performed with the patient supine (Fig. 4.36). The goal of this test is to evaluate how much laxity the patient has when the humeral head is moved out of the socket. The amount of movement can be measured with the same modified Hawkins scale as previously described. It is important to realize that this test is a test of laxity and not of instability. If the humeral head is subluxated by the examiner out the back of the shoulder, it is considered instability only if the patient says that the subluxation is what he or she feels when having shoulder symptoms. Pain alone is not an adequate criterion for making a diagnosis of posterior instability with this test.

The test is performed with the patient supine and the shoulder at the edge of the table or slightly off the table. The shoulder should be relaxed. The patient's arm is abducted approximately 70 degrees and in neutral rotation (see Fig. 4.36). The examiner holds the arm with one hand and uses the other hand to move the shoulder posteriorly. The hand should be placed so that the thumb is on the anterior aspect of the humeral head, and the thumb is used to push the humeral head posteriorly while the other hand elevates the humerus to facilitate a posteriorly directed force. The fingers behind the shoulder feel for the humeral head to subluxate out the back of the joint. The shoulder

Table 4.8 Tests for Posterior Shoulder Instability

Test	Description	Clinical Utility
Posterior drawer test	Assuming the left shoulder is being tested, the examiner grasps the patient's proximal forearm with left hand, flexes the elbow to about 120 degrees, and positions the shoulder into 80–120 degrees of abduction and 20–30 degrees of forward flexion. The examiner holds the scapula with the right hand, with the index and middle fingers on the scapular spine; the thumb lies immediately lateral to the coracoid process, so that its ulnar aspect remains in constant contact with the coracoid while performing the test. With the left hand, the examiner slightly rotates the upper arm medially and flexes it to about 60 or 80 degrees. During this maneuver, the thumb of the examiner's right hand subluxates the humeral head posteriorly.	There are no studies on sensitivity and specificity of this test.
Posterior apprehension sign	This tests posterior instability and subacromial impingement; by flexing the humerus to 90 degrees and internally rotating, it fully reproduced symptoms of instability.	McFarland[26] For apprehension: Sensitivity: 42% Specificity: 99% For pain: Sensitivity: 50% Specificity: 86% For subluxation: Sensitivity: 25% Specificity: 98%
Jerk test	The patient sits with the arm internally rotated and flexed forward to 90 degrees. The examiner grasps the elbow and axially loads the humerus in a proximal direction. While axial loading of the humerus is maintained, the arm is moved horizontally across the body. A positive result is indicated by a sudden jerk as the humeral head slides off the back of the glenoid. When the arm is returned to the original position of 90 degrees of abduction a second jerk may be observed, that of the humeral head returning to the glenoid.	Holovacs et al.[73] reported the test to have sensitivity of 19% and specificity of 95% for labral injury when compared with findings of arthroscopy.

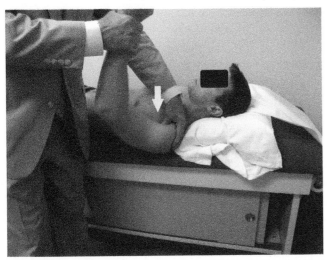

Figure 4.36   The posterior drawer test is performed with the patient supine and with the arm forward flexed approximately 45 degrees and abducted 45 degrees. The examiner translates the humeral head posteriorly with the thumb while lifting the arm forward. *Arrow* shows direction of examiner's force.

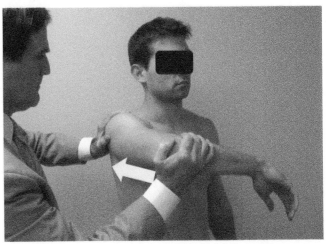

Figure 4.37   The posterior apprehension sign is performed by applying a posteriorly directed force on the arm in flexion and internal rotation as shown. The *arrow* shows the direction of the examiner's force.

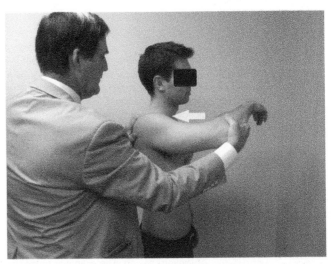

Figure 4.38   The goal of the posterior jerk test is to allow the shoulder to subluxate out the back of the shoulder when the capsule is least tight. With elevation, the arm subluxates, and this subluxation can be better appreciated as the shoulder reduces on extension of the arm. The *arrow* shows the direction of the examiner's force.

is reduced by extending the arm so that the humeral head moves back into the joint.

At one time, it was believed to be pathologic to be able to subluxate the humeral head over the glenoid rim (ie, a modified Hawkins grade 2). Subsequent studies have shown that it is actually more common to be able to subluxate the humeral head over the posterior rim of the shoulder than to not be able to subluxate over the rim.[77] In a study of high school athletes, it was found that 60% of the athletes with asymptomatic shoulders could be subluxated over the glenoid rim with a posterior drawer test. Subsequent study of patients under anesthesia showed that 21% could be subluxated over the glenoid rim posteriorly with a posterior drawer test and that 29% could be subluxated over the rim anteriorly with an anterior drawer test.[76] Consequently, the ability for the shoulder to subluxate upon examination over the rim anteriorly or posteriorly is very common, and unless the subluxation reproduces the symptoms of instability, a Hawkins grade 2 or 3 should be interpreted as normal.

POSTERIOR APPREHENSION SIGN

The posterior apprehension sign was first described by Kessell,[78] who noticed that patients with posterior shoulder instability often held their arms in forward flexion and internal rotation (Fig. 4.37). He described a test in which the examiner holds the arm in flexion and internal rotation and applies a posteriorly directed force on the humerus. A positive test result was if the patient became apprehensive that the shoulder would come out of the socket.

No studies have evaluated the clinical utility of the posterior apprehension test. However, one researcher[26] has suggested that the test is based on faulty observations because in patients with posterior instability, the arm position of flexion, adduction, and internal rotation is not the position where the posterior capsule is loose. The arm position where the capsule is loosest is with the arm abducted approximately 80 degrees and slightly forward flexed. As a result, pushing the arm posteriorly when it is in the flexed

position will not subluxate the shoulder out of the joint. This test needs further study before it can be recommended clinically.

JERK TEST

We were unable to find the original description of the jerk test (Fig. 4.38). The test for glenohumeral instability was described by Matsen and associates[79] as follows:

> The patient sits with the arm internally rotated and flexed forward to 90 degrees. The examiner grasps the elbow and axially loads the humerus in a proximal direction. While axial loading of the humerus is maintained, the arm is moved horizontally across the body. A positive result is indicated by a sudden jerk as the humeral head slides off the back of the glenoid. When the arm is returned to the original position of 90-degree abduction a second jerk may be observed, that of the humeral head returning to the glenoid.

Table 4.9 Tests for Inferior Shoulder Instability

Test	Description	Reliability/Validity
Sulcus sign	The test is performed with the patient upright and the shoulder in the neutral position and relaxed. Stress is applied to the upper arm and not the forearm; this eliminates the effect of the biceps and the triceps brachii. A positive result invariably points to a more complex (multidirectional) instability.	No studies have examined the sensitivity or specificity of the sulcus sign for inferior instability.
Hyperabduction test	To measure the range of passive abduction, the physician stands behind the patient with the forearm pushed down firmly on the shoulder girdle in its lowest position while lifting the relaxed upper limb in abduction with the other hand. During the test, the elbow is flexed at 90 degrees, and the forearm is horizontal. Under these conditions, the shoulder girdle should not move, and any movement is measured by a goniometer.	Sodha et al.[80] Sensitivity: 68% Specificity: 62.3%

To our knowledge, there has never been a peer-reviewed study of the clinical utility of the jerk test.

TESTS FOR INFERIOR SHOULDER INSTABILITY

See Table 4.9.

The superior glenohumeral ligament and coracohumeral ligaments are the primary restraints to translation of the humeral head when the arm is in an adducted position. At 45 degrees or more of abduction, the inferior glenohumeral ligament increasingly assists in preventing inferior instability. The rotator interval and labrum also play roles.[13-17]

There are several tests to gauge inferior instability. It is important to remember that many of these tests are of shoulder laxity only. As a result, these tests can be considered diagnostic only if they provoke a sense of instability and not just pain.

SULCUS SIGN (Video 4-16)

Credit is given to Neer and Foster[71] for first describing the use of the sulcus sign to develop the concept of multidirectional instability (Fig. 4.39). They suggested that by using the sulcus sign, the examiner could determine if the patient had shoulder instability in an inferior direction. In their original description of the test, the result was positive if it demonstrated inferior subluxation of the shoulder joint. However, they did not describe the technique fully, nor did they delineate how to grade the laxity.

The test is best performed with the patient sitting, although it can be done with the patient standing. The examiner pulls inferiorly on the arms and observes how much the humeral head moves inferiorly. The test is positive for instability if the head slides out of the socket, and the patient reports that this reproduces their symptoms. Pain alone with a sulcus sign is not a positive test for inferior instability.

Inferior laxity with a sulcus sign can be roughly measured with the classification system described by Hawkins et al.[76] This system is based on the idea that the examiner can estimate the amount of movement or translation inferiorly of the humeral head on the glenoid.[76] Grade 1 laxity is 0.5 to 1.0 cm, grade 2 is 1.0 to 2.0 cm, and grade 3 is more than 2.0 cm. This scheme of measuring the sulcus has never been

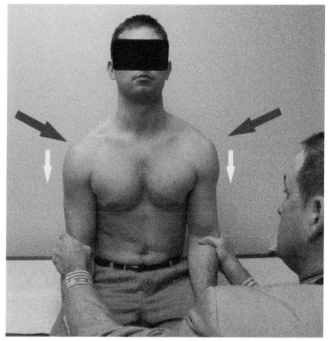

Figure 4.39 The sulcus sign is assessed with the patient sitting or standing, but better relaxation is achieved with the patient sitting. An axial distraction load is placed downward on both arms *(yellow arrows)*, and the amount of displacement of the humeral head inferiorly is estimated *(black arrows)*.

validated, and generally, the observer can only estimate how much movement is occurring with this test.

Another issue with this test is that the interobserver reliability is poor.[81] The grading system has not been validated, and it is common that two observers will have different grades when examining the same individual. Also, although a grade 3 sulcus has been indicative of inferior instability, it has been shown in subjects with no shoulder problems that the prevalence of a grade 3 sulcus sign can be present in 3% of men and 9% of women.[77] This is possible because there is a wide range of shoulder laxities, and in some people, a grade 3 inferior laxity is normal.

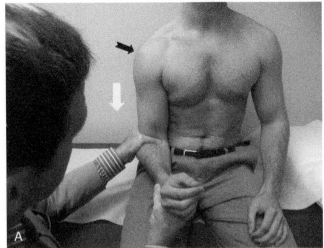

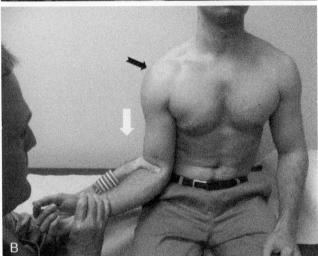

Figure 4.40 Testing for the sulcus sign in internal rotation (**A**) and external rotation (**B**). The *yellow arrow* shows the direction of the examiner's force, and the *black arrow* shows the location of the sulcus sign.

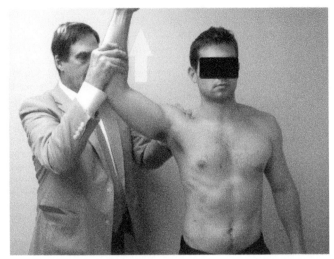

Figure 4.41 The hyperabduction test is performed with the examiner behind the patient and the scapula stabilized with one arm. The examiner raises the arm *(arrow)* until feeling the glenohumeral ligaments tighten. The degree of elevation deemed indicative of inferior instability has not been established.

HYPERABDUCTION TEST

Gagey and Gagey[8] described this test for assessing the laxity of the inferior glenohumeral ligament (IGHL) as follows (Fig. 4.41):

> In order to measure the range of passive abduction, the physician stood behind the patient with his forearm pushed down firmly on the shoulder girdle in its lowest position, while lifting the relaxed upper limb in abduction with his other hand. During the test, the elbow was flexed at 90 degrees and the forearm was horizontal. Under these circumstances, the shoulder girdle should not move. Any movement was recorded with a goniometer.

Normal subjects were found to have between 85 and 90 degrees of abduction, whereas patients with instability had more than 105 degrees of abduction. A positive test result for laxity of the IGHL was a hyperabduction test greater than 105 degrees. However, one study found that in patients with multidirectional instability, only 2% had a positive Gagey sign.[80] The authors concluded that the Gagey sign needs more study before it can be recommended for making the diagnosis of multidirectional instability.

TESTS FOR LABRAL PATHOLOGY

See Table 4.10.

The labrum is a special fibrocartilage that goes around the outer edge of the glenoid. The way it normally attaches to the rim is important when trying to understand the rationale of certain shoulder examinations designed to test the labrum. The labrum is essentially a type of "chock-block" that deepens the socket by providing a bumper around the socket. In some portions of the socket, the labrum blends gradually into the cartilage of the socket, so where the articular cartilage starts and the labral cartilage ends is difficult to discern. In other areas of the socket, the labrum is distinctly different from the glenoid cartilage, so that it appears more like a meniscus in the knee. Last, there are some areas

Because of these issues, a positive sulcus sign should be reserved for individuals who feel an inferior subluxation with sulcus testing.

The sulcus sign has been shown in cadaver studies to be influenced by whether the arm is in internal or external rotation with the elbow bent (Fig. 4.40). When the arm is in external rotation, the tissue superiorly in the shoulder between the subscapularis tendon and the supraspinatus tendon (called the "rotator cuff interval") should tighten with this test, and the sulcus should be diminished compared with when the arm is in internal rotation.[82–84] If the sulcus sign is not diminished in this position, then there is believed to be a lesion of the rotator cuff interval making the shoulder lax to inferior stress. A positive test result has been used to suggest that these tissues should be tightened surgically. Unfortunately, studies have shown that this results in a loss of external rotation of the shoulder. Therefore, using the sulcus sign to test the rotator cuff interval has yet to be accepted as common practice, and its application to treatment is indeterminant.

Table 4.10   Tests for Labral Pathology[a]

Test	Description	Reliability/Validity

Active compression (O'Brien) test	With the physician behind the patient, the patient is asked to forward flex the affected arm 90 degrees with the elbow in full extension. The patient then adducts the arm 10–15 degrees medial to the sagittal plane of the body. The arm is then internally rotated so the thumb is pointed downward. The examiner then applies uniform downward force to the arm. With the arm in the same position, the palm is then fully supinated and the maneuver is repeated. The test result is considered positive if pain is elicited with the first maneuver and is reduced or eliminated with the second maneuver. Pain localized to the acromioclavicular joint or on top of the shoulder is diagnostic of acromioclavicular joint abnormality. Pain or painful clicking described as inside the glenohumeral joint itself is indicative of labral abnormality.	O'Brien et al.[85]
		  Sensitivity: 100%
		  Specificity: 98.5%
		Burkhart et al.[15]
		  Anterior:
		    Sensitivity: 88%
		    Specificity: 42%
		  Posterior:
		    Sensitivity: 32%
		    Specificity: 13%
		  Combined:
		    Sensitivity: 85%
		    Specificity: 41%
		Holovacs et al.[73]
		  Sensitivity: 69%
		  Specificity: 50%
		Stetson and Templin[86]
		  Sensitivity: 67%
		  Specificity: 41%
		McFarland et al.[50]
		  Sensitivity: 47%
		  Specificity: 55%
		  PPV: 10%
		  NPV: 91%
		  Accuracy: 54%

Biceps load test	With the patient supine, an anterior apprehension test is performed. When the patient becomes apprehensive during the external rotation of the shoulder, external rotation is stopped. The patient is then asked to flex the elbow while the examiner resists the flexion with one hand and asks how the apprehension has changed, if at all. If the apprehension is lessened, or if the patient feels more comfortable than before the test, the test is negative for a superior labral, anterior–posterior (SLAP) lesion. If the apprehension has not changed, or if the shoulder becomes more painful, the test is positive. The test is repeated, and the patient is instructed not to pull the whole upper extremity, but to bend the elbow against the examiner's resistance. The examiner should be sitting adjacent to the shoulder to be examined at the same height as the patient and should also face the patient at a right angle.	Kim et al.[87]
		  Sensitivity: 90.9%
		  Specificity: 96.9%

Biceps load test II	This test is conducted with the patient in the supine position. The examiner sits adjacent to the patient on the same side as the shoulder and grasps the patient's wrist and elbow gently. The arm to be examined is elevated to 120 degrees and externally rotated to its maximal point, with the elbow in 90 degrees of flexion and the forearm in the supinated position. The patient is asked to flex the elbow while resisting the elbow flexion by the examiner. The test result is considered positive if the patient experiences more pain from the resisted elbow flexion regardless of the degree of pain before the elbow flexion maneuver. The test result is negative if pain is not elicited by the resisted flexion or if the preexisting pain during the elevation and external rotation of the arm is unchanged or diminished by resisted elbow flexion.	Kim et al.[87]
		  Sensitivity: 89.7%
		  Specificity: 96.6%

Continued on following page

Table 4.10   Tests for Labral Pathology (Continued)

Test	Description	Reliability/Validity

New pain provocation test	With the patient in a seated position, the abduction angle of the upper arm is maintained at 90–100 degrees, and the shoulder is rotated externally by the examiner. This maneuver is similar to the anterior apprehension test. The new pain provocation test is performed with the forearm in two different positions: maximum pronation and maximum supination. The test result is described as positive for a superior labral tear when pain is provoked only with the forearm in the pronated position or when pain is more severe in this position (pronated) than with the forearm supinated.	Mimori et al.[88]
		  Sensitivity: 100%
		  Specificity: 90%

Crank test	The crank test is performed with the patient in the upright position with the arm elevated to 160 degrees in the scapular plane. Joint load is applied along the axis of the humerus with one hand while the other performs humeral rotation. A positive test result is determined by (1) pain during the maneuver usually during external rotation with or without click, or (2) reproduction of the symptoms usually pain or catching felt by the patient during athletic or work activities. The test should be repeated in the supine position where the patient is usually more relaxed.	Liu et al.[89]
		  Sensitivity: 91%
		  Specificity: 93%
		Liu et al.[72]
		  When combined with sulcus sign, apprehension and relocation tests in predicting labral tears:
		  Sensitivity: 90%
		  Specificity: 93%
		Mimori et al.[88]
		  Sensitivity: 83%
		  Specificity: 100%
		Stetson and Templin[90]
		  Sensitivity: 64%
		  Specificity: 67%
		Stetson and Templin[86]
		  For superior labral tears:
		  Sensitivity: 64%
		  Specificity: 56%

Anterior slide test	The patient is examined either standing or sitting, with hands on hips and thumbs pointing posteriorly. One of the examiner's hands is placed across the top of the shoulder from the posterior direction, with the last segment of the index finger extending over the anterior aspect of the acromion at the glenohumeral joint. The examiner's other hand is placed behind the elbow and a forward and slightly superiorly directed force is applied to the elbow and upper arm. The patient is asked to push back against this force. Pain localized to the front of the shoulder under the examiner's hand, and/or a pop or click in the same area, is considered to be a positive test result. This test result is also positive if the athlete reports a subjective feeling that this testing maneuver reproduces the symptoms that occur during overhead activity.	Kibler[91]
		  Sensitivity: 78.4%
		  Specificity: 91.5%
		McFarland et al.[50]
		  Sensitivity: 8%
		  Specificity: 84%
		  PPV: 5%
		  NPV: 90%
		  Accuracy: 77%

Compression-rotation test	The test is performed by placing an axial load on the humerus with arm abducted 90 degrees and the elbow flexed 90 degrees. The arm is then rotated, and a positive test is a click or catch. The test is predicated upon the same ideas of the McMurray test of the knee, but in reality, the labrum does not act like a meniscus, and this test is not sensitive for labrum tears.	Holovacs et al.[73]
		  Sensitivity: 80%
		  Specificity: 19%
		McFarland et al.[50]
		  Sensitivity: 24%
		  Sensitivity: 76%
		  PPV: 9%
		  NPV: 90%
		  Accuracy: 71%

Table 4.10   Tests for Labral Pathology (Continued)

Test	Description	Reliability/Validity
Dynamic shear test	With the examiner standing behind the patient, the patient's arm is placed in abduction of approximately 70 degrees, and an anteriorly directed force is applied on the posterior shoulder. The arm is raised from 70 to 120 degrees. In a positive test result, the patient experiences pain, particularly in the posterior and superior shoulder.	Ben Kibler et al.[92] For labral tears: Sensitivity: 72% Specificity: 98% PPV: 97% NPV: 77% +LR: 31.6 Accuracy: 0.84 Cook et al.[93] For labral tears: Sensitivity: 89% Specificity: 30% PPV: 69% NPV: 60% Accuracy: 1.3 Sodha et al.[94] Sensitivity: 85.7% Specificity: 51.9% PPV: 1.8% NPV: 99.7% LR: 6.4 Accuracy: 54.4%
Clunk test	The patient lies supine. The examiner places one hand on the posterior aspect of the shoulder over the humeral head while holding the humerus above the elbow and fully abducts the arm over the patient's head. The examiner then pushes anteriorly with the hand over the humeral head while the other hand rotates the humerus into lateral rotation. A clunk or grinding sound indicates a positive test result and is indicative of a tear of the labrum. This test may also cause apprehension if anterior instability is present.	There are no studies assessing the sensitivity and specificity of the maneuver.[b]

[a]See also Instability Tests, some of which evaluate labral pathology.
[b]It is interesting to note that Hawkins et al.[95] described a palpable and often audible "clunk" to mean shoulder relocation in glenohumeral instability. There has been no validation of the test for this indication either.
LR, likelihood ratio; *NPV,* negative predictive value; *PPV,* positive predictive value.

where it is normal to have the labrum not attached to the glenoid at all and some areas where the labrum is absent (Fig. 4.42). As a general rule, the labrum in the inferior half of the socket blends in with the articular cartilage, but in the upper or superior half of the socket, the labrum can be more like a meniscus, not attached to the glenoid at all or even absent.

This variation in the anatomy has contributed to many misconceptions of how the examination of the shoulder works. The first misconception is that because the labrum looks like a meniscus in some areas, it can cause clicking and catching. The reality is that labrum tears produce clicks only about 5% of the time.[50] A labral tear that causes locking, as seen in the knee with a meniscus, is almost unheard of in the shoulder.

The second misconception is that examinations for the labrum study the whole labrum, but this is false because most physical examination tests are designed to study only certain portions of the labrum. This is important to realize because many studies of examination techniques for labral tears include tests of different portions of the labrum but claim to be clinically helpful for nearly any labral tear. For example, labral tears in the anterior and inferior part of the socket (where detachments of the labrum are known as Bankart lesions and where the humeral head dislocates in anterior shoulder instability) are studied with different physical examination tests than labral tears in the posterior and inferior glenoid. Similarly, because the superior labrum serves as the attachment site of the biceps tendon, the physical examination tests for this portion of the labrum are entirely different than tests for other portions of the labrum. The theory is that tests that put tension on the biceps tendon should cause pain in the shoulder, which is typically described as "deep in the shoulder," or in the posterior and superior portion of the shoulder. Unfortunately, these tests of the superior labrum rely on the patient to report the location of pain, and other lesions in the shoulder can produce pain with these physical examination tests.

No single test will convincingly make the diagnosis of a superior labral tear (called a superior labrum anterior posterior [SLAP] lesion) (Fig. 4.43).[96-99] As a result, many tests have been described for SLAP lesions and have popular appeal but not diagnostic accuracy. Also, combinations of tests do not seem to increase the diagnostic accuracy of

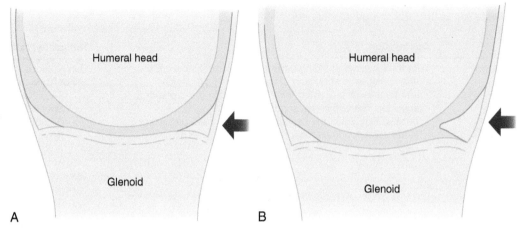

Figure 4.42 Drawing of the two types of labrum attachment to bone. **A,** The labrum below the equator of the glenoid blends imperceptibly with the articular cartilage in most cases. **B,** In the upper half of the glenoid, the labrum attachment is to the rim of the labrum only, leaving a free edge similar to the meniscus in the knee.

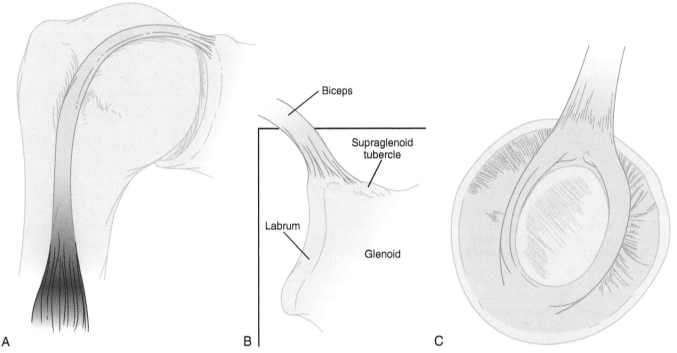

Figure 4.43 Drawings of (A) normal biceps attachment, which is shown grossly (**A**), and a coronal view showing the attachment to the superior glenoid tubercle and to the labrum (**B**). **C,** In a type II superior labral, anterior–posterior (SLAP) lesion, the biceps attachment to the superior glenoid tubercle and the labrum attachment to the glenoid are torn. (Fig C redrawn from Snyder SJ, Karzel RP, Del Pizzo W, Ferkel RD, Friedman MJ. SLAP lesions of the shoulder. *Arthroscopy.* 1990;6(4):274-9.)

the examinations for SLAP lesion. The only test that can make the diagnosis of a SLAP lesion with assurance is arthroscopy of the shoulder; the most common indication for arthroscopy is failure of nonoperative treatment of a suspected SLAP lesion.

ACTIVE COMPRESSION (O'BRIEN) TEST (Video 4-17)

O'Brien et al.[85] introduced a test for diagnosing superior labral tears and AC joint abnormalities. They termed this examination "the active compression test" and described it as follows (Fig. 4.44):

This test was conducted with the physician standing behind the patient. The patient was asked to forward flex the affected arm 90 degrees with the elbow in full extension. The patient then abducted the arm 10 to 15 degrees medial to the sagittal plane of the body. The arm was internally rotated so that the thumb pointed downward. The examiner then applied uniform downward force to the arm. With the arm in the same position, the palm was then fully supinated and the maneuver was repeated. The test was considered positive if pain was elicited with the first maneuver and was reduced or eliminated with the second maneuver. Pain localized to the AC joint or on top of the shoulder was diagnostic of AC joint abnormality. Pain or painful clicking described as inside the glenohumeral joint itself was indicative of labral abnormality.

Although the active compression test is commonly cited as a test for SLAP lesions, its clinical utility for that purpose

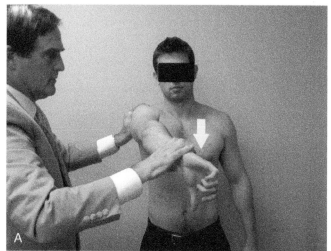

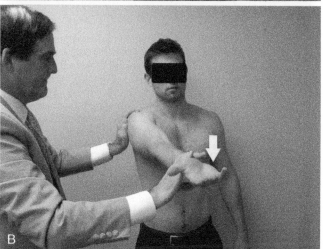

Figure 4.44 A, The active compression test is performed with the patient standing and the arm forward flexed 90 degrees and adducted 10 degrees and the thumb pointing down. The examiner places a downward force on the arm, and the patient should report pain either deep in the joint (superior labral, anterior–posterior [SLAP] tear) or at the acromioclavicular joint. **B,** The test is repeated with the arm in the same position but with the patient's hand facing up. With the arm in this position, the pain should be decreased. *Arrows* shows direction of examiner's force.

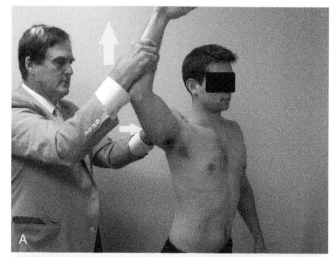

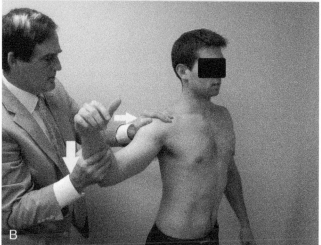

Figure 4.45 The dynamic shear test is performed similarly to an anterior apprehension test with the examiner behind the patient. **A,** The arm is placed in abduction and external rotation while the examiner applies an anteriorly directed force on the shoulder from the back. **B,** The arm is then elevated between 70 and 120 degrees, which should cause pain deep in the joint or in the posterior-superior part of the joint. *Arrows* show direction of examiner's force.

remains in question. This test requires the patient to state where the pain is located, and often the patient cannot localize the pain or the pain is not deep in the joint. Studies have shown that this test has higher clinical usefulness for making the diagnosis of AC joint abnormalities than for SLAP lesions because it is easier to verify the location of the pain.[17] Although O'Brien and Pagnani reported that the active compression test had a sensitivity of 100% and a specificity of 95% for making the diagnosis of SLAP tears, these results have not been replicated in subsequent studies.[85] Although this is a popular test, it does not increase the odds of making the correct diagnosis for SLAP tears. McFarland et al.[98] found that this test has a sensitivity of 32% to 100%, specificity of 11% to 98.5%, PPV of 10% to 100%, and NPV of 14% to 100%. Stetson and Templin[86] found a sensitivity of 54%, specificity of 31%, PPV of 34%, and NPV of 50% for diagnosis of SLAP tears. Guanche and Jones[100]

reported a sensitivity of 63%, specificity of 73%, PPV of 87%, and NPV of 40% for diagnosing SLAP tears. Thus, no study found this test to be valuable for diagnosis of SLAP tears.

DYNAMIC SHEAR TEST

The dynamic shear test was first described by Cheung and O'Driscoll[101] at a meeting and published in abstract form only. The test is designed to determine the presence of a SLAP lesion and is performed with the patient standing with the examiner behind the patient (Fig. 4.45). The arm is placed in abduction of approximately 70 degrees, and the examiner applies an anteriorly directed force on the posterior shoulder. The examiner then raises the arm from 70 to 120 degrees, and if the patient experiences pain, particularly in the posterior and superior shoulder, it is considered a positive test result. This test can be difficult to perform in patients who have anterior shoulder instability because it is very similar to an anterior apprehension sign.

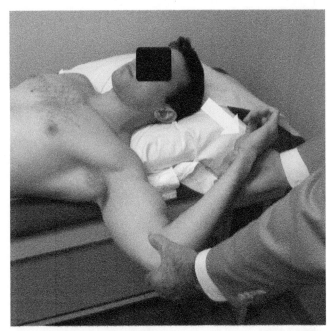

Figure 4.46 The biceps load test is performed with the patient supine or sitting and the arm abducted. The patient is asked to try to bring the wrist toward the head against resistance. The *arrow* shows the direction of the examiner's force.

This test has been the subject of three studies. First, Kibler and coworkers[92] reported a positive likelihood ratio for this test as high as 31.6 and, thus, that a patient with a positive test result has a very high probability of having a SLAP lesion. However, Cook and others[93] found that it had a likelihood ratio of less than 2, suggesting it is not useful at all. Finally, Sodha and associates[94] found that the dynamic shear test had a likelihood ratio of 6.5 when the patient had an isolated SLAP lesion but only 1.5 when there were coexisting shoulder lesions. This test has promise for making the diagnosis of SLAP lesions, but similar to many tests for SLAP lesions, coexisting shoulder lesions can confound the results.

BICEPS LOAD TEST

Kim and others[87] described the biceps load test for evaluating the integrity of the superior glenoid labrum in shoulders with recurrent anterior dislocations as follows (Fig. 4.46):

> The test is performed with the patient in the supine position. The examiner sits adjacent to the patient on the same side as the affected shoulder and gently grasps the patient's wrist and elbow. The arm to be examined is abducted at 90 degrees, with the forearm in the supinated position. The patient is allowed to relax, and an anterior apprehension test is performed. When the patient becomes apprehensive during the external rotation of the shoulder, external rotation is stopped. The patient is then asked to flex the elbow while the examiner resists the flexion with one hand and asks how the apprehension has changed, if at all. If the apprehension is lessened, or if the patient feels more comfortable than before the test, the test is negative for a SLAP lesion. If the apprehension has not changed, or if the shoulder becomes more painful, the test is positive. The test is repeated and the patient is instructed

not to pull the whole upper extremity, but to bend the elbow against the examiner's resistance. The examiner should be sitting adjacent to the shoulder to be examined at the same height as the patient, and he or she should also face the patient at a right angle. The direction of the examiner's resistance should be on the same plane as the patient's arm so as not to change the degree of abduction and rotation of the shoulder. The forearm should be kept in the supinated position during the test (Video 4-18).

The authors noted that the test had a sensitivity of 90.9%, specificity of 96.9%, PPV of 83%, and NPV of 98% when compared with arthroscopy. There are no other published studies of its validity, reliability, specificity, or sensitivity.

BICEPS LOAD TEST II

Kim and coworkers[102] also described a modified version of the biceps load test as follows:

> This test is conducted with the patient in the supine position. The examiner sits adjacent to the patient on the same side as the shoulder and grasps the patient's wrist and elbow gently. The arm to be examined is elevated to 120 degrees and externally rotated to its maximal point, with the elbow in 90 degree flexion and the forearm in the supinated position. The patient is asked to flex the elbow while resisting the elbow flexion by the examiner. The test is considered positive if the patient complains of more pain from the resisted elbow flexion regardless of the degree of pain before the elbow flexion maneuver. The test is negative if pain is not elicited by the resisted elbow flexion or if the pre-existing pain during the elevation and external rotation of the arm is unchanged or diminished by resisted elbow flexion (Video 4-19).

The authors found the test to have a sensitivity of 89.7%, specificity of 96.6%, and NPV of 95.5% when compared with arthroscopy. Compared with the first biceps load test described earlier, the PPV improved to 92.1%. No other studies have evaluated its validity, reliability, sensitivity, or specificity.

NEW PAIN PROVOCATION TEST (Video 4-20)

Mimori and associates[88] described the new pain provocation test for superior labral tears of the shoulder as follows (Fig. 4.47):

> The new pain provocation test was performed with the patient in the sitting position. During testing, the abduction angle of the upper arm was maintained at 90 to 100 degrees, and the shoulder was rotated externally by the examiner. This maneuver is similar to the anterior apprehension test. The new pain provocation test was performed with the forearm in two different positions: maximum pronation and maximum supination.

The test result is described as positive for a superior labral tear when pain is provoked only with the forearm in the pronated position or when pain is more severe in this position (pronated) than with the forearm supinated.

The authors found the test to have a sensitivity of 100%, specificity of 90%, and accuracy of 97% compared with MRI/arthrography (in 22 patients) or arthroscopy (in 15 patients). No other studies have evaluated its validity, reliability, sensitivity, or specificity for SLAP lesions.

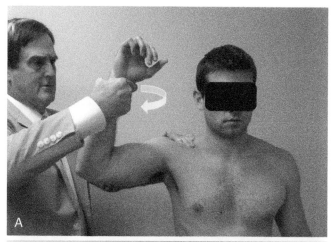

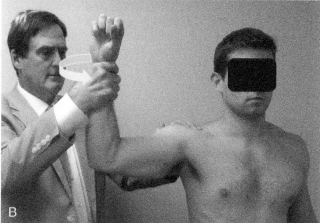

Figure 4.47 The new pain provocation test is performed with the examiner standing behind the patient and the arm in a position similar to the anterior apprehension test. The patient is asked to resist pronation (**A**) and supination (**B**) of the forearm. The *arrows* show the direction of the examiner's force.

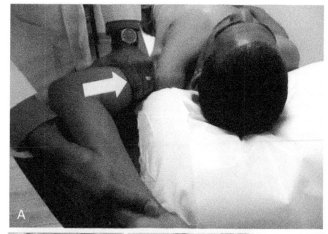

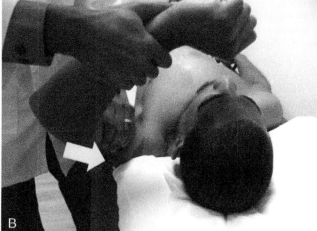

Figure 4.48 The crank test is performed with the patient supine and the arm in maximum elevation. With an axial force down the arm, the examiner exernally (**A**) and internally (**B**) rotates the arm. *Arrows* show direction of examiner's force.

CRANK TEST

Liu and Henry[72] used the crank test to assist in predicting the presence of labral tears (Fig. 4.48). They described the test as follows:

> The crank test is performed with the patient in the upright position with the arm elevated to 160 degrees in the scapular plane. Joint load is applied along the axis of the humerus with one hand while the other performs humeral rotation. A positive test is determined either by (1) pain during the maneuver (usually during external rotation) with or without click or (2) reproduction of the symptoms, usually pain or catching felt by the patient during athletic or work activities. This test should be repeated in the supine position, where the patient is usually more relaxed. Frequently, a positive crank test in the upright position will also be positive in the supine position (Video 4-21).

This test differs from the dynamic shear test in that the arm is not brought up and down in elevation in this test. When comparing the results from the crank test with findings from arthroscopy, the authors found the test to have a sensitivity of 91%, specificity of 93%, PPV of 94%, and NPV of 90%.[72] These results have not been replicated by independent study.

In a later study, the authors found that combining the crank test with the sulcus sign, apprehension, and relocation tests produced a sensitivity of 90% and specificity of 85% in predicting labral tears when compared with arthroscopy.[89]

Mimori and others[88] found the crank test to have a sensitivity of 83% and specificity of 100% when compared with arthroscopy. Stetson and Templin[90] reported a sensitivity of 64%, specificity of 67%, and PPV of 53% when compared with arthroscopy.

Stetson and Templin[86] also compared the crank test, O'Brien test, and MRI with arthroscopy for evaluating superior labral tears. The crank test had a sensitivity of 46%, specificity of 56%, PPV of 41%, and NPV of 61%. The O'Brien test had a sensitivity of 54%, specificity of 31%, PPV of 34%, and NPV of 50%. This showed physical examination using these tests to be poor compared with imaging.

ANTERIOR SLIDE TEST (Video 4-22)

Kibler[91] described the anterior slide test for diagnosing labral tears as follows (Fig. 4.49):

> The patient is examined either standing or sitting, with their hands on the hips with thumbs pointing posteriorly. One of

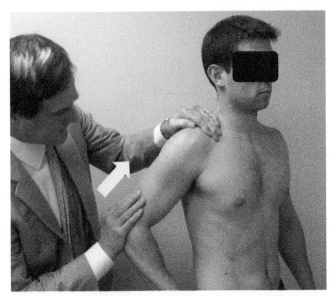

Figure 4.49 The anterior slide test is performed by the examiner applying an axial force up the arm as shown. The *arrow* shows the direction of the examiner's force. A positive test result is pain or a click deep in the shoulder.

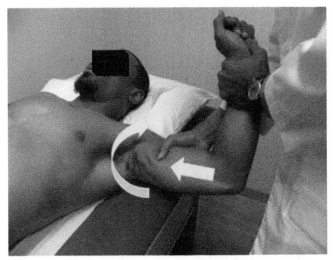

Figure 4.50 The compression-rotation test is performed with the patient supine. The examiner directs a compressive force on the joint while grinding the joint in a rotational manner. The *arrow* shows the direction of the examiner's force.

the examiner's hands is placed across the top of the shoulder from the posterior direction, with the last segment of the index finger extending over the anterior aspect of the acromion at the glenohumeral joint. The examiner's other hand is placed behind the elbow and a forward and slightly superiorly directed force is applied to the elbow and upper arm. The patient is asked to push back against this force. Pain localized to the front of the shoulder under the examiner's hand, and/or a pop or click in the same area, was considered to be a positive test. This test is also positive if the athlete reports a subjective feeling that this testing maneuver reproduces the symptoms that occur during overhead activity.

The author found the test to have a sensitivity of 78.4% and specificity of 91.5% when compared with arthroscopy. A further study[50]found that it had a sensitivity of 8%, specificity of 84%, and accuracy of 77%. The authors concluded that this test was not useful for making the diagnosis of SLAP tears.

COMPRESSION-ROTATION TEST

Snyder and coworkers[103] described the compression-rotation test for diagnosing labral tears as follows (Fig. 4.50):

> The compression–rotation test is performed with the patient supine, the shoulder abducted 90 degrees and the elbow flexed at 90 degrees. A compression force is applied to the humerus, which is then rotated, in an attempt to trap the torn labrum. Labral tears may be felt to catch and snap during the test, as meniscal tears do with MacMurray's test (Video 4-23).

This test is based on the faulty concept that a labral tear behaves like a meniscus tear by causing catching or locking of the joint; however, labral tears rarely cause clicking, and locking from labral tears is almost unheard of. Holovacs et al.[73] reported the test to have a sensitivity of 80% and specificity of 19% for labral pathology when compared with arthroscopy.

McFarland et al.[50] compared the active compression, anterior slide, and compression–rotation tests for SLAP lesions with findings from arthroscopy. They identified the active compression test as the most sensitive at 47%, with the highest PPV of 10%, and the anterior slide as the most specific test at 84%. They noted that clicking or pain location were not reliable portions of the tests. They concluded that none of these three tests was diagnostic of SLAP lesions, and that results from these tests should be interpreted with caution.

CLUNK TEST

Andrews and Gillogly[104] are credited with developing the clunk test (Fig. 4.51). They described it as follows:

> The patient lies supine. The examiner places one hand on the posterior aspect of the shoulder over the humeral head while holding the humerus above the elbow and fully abducts the arm over the patient's head. The examiner then pushes anteriorly with the hand over the humeral head while the other hand rotates the humerus into lateral rotation. A clunk or grinding sound indicates a positive test and is indicative of a tear of the labrum. This test may also cause apprehension if anterior instability is present.

No studies have assessed the validity, reliability, sensitivity or specificity, of this maneuver.

It is interesting to note that Hawkins and McCormack[105] described a palpable and often audible "clunk" to mean shoulder relocation in posterior glenohumeral instability. There has been no validation of the test for this indication either.

TESTS OF THE AC JOINT

See Table 4.11.

The AC joint is a frequent source of shoulder pain and is one of the few sites of shoulder pathology in which pain can radiate up into the trapezius muscle. The main causes of damage to the AC joint include direct trauma from a fall or

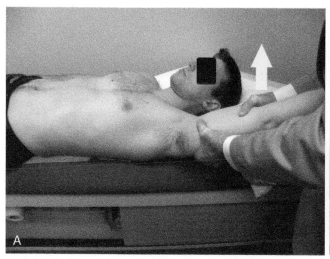
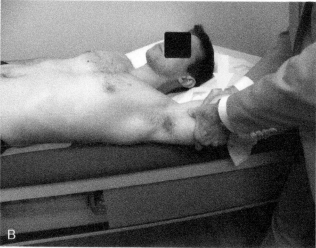

Figure 4.51   The clunk test is performed by fully elevating the arm and translating the humeral head (A) anteriorly and (B) posteriorly on the glenoid. The *arrow* shows the direction of the examiner's force.

Table 4.11   Tests of the Acromioclavicular Joint

Test	Description	Reliability/Validity
Crossed-arm adduction (Apley scarf) test	The test is performed by passively adducting the arm across the body, horizontally approximating the elbow to the contralateral shoulder. Pain at the acromioclavicular joint constitutes a positive test result.	There are no studies assessing the test's sensitivity, specificity, PPV, NPV, or reliability.
Active compression (O'Brien) test	With the physician behind the patient, the patient is asked to forward flex the affected arm 90 degrees with the elbow in full extension. The patient then adducts the arm 10–15 degrees medial to the sagittal plane of the body. The arm is then internally rotated so the thumb is pointed downward. The examiner then applies uniform downward force to the arm. With the arm in the same position, the palm is then fully supinated and the maneuver is repeated. The test result is considered positive if pain is elicited with the first maneuver and is reduced or eliminated with the second maneuver. Pain localized to the acromioclavicular joint or on top of the shoulder is diagnostic of acromioclavicular joint abnormality. Pain or painful clicking described as inside the glenohumeral joint itself is indicative of labral abnormality.	O'Brien et al.[85] For detecting acromioclavicular joint pathology: Sensitivity: 100% Specificity: 96.6% For detecting both acromioclavicular joint pathology and labral tears: Sensitivity: 100% Specificity: 95.2% Chronopoulos et al.[106] Sensitivity: 41% Specificity: 95% Walton et al.[107] Sensitivity: 16% Specificity: 90%
Resisted arm extension test	This test is performed by having the patient forward flex the arm 90 degrees with the elbow bent 90 degrees. The patient is then asked to horizontally extend the arm against resistance by the examiner. A positive test result is pain that localizes to the acromioclavicular joint.	Chronopoulos et al.[106] Sensitivity: 72% Specificity: 85% PPV: 20% NPV: 98% Accuracy: 84%

LR, likelihood ratio; *NPV*, negative predictive value; *PPV*, positive predictive value.

blow or chronic injuries from overuse stress. The exercises that most commonly aggravate the AC joint include bench presses, dips, and pushups. The joint is composed medially of the distal end of the clavicle and laterally of the acromion of the scapula. It is a diarthrodial joint, which usually contains an articular disc. The joint capsule is quite thin but surrounded by strong ligamentous support.

When examining the AC joint, it is important to have the patient undress to see the other side (Fig. 4.52). It is often helpful to ask the patient to point to the location of the pain (called a "one finger test"), and often they point directly to the AC joint (Fig. 4.53). Localized tenderness at the AC joint is almost necessary to confirm the diagnosis of a symptomatic AC joint.

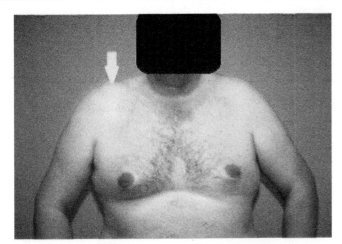

Figure 4.52 Comparison of sides for identifying acromioclavicular joint pathology. The *arrow* shows swelling caused by dislocation of the acromioclavicular joint.

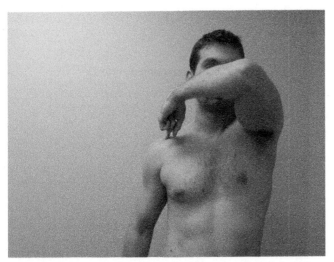

Figure 4.53 The one-finger test for acromioclavicular joint problems is performed by asking the patient to use one finger to point to the location where the pain is the worst.

Also, it is important when performing the AC joint tests to verify the location of the pain with the patient. Some of these tests may cause pain in the posterior shoulder (eg, when the patient has stiffness) and not in the AC joint, so this should not be considered a positive test result. Similarly, the pain may be into the deltoid muscle, and that too is not considered a positive test result.

CROSSED-ARM ADDUCTION (APLEY SCARF TEST)

The Apley scarf test, also known as the AC joint test and the crossed-arm adduction test, was first described by A. G. Apley in the late 1940s to determine the integrity of the AC joint. The test is performed by passively adducting the arm across the body, horizontally approximating the elbow to the contralateral shoulder (Fig. 4.54). Pain at the AC joint constitutes a positive test[22,54,88] (Video 4-24). Chronopoulos and others[106] examined the clinical accuracy of several physical examination tests, including the crossed-arm adduction test, resisted extension test, and active compression test. The diagnosis was based on localized AC joint pain, local tenderness at the AC joint, and pain resolution with a diagnostic

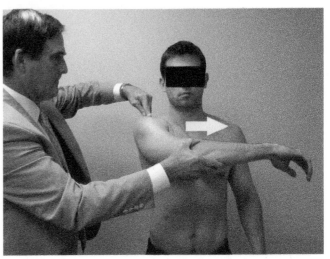

Figure 4.54 The crossed-arm adduction test is performed with the elbow extended and the arm flexed 90 degrees. When the arm is pushed across the body in adduction, the pain should localize to the acromioclavicular joint being palpated by the examiner. The *arrow* shows the direction of the examiner's force.

injection and arthroscopic findings. The crossed-arm adduction test had reasonable sensitivity and specificity, but the active compression test had higher clinical utility for AC conditions.

ACTIVE COMPRESSION TEST

The active compression test developed by O'Brien et al.[85] can be used to diagnose and differentiate AC pathology and labral tears (see Fig. 4.44). A detailed description of this test can be found in the tests for the labrum section of this chapter. In their original study, O'Brien et al.[85] found that, when compared with various combinations of radiography, MRI, and clinical data, the test had a sensitivity of 100%, specificity of 96.6%, PPV of 88.7%, and NPV of 100% for detecting AC joint pathology. For determining both AC joint pathology and labral tears, the authors showed the test had a sensitivity of 100%, specificity of 95.2%, PPV of 91.5%, and NPV of 100%.

Chronopoulos and associates[106] found the active compression test had a sensitivity of 41%, specificity of 95%, PPV of 29%, and NPV of 97%. They noted an overall accuracy of 92% for AC joint pathology. Walton and coworkers[107] found the active compression test had a sensitivity of 16%, specificity of 90%, PPV of 62%, and NPV of 52%. They noted an overall accuracy of 53% for AC joint pathology.

RESISTED ARM EXTENSION TEST

The resisted arm extension test was described by Jacob and Sallay[108] in 1997. This test is performed by having the patient forward flex the arm 90 degrees with the elbow bent 90 degrees (Fig. 4.55). The patient is then asked to horizontally extend the arm against resistance by the examiner. A positive test is pain that localizes to the AC joint.

The only study of this test to date was by Chronopoulos and others[106] who reported a sensitivity of 72%, specificity of 85%, PPV of 20%, NPV of 98%, and accuracy of 84%. Interestingly, this test performed better than the crossed-arm adduction test in confirming the diagnosis of symptomatic AC joint pathology.[106]

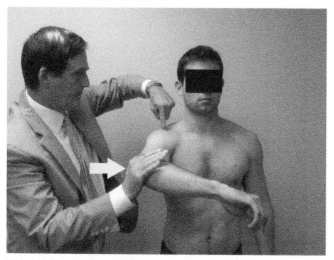

Figure 4.55 The resisted arm extension test is performed by having the patient forward flex the arm 90 degrees and flex the elbow 90 degrees. The patient is then asked to extend the arm horizontally against resistance by the examiner *(arrow)*. A positive test result is pain localized at the acromioclavicular joint.

AUTHOR'S PREFERRED APPROACH

One of the most commonly missed diagnoses is a stiff or frozen shoulder. When patients do not have symmetric motion, they are limited because of pain, joint contracture, or weakness. Loss of motion without pain is a nerve injury until proven otherwise. The most important observation is that the motion is asymmetric and not what type of dyskinesis the abnormal motion might represent.

Although scapular motion is complicated, the main goal when examining the shoulder blade is to see if it wings or if there is asymmetry of motion (called dyskinesis). When evaluating scapular motion, these tests of scapular function are not diagnostic of any one entity and are to be interpreted with caution.

Pain in the anterior shoulder into the front of the arm is often called "biceps pain" by patients, but in reality, the pain in the front of the shoulder can be caused by any number of conditions, including rotator cuff pathology, stiff shoulder, labrum tears, and arthritis. Do not rely on anterior shoulder pain being diagnostic of biceps tendon pathology.

It is now realized that rotator cuff disease results more from aging of the rotator cuff tendons or too much stress on the tendons rather than "impingement" of the rotator cuff against other structures such as the acromion. Pain in the anterior and lateral shoulder can be caused by many different shoulder pathologies and should no longer routinely be called "impingement."

The most reliable sign of rotator cuff pathology is weakness when testing that muscle: abduction for the supraspinatus, external rotation with the arm at the side for the infraspinatus, and a lift-off sign for the subscapularis tendon.

Athletic individuals with pain in the shoulder often are said to have multidirectional instability, but rarely will they say that they feel their shoulder subluxating. The truth is that the cause of pain in the overhead athlete is not currently known. These patients often are "loose jointed," but it is inappropriate to label them as having "multidirectional instability." These individuals are best described as having "shoulder hyperlaxity with pain" or "failed athlete shoulder." In reality, the sulcus sign is misinterpreted by many practitioners who see patients with shoulder pathologies. A sulcus sign reflects laxity only, and it is rare for a patient to report that a sulcus sign reproduces a sense of instability. Pain alone with a sulcus sign does not indicate inferior instability.

It is important not to confuse "laxity" with "instability." Because the shoulder joint has a lot of laxity, in many relaxed individuals, it is normal for the examiner to be able to subluxate the humeral head over the glenoid rim. This is not to be confused with instability.

The anterior apprehension sign and the relocation sign are two of the most clinically useful tests for making an accurate diagnosis of traumatic anterior shoulder instability. This is true only if the patient reports apprehension that the shoulder might come out of the socket, and pain alone is not adequate for making the diagnosis of instability. One of the most difficult examinations of the shoulder is determining the existence of posterior shoulder instability. In these individuals, subluxating the shoulder over the rim with a posterior drawer test should reproduce their symptoms. Often, MRI scanning is needed to confirm the diagnosis.

Making a diagnosis of a SLAP tear remains a challenge, and no one physical examination test can convincingly make the diagnosis. The dynamic shear test has potential as a good test for isolated SLAP lesions, but other coexisting pathologies make it less reliable. Although it is good to know that many tests exist for making the diagnosis of SLAP tears, in my practice, I use the dynamic shear and pain with a resisted lift-off test as signs suspicious for SLAP lesions.

When a patient says the pain in the shoulder comes up into the trapezius from the shoulder, the first thing to consider is the AC joint and the second is the cervical spine. The tests for symptomatic AC joint pathology are not as important as the presence of tenderness directly on the AC joint. It is uncommon for these test results to be positive without a tender AC joint.

CONCLUSION

Many physical examination tests of the shoulder have been described. It is important to know how to perform these tests properly and to understand the sensitivity and specificity of each test when examining patients. The usefulness of these tests is enhanced when they are performed in conjunction with a careful history. The overall sensitivity and specificity of the individual tests may be enhanced by using them in combination rather than relying on the results of a single test. When used in this manner, physical examination of the shoulder can be extremely helpful in guiding appropriate treatment and eliminating unnecessary imaging studies.

REFERENCES

1. Han SH, Oh KS, Han KJ, et al. Accuracy of measuring tape and vertebral-level methods to determine shoulder internal rotation. *Clin Orthop Relat Res.* 2012;470:562-566.

2. Saha AK. The classic. Mechanism of shoulder movements and a plea for the recognition of "zero position" of glenohumeral joint. *Clin Orthop Relat Res.* 1983;173:3-10.

3. Kibler WB. Role of the scapula in the overhead throwing motion. *Contemp Orthop.* 1991;22:525-532.

4. Poppen NK, Walker PS. Normal and abnormal motion of the shoulder. *J Bone Joint Surg Am.* 1976;58:195-201.

5. Salaffi F, Ciapetti A, Carotti M, et al. Clinical value of single versus composite provocative clinical tests in the assessment of painful shoulder. *J Clin Rheumatol.* 2010;16(3):105-108.

6. Silliman JF, Hawkins RJ. Current concepts and recent advances in the athlete's shoulder. *Clin Sports Med.* 1991;10:693-705.

7. Speer KP. Anatomy and pathomechanics of shoulder instability. *Clin Sports Med.* 1995;14:751-760.

8. Gagey OJ, Gagey N. The hyperabduction test. An assessment of the laxity of the inferior glenohumeral ligament. *J Bone Joint Surg Br.* 2001;83:69-74.

9. Naredo E, Aguado P, De Miguel E, et al. Painful shoulder: comparison of physical examination and ultrasonographic findings. *Ann Rheum Dis.* 2002;61:132-136.

10. Park HB, Yokota A, Gill HS, et al. Diagnostic accuracy of clinical tests for the different degrees of subacromial impingement syndrome. *J Bone Joint Surg Am.* 2005;87:1446-1455.

11. Itoi E, Minagawa H, Yamamoto N, et al. Are pain location and physical examinations useful in locating a tear site of the rotator cuff? *Am J Sports Med.* 2006;34:256-264.

12. Bryant L, Shnier R, Bryant C, et al. A comparison of clinical estimation, ultrasonography, magnetic resonance imaging, and arthroscopy in determining the size of rotator cuff tears. *J Shoulder Elbow Surg.* 2002;11:219-224.

13. An YH, Friedman RJ. Multidirectional instability of the glenohumeral joint. *Orthop Clin North Am.* 2000;31:275-285.

14. Arroyo JS, Hershon SJ, Bigliani LU. Special considerations in the athletic throwing shoulder. *Orthop Clin North Am.* 1997;28:69-78.

15. Burkhart SS, Morgan CD, Kibler WB. Shoulder injuries in overhead athletes. The "dead arm" revisited. *Clin Sports Med.* 2000;19:125-158.

16. Cleeman E, Flatow EL. Shoulder dislocations in the young patient. *Orthop Clin North Am.* 2000;31:217-229.

17. Doukas WC, Speer KP. Anatomy, pathophysiology, and biomechanics of shoulder instability. *Orthop Clin North Am.* 2001;32:381-391, vii.

18. Jenp YN, Malanga GA, Growney ES, et al. Activation of the rotator cuff in generating isometric shoulder rotation torque. *Am J Sports Med.* 1996;24:477-485.

19. Jobe FW, Jobe CM. Painful athletic injuries of the shoulder. *Clin Orthop Relat Res.* 1983;173:117-124.

20. Boettcher CE, Ginn KA, Cathers I. Which is the optimal exercise to strengthen supraspinatus? *Med Sci Sports Exerc.* 2009;41:1979-1983.

21. Itoi E, Kido T, Sano A, et al. Which is more useful, the "full can test" or the "empty can test," in detecting the torn supraspinatus tendon? *Am J Sports Med.* 1999;27:65-68.

22. Malanga GA, Jenp YN, Growney ES, et al. EMG analysis of shoulder positioning in testing and strengthening the supraspinatus. *Med Sci Sports Exerc.* 1996;28:661-664.

23. Jobe FW, Moynes DR. Delineation of diagnostic criteria and a rehabilitation program for rotator cuff injuries. *Am J Sports Med.* 1982;10:336-339.

24. Blackburn TA, McLeod WD, White B. EMG analysis of posterior rotator cuff exercise. *Athl Train.* 1990;25:40-45.

25. Bak K, Sorensen AK, Jorgensen U, et al. The value of clinical tests in acute full-thickness tears of the supraspinatus tendon: does a subacromial lidocaine injection help in the clinical diagnosis? A prospective study. *Arthroscopy.* 2010;26:734-742.

26. McFarland EG. Instability and laxity. In: Kim TK, Park HB, El Rassi G, eds. *Examination of the Shoulder: The Complete Guide.* New York: Thieme; 2006:162-212.

27. Magee DJ. Shoulder. In: *Orthopedic Physical Assessment.* 3rd ed. Philadelphia: W.B. Saunders Company; 1997:175-246.

28. Kelly BT, Kadrmas WR, Kirkendall DT, et al. Optimal normalization tests for shoulder muscle activation: an electromyographic study. *J Orthop Res.* 1996;14:647-653.

29. Bartsch M, Greiner S, Haas NP, et al. Diagnostic values of clinical tests for subscapularis lesions. *Knee Surg Sports Traumatol Arthrosc.* 2010;18:1712-1717.

30. Miller CA, Forrester GA, Lewis JS. The validity of the lag signs in diagnosing full-thickness tears of the rotator cuff: a preliminary investigation. *Arch Phys Med Rehabil.* 2008;89:1162-1168.

31. Barth JRH, Burkhart SS, De Beer JF. The bear-hug test: a new and sensitive test for diagnosing a subscapularis tear. *Arthroscopy.* 2006;22:1076-1084.

32. Gerber C, Krushell RJ. Isolated rupture of the tendon of the subscapularis muscle. Clinical features in 16 cases. *J Bone Joint Surg Br.* 1991;73:389-394.

33. Stefko JM, Jobe FW, VanderWilde RS, et al. Electromyographic and nerve block analysis of the subscapularis liftoff test. *J Shoulder Elbow Surg.* 1997;6:347-355.

34. Hertel R, Ballmer FT, Lambert SM, et al. Lag signs in the diagnosis of rotator cuff rupture. *J Shoulder Elbow Surg.* 1996;5:307-313.

35. Odom CJ, Taylor AB, Hurd CE, et al. Measurement of scapular asymmetry and assessment of shoulder dysfunction using the Lateral Scapular Slide Test: a reliability and validity study. *Phys Ther.* 2001;81:799-809.

36. Wright AA, Wassinger CA, Frank M, et al. Diagnostic accuracy of scapular physical examination tests for shoulder disorders: a systematic review. *Br J Sports Med.* 2013;47:886-892.

37. Rabin A, Irrgang JJ, Fitzgerald GK, et al. The intertester reliability of the Scapular Assistance Test. *J Orthop Sports Phys Ther.* 2006;36:653-660.

38. Kibler WB, Sciascia A. Current concepts: scapular dyskinesis. *Br J Sports Med.* 2010;44:300-305.

39. Kibler WB, Ludewig PM, McClure PW, et al. Clinical implications of scapular dyskinesis in shoulder injury: the 2013 consensus statement from the Scapular Summit. *Br J Sports Med.* 2013;47:877-885.

40. Kibler WB, Uhl TL, Maddux JWQ, et al. Qualitative clinical evaluation of scapular dysfunction: a reliability study. *J Shoulder Elbow Surg.* 2002;11:550-556.

41. Uhl TL, Kibler WB, Gecewich B, et al. Evaluation of clinical assessment methods for scapular dyskinesis. *Arthroscopy.* 2009;25:1240-1248.

42. Kibler WB, McMullen J. Scapular dyskinesis and its relation to shoulder pain. *J Am Acad Orthop Surg.* 2003;11:142-151.

43. Kibler WB. The role of the scapula in athletic shoulder function. *Am J Sports Med.* 1998;26:325-337.

44. Rayan GM, Jensen C. Thoracic outlet syndrome: provocative examination maneuvers in a typical population. *J Shoulder Elbow Surg.* 1995;4:113-117.

45. Sanders RJ, Hammond SL, Rao NM. Diagnosis of thoracic outlet syndrome. *J Vasc Surg.* 2007;46:601-604.

46. Kibler WB, Sciascia A, Wilkes T. Scapular dyskinesis and its relation to shoulder injury. *J Am Acad Orthop Surg.* 2012;20:364-372.

47. Calis M, Akgun K, Birtane M, et al. Diagnostic values of clinical diagnostic tests in subacromial impingement syndrome. *Ann Rheum Dis.* 2000;59:44-47.

48. Bennett WF. Specificity of the Speed's test: arthroscopic technique for evaluating the biceps tendon at the level of the bicipital groove. *Arthroscopy.* 1998;14:789-796.

49. Gill HS, El Rassi G, Bahk MS, et al. Physical examination for partial tears of the biceps tendon. *Am J Sports Med.* 2007;35:1334-1340.

50. McFarland EG, Kim TK, Savino RM. Clinical assessment of three common tests for superior labral anterior-posterior lesions. *Am J Sports Med.* 2002;30:810-815.

51. Ludington NA. Rupture of the long head of the biceps flexor cubiti muscle. *Ann Surg.* 1923;77:358-363.

52. Yergason RM. Supination sign. *J Bone Joint Surg Am.* 1931;13:160.

53. Crenshaw AH, Kilgore WE. Surgical treatment of bicipital tenosynovitis. *J Bone Joint Surg Am.* 1966;48:1496-1502.

54. MacDonald PB, Clark P, Sutherland K. An analysis of the diagnostic accuracy of the Hawkins and Neer subacromial impingement signs. *J Shoulder Elbow Surg.* 2000;9:299-301.

55. Braman JP, Zhao KD, Lawrence RL, et al. Shoulder impingement revisited: evolution of diagnostic understanding in orthopedic surgery and physical therapy. *Med Biol Eng Comput.* 2013;52:211-219.

56. McFarland EG, Maffulli N, Del Buono A, et al. Impingement is not impingement: the case for calling it "Rotator Cuff Disease." *Muscles Ligaments Tendons J.* 2013;3:196-200.

57. Murrell GAC, Walton JR. Diagnosis of rotator cuff tears. *Lancet.* 2001;357:769-770.

58. Neer CS II. Anterior acromioplasty for the chronic impingement syndrome in the shoulder: a preliminary report. *J Bone Joint Surg Am.* 1972;54:41-50.

59. Kim TK, McFarland EG. Internal impingement of the shoulder in flexion. *Clin Orthop Relat Res.* 2004;421:112-119.

60. Hawkins RJ, Kennedy JC. Impingement syndrome in athletes. *Am J Sports Med.* 1980;8:151-157, discussion 157-158.

61. Kirkley A, Litchfield RB, Jackowski DM, et al. The use of the impingement test as a predictor of outcome following subacromial decompression for rotator cuff tendinosis. *Arthroscopy.* 2002;18:8-15.

62. Hawkins RJ, Schutte JP. The assessment of glenohumeral translation using manual and fluoroscopic techniques. *Orthop Trans.* 1988;12:727-728.

63. Yocum LA. Assessing the shoulder. *Clin Sports Med.* 1983;2:281-289.

64. Silva L, et al. Accuracy of physical examination in subacromial impingement syndrome. *Rheumatology.* 2008;47:679-683.

65. Burkart AC, Debski RE. Anatomy and function of the glenohumeral ligaments in anterior shoulder instability. *Clin Orthop Relat Res.* 2002;400:32-39.

66. Rowe CR, Zarins B. Recurrent transient subluxation of the shoulder. *J Bone Joint Surg Am.* 1981;63:863-872.

67. Speer KP, Hannafin JA, Altchek DW, et al. An evaluation of the shoulder relocation test. *Am J Sports Med.* 1994;22:177-183.

68. Farber AJ, Castillo RC, Clough M, et al. Clinical assessment of three common tests for traumatic anterior shoulder instability. *J Bone Joint Surg Am.* 2006;88:1467-1474.

69. Jobe FW, Bradley JP. The diagnosis and nonoperative treatment of shoulder injuries in athletes. *Clin Sports Med.* 1989;8:419-438.

70. Gross ML, Distefano MC. Anterior release test. A new test for occult shoulder instability. *Clin Orthop Relat Res.* 1997;339:105-108.

71. Neer CS 2nd, Foster CR. Inferior capsular shift for involuntary inferior and multidirectional instability of the shoulder. A preliminary report. *J Bone Joint Surg Am.* 1980;62:897-908.

72. Liu SH, Henry MH, Nuccion SL. A prospective evaluation of a new physical examination in predicting glenoid labral tears. *Am J Sports Med.* 1996;24:721-725.

73. Holovacs TF, Osbahr DC, Singh H, et al. *The sensitivity and specificity of the physical examination to detect glenoid labrum tears.* Presented at the Specialty Day Meeting of the American Shoulder and Elbow Society. Orlando, FL, March 18, 2000.

74. Matsen FA III, Kirby RM. Office evaluation and management of shoulder pain. *Orthop Clin North Am.* 1982;13:453-475.

75. Gerber C, Ganz R. Clinical assessment of instability of the shoulder. With special reference to anterior and posterior drawer tests. *J Bone Joint Surg Br.* 1984;66:551-556.

76. Hawkins RJ, Schutte JP, Janda DH, et al. Translation of the glenohumeral joint with the patient under anesthesia. *J Shoulder Elbow Surg.* 1996;5:286-292.

77. McFarland EG, Campbell G, McDowell J. Posterior shoulder laxity in asymptomatic athletes. *Am J Sports Med.* 1996;24:468-471.

78. Kessel L, ed. *Clinical Disorders of the Shoulder.* New York: Churchill Livingstone; 1982.

79. Matsen FA III, Thomas SC, Rockwood CA Jr, et al. Glenohumeral instability. In: Rockwood CA Jr, Matsen FA III, eds. *The Shoulder.* 2nd ed. Philadelphia: W.B. Saunders; 1998:611-754.

80. Sodha S, Johnson C, Garzon-Muvdi J, et al. *Clinical Assessment of Three Tests for the Diagnosis of Multidirectional Shoulder Instability.* Presented at The Americal College of Sports Medicine (ACSM) annual meeting. San Diego, CA, May 26-30, 2015.

81. Levy AS, Lintner S, Kenter K, et al. Intra- and interobserver reproducibility of the shoulder laxity examination. *Am J Sports Med.* 1999;27:460-463.

82. Harryman DT II, Sidles JA, Harris SL, et al. The role of the rotator interval capsule in passive motion and stability of the shoulder. *J Bone Joint Surg Am.* 1992;74:53-66.

83. Sharkey NA, Marder RA. The rotator cuff opposes superior translation of the humeral head. *Am J Sports Med.* 1995;23:270-275.

84. Warner JJP, Deng XH, Warren RF, et al. Static capsuloligamentous restraints to superior-inferior translation of the glenohumeral joint. *Am J Sports Med.* 1992;20:675-685.

85. O'Brien SJ, Pagnani MJ, Fealy S, et al. The active compression test: a new and effective test for diagnosing labral tears and acromioclavicular joint abnormality. *Am J Sports Med.* 1998;26:610-613.

86. Stetson WB, Templin K. The crank test, the O'Brien test, and routine magnetic resonance imaging scans in the diagnosis of labral tears. *Am J Sports Med.* 2002;30:806-809.

87. Kim SH, Ha KI, Han KY. Biceps load test: a clinical test for superior labrum anterior and posterior lesions in shoulders with recurrent anterior dislocations. *Am J Sports Med.* 1999;27:300-303.

88. Mimori K, Muneta T, Nakagawa T, et al. A new pain provocation test for superior labral tears of the shoulder. *Am J Sports Med.* 1999;27:137-142.

89. Liu SH, Henry MH, Nuccion S, et al. Diagnosis of glenoid labral tears. A comparison between magnetic resonance imaging and clinical examinations. *Am J Sports Med.* 1996;24:149-154.

90. Stetson WB, Templin KT. *Sensitivity of the crank test vs. the O'Brien test in detecting SLAP lesions of the shoulder.* Presented at the Specialty Day Meeting of the American Shoulder and Elbow Society. Anaheim, CA, February 7, 1999.

91. Kibler WB. Specificity and sensitivity of the anterior slide test in throwing athletes with superior glenoid labral tears. *Arthroscopy.* 1995;11:296-300.

92. Ben Kibler W, Sciascia AD, Hester P, et al. Clinical utility of traditional and new tests in the diagnosis of biceps tendon injuries and superior labrum anterior and posterior lesions in the shoulder. *Am J Sports Med.* 2009;37:1840-1847.

93. Cook C, Beaty S, Kissenberth MJ, et al. Diagnostic accuracy of five orthopedic clinical tests for diagnosis of superior labrum anterior posterior (SLAP) lesions. *J Shoulder Elbow Surg.* 2012;21:13-22.

94. Sodha S, Joseph J, Borade A, et al. *Clinical assessment of the dynamic shear test for SLAP lesions.* Presented at The American Orthopaedic Society for Sports Medicine (AOSSM) annual meeting. Orlando, FL, July 9-12, 2015.

95. Hawkins RJ, Abrams JS, Schutte JP. Multidirectional instability of the shoulder: an approach to diagnosis. *Orthop Trans.* 1987;11:246.

96. Hegedus EJ, Goode A, Campbell S, et al. Physical examination tests of the shoulder: a systematic review with meta-analysis of individual tests. *Br J Sports Med.* 2008;42:80-92.

97. Hegedus EJ, Goode AP, Cook CE, et al. Which physical examination tests provide clinicians with the most value when examining the shoulder? Update of a systematic review with meta-analysis of individual tests. *Br J Sports Med.* 2012;46:964-978.

98. McFarland EG, Tanaka MJ, Garzon-Muvdi J, et al. Clinical and imaging assessment for superior labrum anterior and posterior lesions. *Curr Sports Med Rep.* 2009;8:234-239.

99. Sandrey MA. Special physical examination tests for superior labrum anterior-posterior shoulder tears: an examination of clinical usefulness. *J Athl Train.* 2013;48:856-858.

100. Guanche CA, Jones DC. Clinical testing for tears of the glenoid labrum. *Arthroscopy.* 2003;19:517-523.

101. Cheung EV, O'Driscoll SW. *The dynamic labral shear test for superior labral anterior posterior tears of the shoulder.* Podium presentation at the 76th Annual Meeting of the American Academy of Orthopaedic Surgeons. San Diego, CA, February 14-17, 2007.

102. Kim SH, Ha KI, Ahn JH, et al. Biceps load test II: a clinical test for SLAP lesions of the shoulder. *Arthroscopy.* 2001;17:160-164.

103. Snyder SJ, Karzel RP, Del Pizzo W, et al. SLAP lesions of the shoulder. *Arthroscopy.* 1990;6:274-279.

104. Andrews JR, Gillogly S. Physical examination of the shoulder in throwing athletes. In: Zarins B, Andrews JR, Carson WG Jr, eds. *Injuries to the Throwing Arm.* Philadelphia: W.B. Saunders; 1985:51-65.

105. Hawkins RJ, McCormack RG. Posterior shoulder instability. *Orthopedics.* 1988;11:101-107.

106. Chronopoulos E, Kim TK, Park HB, et al. Diagnostic value of physical tests for isolated chronic acromioclavicular lesions. *Am J Sports Med.* 2004;32:655-661.

107. Walton J, Mahajan S, Paxinos A, et al. Diagnostic values of tests for acromioclavicular joint pain. *J Bone Joint Surg Am.* 2004;86:807-812.

108. Jacob AK, Sallay PI. Therapeutic efficacy of corticosteroid injections in the acromioclavicular joint. *Biomed Sci Instrum.* 1997;34:380-385.

5 Physical Examination of the Elbow

Kenneth D. Montgomery, MD | Matthew S. Mendez-Zfass, MD | Andrew Willis, MD

INTRODUCTION

A thorough history should be ascertained before a physical examination is performed on a patient with an upper extremity complaint. The upper extremity injury history should include the severity, duration, description, and onset of symptoms and effect on sport or performance as well as hand dominance, sport or profession, and associated conditions. Following the history, a visual inspection of the extremity for signs of trauma, side-to-side differences, and muscle wasting is undertaken before any physical examination maneuvers. Moreover, a basic understanding of anatomy is necessary before performing a physical examination of the upper extremity. Although not sufficient to make a diagnosis, it is critical to understand the basic anatomic structures and their healthy function before probing the extremity for signs of disease.

ANATOMY

THE ELBOW JOINT

The elbow joint is a complex synovial-hinged joint that consists of three separate articulations: the ulnohumeral, radiocapitellar, and proximal radioulnar joints. These three articulations allow the elbow 2 degrees of freedom, flexion and extension, as well as supination and pronation. In addition, the bony congruency of these three articulations, when combined with the surrounding ligamentous, capsular, and dynamic structures, serves to provide stability to the elbow throughout physiologic forces and ranges of motion. In contradistinction to the knee, there are no intraarticular cruciate joints that provide stability to the elbow.

OSSEOUS ANATOMY

The distal humeral and proximal radioulnar osseous anatomy is congruent and provides a degree of inherent stability to the elbow joint. The humerus fans out distally to lateral and medial epicondyles that serve as attachment points for the collateral ligaments. The distal humerus has 6 to 8 degrees of valgus tilt and 3 to 8 degrees of internal rotation when comparing the epicondylar axis and the humeral shaft. Additionally, the distal humeral articular surface is angled approximately 30 degrees anterior to the humeral shaft axis.

Continuing distally from the epicondyles, the distal humerus has two condyles that form the articular surfaces laterally and medially. The lateral condyle forms the articular surface of the capitellum that articulates with the radial head.

On the medial side, the articular portion of the more prominent medial condyle is the trochlea or "pulley" that articulates with the proximal ulna to create the ulnohumeral joint.[1] (Fig. 5.1) The lateral ridge of the trochlea is slightly more prominent than the medial ridge that gives the elbow the slight valgus angle that can be seen on radiographs (Fig. 5.2).

The concave radial head and the convex capitellum create the radiocapitellar joint. The bony congruency of the radiocapitellar joint, as well as the radial head in the lesser sigmoid notch of the ulna, provides approximately 240 degrees of radial head rotation.

The trochlea articulates with the greater sigmoid notch of the ulna that consists of the olecranon posteriorly and the coronoid anteriorly. (Fig. 5.3) During extension, the olecranon "screws out" creating a valgus carrying angle, and during flexion, the olecranon "screws in," creating a normal varus angle.[1-3]

LIGAMENTOUS ANATOMY

In addition to osseous congruency, the main sources of stability to the elbow are the ulnar (medial) collateral ligamentous complex, lateral collateral ligamentous complex, anterior ligament, posterior ligament, joint capsule, muscles, and tendons.

The ulnar collateral (medial) ligamentous complex runs from the medial condyle of the humerus to the sublime tubercle on the ulna. The ulnar collateral ligamentous complex can be further subdivided into three distinct bands: the anterior bundle, posterior bundle, and transverse ligaments (Fig. 5.4). The anterior bundle runs from the medial humeral condyle to the medial side of the coronoid process of the ulna. These fibers are the most important for providing resistance to valgus instability.[1,4-13] The posterior bundle runs from the medial condyle of the humerus to the medial portion of the olecranon process of the ulna. There are also transverse fibers running from the olecranon to the coronoid process of the ulna. These transverse fibers reinforce the underlying articular capsule but do not play any role in ligamentous stability.[4-6,8-11,13-15] Anatomic studies have demonstrated that the anterior bundle actually consists of an anterior band and a posterior band that have reciprocal

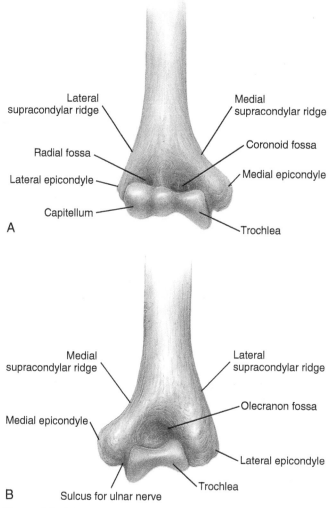

Figure 5.1   Distal humerus anatomy. **A,** Anterior View. **B,** Posterior View. (Miyasaka KC. Anatomy of the elbow. *Orthop Clin North Am.* 1999;30:1-13.)

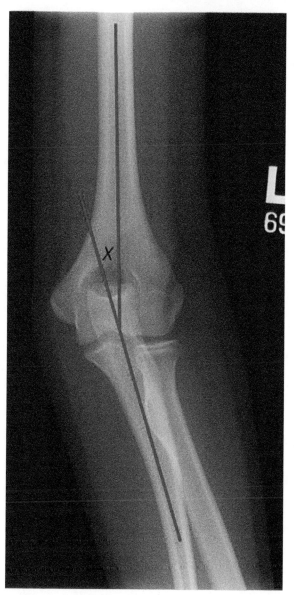

Figure 5.2   Radiographic anatomy of the distal humeral carrying angle *(X).* (Reprinted with permission from Goldfarb CA, Megan J, Patterson M, et al. Elbow radiographic anatomy: measurement techniques and normative data. *J Shoulder Elbow Surg.* 2012;21:1236-1246.)

functions in providing elbow stability depending on the degree of elbow flexion.[11]

The anterior band is the most important medial stabilizer from full extension to 85 degrees of flexion. The posterior band provides stability and is tensioned at elbow flexion greater than 55 degrees, and the posterior oblique ligament provides stability and is taught at flexion greater than 90 degrees.[16]

The ulnar collateral ligament (UCL) consists of three portions. The anterior bundle is anatomically most discrete, and functionally it provides the most stability to the medial aspect of the joint. It arises from the lateral 80% of the medial epicondyle to insert on the medial edge of the coronoid process on the sublime tubercle.

The anterior ligament provides 70% of the valgus stability at the elbow, except in full extension where the radial head and anterior capsule provide the majority of valgus stability. The posterior portion of the UCL is a fan-shaped thickening of the posterior capsule, which originates from the posterior aspect of the medial epicondyle to insert on the medial semilunar notch. This structure does not provide significant valgus stability until the arm is flexed beyond 90 degrees.[9-11]

The transverse oblique segment is composed of horizontally arranged medial capsule fibers that traverse from the tip of the olecranon to the coronoid process. No contribution to stability is derived from this portion of the UCL complex as both its origin and insertion lie on the ulna.

The lateral collateral (radial) ligamentous complex runs from the lateral condyle of the humerus to the annular ligament with some fibers extending to the radial neck. The lateral collateral ligament complex consists of three components: the annular ligament, the radial collateral ligament (RCL), and the lateral ulnar collateral ligament (LUCL) (Fig. 5.5). To avoid confusion, O'Driscoll suggests thinking of the lateral collateral ligament complex of consisting of a radial part (RCL), an annular part (the annular ligament), and an ulnar part (LUCL).[17]

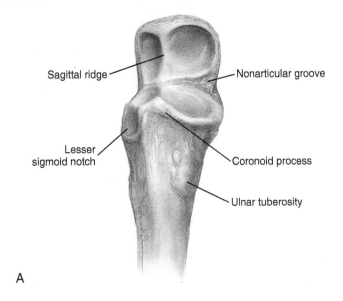

Sagittal ridge

Nonarticular groove

Lesser
sigmoid notch

Coronoid process

Ulnar tuberosity

A

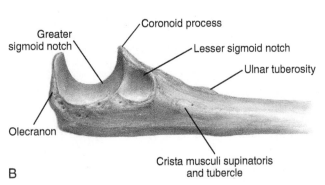

Greater
sigmoid notch

Coronoid process

Lesser sigmoid notch

Ulnar tuberosity

Olecranon

Crista musculi supinatoris
and tubercle

B

Figure 5.3 Proximal ulna osseous anatomy. **A,** AP view. **B,** Lateral View. (Miyasaka KC. Anatomy of the elbow. *Orthop Clin North Am.* 1999;30:1-13.)

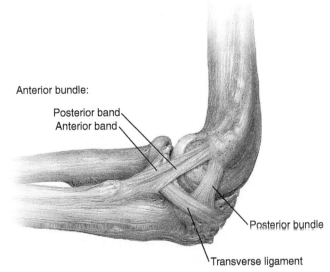

Anterior bundle:

Posterior band
Anterior band

Posterior bundle

Transverse ligament

Figure 5.4 Ulnar collateral (medial) ligament complex. The posterior bundle, anterior bundle, and transverse ligament can be seen. (Lynch JR, Waitayawinyu T, Hanel DP, et al. Medial collateral ligament injury in the overhand-throwing athlete. *J Hand Surg Am.* 2008; 33:430-437.)

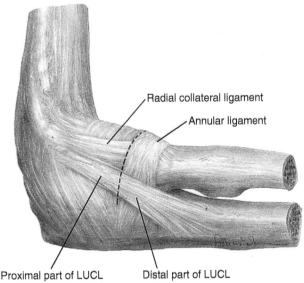

Radial collateral ligament

Annular ligament

Proximal part of LUCL   Distal part of LUCL

Figure 5.5 Lateral ulnar ligamentous complex. The lateral ulnar collateral ligament (LUCL), annular ligament, and radial collateral ligament can all be seen. (Lynch JR, Waitayawinyu T, Hanel DP, et al. Medial collateral ligament injury in the overhand-throwing athlete. *J Hand Surg Am.* 2008;33:430-437.)

The annular ligament almost completely surrounds the radial head, allowing radial rotation and stability of the radial head in the lesser sigmoid notch. The RCL is fan shaped and originates on the lateral epicondyle and inserts into and blends with the annular ligament. The LUCL originates from the lateral humeral epicondyle to insert on the tubercle of the supinator crest. The LUCL is a key component in preventing posterolateral and varus instability.[17,18]

The anterior aspect of the elbow capsule is comparatively thick and performs a role in affording stability against hyperextension of the elbow. The posterior capsule also has thickened bands that are often considered the posterior ligament.

ELBOW AND FOREARM MUSCULATURE

The biceps brachii has two origins called the short and long heads. The origin of the long head is the supraglenoid tubercle and is intimately associated with the shoulder joint. The long head may be diseased and a pain generator in patients presenting with shoulder pain. The origin of the short head is from the coracoid process of the scapula. The two heads join on top of the brachialis muscle on the anterior portion of the arm. The insertion of the biceps is at the radial tuberosity and the biceps aponeurosis, which blends with the forearm flexor sheath on the medial forearm. The major action of the biceps is supination of the forearm and elbow flexion. The biceps brachii receives its innervation from the musculocutaneous nerve from the C5 and C6 nerve roots.

The brachialis muscle originates on the anterior aspect of the humerus distal to the deltoid and coracobrachialis muscle insertions. The insertion is on the ulnar tuberosity situated on the lateral aspect of the proximal ulna. The brachialis is a flexor of the elbow, and its function does not depend on the degree of forearm supination or pronation. It is also receives innervation by the musculocutaneous nerve.

The supinator has multiple origins. It originates from the lateral, posterior aspect of the ulna distal to the olecranon, the lateral humeral epicondyle, the radial collateral ligament of the elbow, and the annular ligament of the radial head. It inserts onto the proximal lateral radius. Supination of the forearm with respect to the arm is the major function of this muscle. It is most effectively tested with the elbow fully flexed, which places the biceps at a mechanical disadvantage. The radial nerve innervates the supinator muscle from the root levels C6 and C7.

The brachioradialis muscle originates from the supracondylar ridge and lateral intermuscular septum on the lateral aspect of the humerus. It inserts near the radial styloid at the distal radial aspect of the radius. The major action of the brachioradialis is elbow flexion with the forearm in neutral rotation (thumb-up position). The radial nerve innervates the brachioradialis from the root levels C5 and C6. The triceps brachii muscle has three heads: the long head, medial head, and lateral head. The long head originates from the infraglenoid tubercle of the scapula. The medial head originates from the medial intermuscular septum and adjacent part of the distal humerus below the radial groove. The lateral head originates from the lateral intermuscular septum and the adjacent humerus proximal and lateral to the radial groove. The three heads join in the posterior aspect of the arm and insert at the proximal olecranon of the ulna. The major action of the triceps brachii is extension of the elbow. The radial nerve innervates the triceps muscle from the root levels C6, C7, and C8.

The anconeus muscle is a small muscle originating on the lateral epicondyle of the humerus; it inserts onto the lateral aspect of the olecranon of the ulna. Its major action is extension of the elbow. The radial nerve innervates the anconeus muscle from the root levels C7 and C8.

The pronator quadratus (PQ), as the name indicates, is a quadrangular shaped muscle with origin and insertion on the distal ulna and radius, respectively. The PQ assists pronation of the forearm and is the last muscle innervated by the anterior interosseous nerve (AIN), the root level most commonly sited at C7 and C8.

The palmaris longus (PL) is absent in a certain percentage of the population. The PL origin is at the medial epicondyle of the humerus from the common flexor tendon, and the insertion is at the palmar aponeurosis of the hand. Because it inserts on the palmar aponeurosis, it is not contained within the carpal tunnel. The major action of the PL is minor assistance wrist flexion. The median nerve innervates the PL, and the root levels are C7 and C8 and, occasionally, T1.

The flexor carpi radialis (FCR) is medial to the pronator teres and lateral to the PL and flexor carpi ulnaris. The FCR muscle's origin is at the medial humeral epicondyle from the common flexor tendon, and the insertion is at the second and third metacarpal bones in the hand. The FCR does not go deep to the flexor retinaculum at the wrist; therefore, like the PL, it is not within the carpal tunnel. The major action of the FCR is wrist flexion with a slight pronation component. The major innervation is from the median nerve from the root levels C6 and C7.

The flexor carpi ulnaris (FCU) has two heads of origin from the common flexor tendon off of the medial humeral epicondyle and from the proximal posterior surface of the ulna just medial to the origin of the extensor carpi ulnaris. The major action of the FCU is wrist flexion with ulnar deviation. The major innervation is from the ulnar nerve from the root levels C8 and T1.

The flexor digitorum superficialis (FDS) also has two heads of origin from the medial to the humeral epicondyle at the common flexor tendon to the coronoid process and from the lateral radius just distal to the insertion of the supinator. The median nerve and the ulnar artery both lie deep to this muscle and pass between the two heads of the FDS. The FDS muscle gives rise to four flexor tendons in the distal forearm. These four tendons pass deep to the flexor retinaculum at the wrist, and therefore the FDS lies within the carpal tunnel at the wrist. The four tendons then continue on to the index, middle, ring, and small fingers and insert on their respective middle phalanges. Importantly, each tendon splits (decussates) just proximal to the final insertion to allow the tendon of the flexor digitorum profundus to pass through. The major action of the muscle is flexion of the proximal interphalangeal joints (PIPJs). In addition, this muscle can aid in flexion at the metacarpophalangeal (MCP) and wrist joints. The median nerve innervates the FDS from the root levels C7, C8, and T1.

The flexor digitorum profundus (FDP) has extensive origin from the anterior and medial ulna and adjacent interosseous membrane. The FDP muscle then gives rise to four tendons that pass deep to the flexor retinaculum at the wrist. Like the FDS, the FDP tendons lie within the carpal tunnel. The final insertion is on the volar base of the proximal aspect of the distal phalanges of the index, middle, ring, and small fingers. Recall that the FDP tendons past through the split tendons of the FDS muscle. The major action of the FDP is flexion of the distal phalanx. The FDP can also secondarily aid more proximal phalangeal flexion and wrist flexion. The FDP has dual innervation from both the anterior interosseous nerve (branch off of the median nerve) and the ulnar nerve. The radial portion of the FDP to the index and middle digits are innervated by the anterior interosseous nerve, whereas the ulnar portion to the ring and small digits are innervated by the ulnar nerve. The root levels innervating the FDP are C7 and C8.

The flexor pollicis longus (FPL) originates just lateral to the FDP on the interosseous membrane and the adjacent radial bone. The anterior interosseous nerve runs between the FPL and FDP and provides innervation to these muscles. The insertion of the FPL is at the volar base of the distal phalanx of the thumb. The FPL tendon passes within the carpal tunnel and is the most laterally situated tendon. The major action of the FPL is flexion of the interphalangeal joint of the thumb. The FPL can secondarily flex the MCP joint of the thumb. It is innervated by the anterior interosseous nerve from root levels C7 and C8.

EXTENSOR GROUP

The extensor tendons of the wrist are best remembered and studied by focusing on the six dorsal extensor compartments in which they travel. The compartments are tunnels on the dorsum of the wrist that contain the extensor tendons. The extensor retinaculum covers these tunnels and prevents tendon subluxation.

The extensor carpi radialis longus (ECRL) originates at the lateral supracondylar ridge of the humerus, the adjacent intermuscular septum, and the lateral humeral epicondyle. It inserts at the base of the second metacarpal bone. The major action of the ECRL is extension of the wrist with a lateral or radial deviation. The innervation of the ECRL is from the radial nerve, root levels C7 and C8. The extensor carpi radialis brevis (ECRB) and the ECRL share a common tendon sheath and extensor compartment at the wrist. The ECRB inserts at the base of the third metacarpal. The major action of the ECRB is wrist extension. The radial nerve innervates the ECRB from the root levels C7 and C8. ECRB travels with ECRL in the first dorsal compartment.

The extensor pollicis brevis (EPB) originates on the posterior surface of the radius and the adjacent intermuscular septum. The insertion is at the base of the proximal phalanx of the thumb. The radial nerve innervates the EPB from root levels C7 and C8. Its major action is extension of the interphalangeal joint of the thumb. EPB runs in the second dorsal compartment.

The abductor pollicis longus (APL) originates on the proximal ulna, adjacent intermuscular septum, and the radius, just distal and posterior to the insertion of the supinator. The insertion of the APL is at the base of the first metacarpal. The major action of the APL is abduction of the thumb. The radial nerve innervates the APL from the root levels C7 and C8. The APL travels in the second dorsal compartment with the EPB.

The extensor pollicis longus (EPL) originates distal to the APL on the intermuscular septum and the ulna just lateral to the origin of the extensor carpi ulnaris. The insertion of the EPL is the proximal end of the distal phalanx of the thumb. Its major action is extension of the interphalangeal joint of the thumb. A secondary action of the EPL is wrist extension with radial deviation. The radial nerve innervates the EPL from root levels C7 and C8. The EPL travels in the third dorsal compartment and becomes prominent with thumb extension because of its acute radial turn.

The extensor indicis (EI) originates on the distal posterior radius and inserts on the extensor surface of the index finger at the middle and distal phalanx. Its major action is extension of the index finger. The EI is the last muscle innervated by the radial nerve from root levels C7 and C8. EI runs in the fourth dorsal compartment.

The extensor digitorum communis (EDC) originates from the common extensor tendon at the lateral humeral epicondyle and inserts into the middle and distal phalanges of the index, middle, ring, and small fingers. Its major action is extension of these digits. The radial nerve innervates the EDC from the root levels C7 and C8. The EDC tendons travel with the EI in the fourth dorsal compartment.

The extensor digiti minimi (EDM), also referred to as the extensor digiti quinti (EDQ), is a small muscle originating at the common extensor tendon of the lateral humeral epicondyle and runs immediately adjacent to the EDC. It inserts at the middle and distal phalanx of the small finger. The major action is to extend the small finger. The radial nerve innervates the EDM from the root levels C7 and C8. The EDM runs in the fifth dorsal compartment.

The extensor carpi ulnaris (ECU) originates from the lateral humeral epicondyle at the common extensor tendon and from the posterior surface of the proximal ulna. The ECU is the most medial muscle in the extensor group. It inserts at the base of the fifth metacarpal bone. The major action is extension of the wrist with ulnar deviation. The radial nerve innervates the ECU from the root levels C7 and C8. The ECU runs in the sixth dorsal compartment.

NERVES IN THE UPPER EXTREMITY

Four major nerves enter and innervate the upper extremity.

MUSCULOCUTANEOUS NERVE

The musculocutaneous nerve enters the arm as an extension of the lateral cord of the brachial plexus containing nerve fibers from cervical roots C5 and C6. The nerve enters the muscle belly of the coracobrachialis muscle and lies in the arm between the biceps and the brachialis muscles, innervating both. This nerve ends as a cutaneous nerve supplying the lateral forearm called the *lateral antebrachial cutaneous nerve (LABCN)*.

MEDIAN NERVE

The median nerve is formed by nerve fibers from the lateral and medial cords of the brachial plexus containing nerve fibers from the cervical root levels C6–T1. This nerve enters the arm running with the ulnar nerve and the brachial artery and travels within the forearm just medial to the biceps tendon insertion and anterior to the elbow joint. The median nerve dives deep to the pronator teres (PT), between its two heads, and runs between the FDS and FDP muscles. The median nerve innervates the PT, PL, FDS, and FCR in the forearm. The median nerve gives off a branch, the AIN, just after crossing the elbow joint. The AIN runs deep to the FDP and innervates the FDP to digits 1 and 2, FPL, and PQ. The median nerve continues between the tendons of the FDS and FDP at the wrist, just radial (lateral) to the superficialis tendon, ulnar (medial) to the FCR, and just deep (and lateral) to the PL tendon. The median nerve gives off the palmar cutaneous branch just proximal to the flexor retinaculum. It then passes deep to the flexor retinaculum and supplies the (superficial head) flexor pollicis brevis (FPB), abductor pollicis brevis (APB), opponens pollicis (OP), and lumbricals 1 and 2.

ULNAR NERVE

The ulnar nerve enters the arm as the extension of the medial cord of the brachial plexus with nerve fibers from the cervical root levels C8 and T1. The nerve enters the arm slightly posterior to the brachial artery, innervating no muscles in the arm, and passes posterior to the medial humeral condyle in the ulnar groove. In the forearm, the ulnar nerve lies between the FCU and FDP and innervates the FDP to digits 3 and 4 and the FCU. Next, the ulnar nerve crosses the wrist joint medial to the FCU tendon and lateral to the ulnar artery. Once in the hand, the ulnar nerve passes medial to the pisiform bone, splitting into the superficial and deep palmar branches. These two branches enter the canal of Guyon together but exit to different end points. The space between the pisiform and the hook of the hamate forms the walls of Guyon canal. The roof of Guyon canal is the distal extension of the FCU tendon, and the floor is the pisohamate ligament. The superficial palmar branch supplies skin sensation to the medial half of the fourth and all of the fifth digits. The deep palmar branch travels (medial side) around the hook of the hamate and travels laterally to innervate the lumbricals 4 and 5, all interosseous muscles, all hypothenar muscles, the deep head of the FPB, and the adductor pollicis.

RADIAL NERVE

The radial nerve is the extension of the posterior cord of the brachial plexus with nerve fibers from the root levels C5–C8. It enters the upper arm through the quadrangular space (borders teres major, minor, long head of the triceps, and the humerus). In general, the radial nerve innervates all extensor muscles of the elbow, wrist, and fingers. The radial nerve has cutaneous innervation to the back of the arm, forearm, and hand. Once in the arm, the radial nerve lies against the humerus, traveling distally and laterally in the spiral groove of the humerus between the lateral and medial heads of the triceps. In the distal arm, the radial nerve lies between the anterior brachialis muscle and the posterior brachioradialis and ECRL muscles.

At the elbow, the radial nerve courses anterior to the lateral condyle of the humerus and splits into superficial and deep branches before entering the belly of the supinator. The superficial branch travels under the brachioradialis muscle becoming subcutaneous lateral to the tendon in the distal forearm. The superficial branch provides cutaneous innervation to the dorsum of the lateral hand and base of the thumb. The deep branch travels distally between the superficial and the deep extensor muscle groups. After innervating the supinator muscle, the radial nerve is called the *posterior interosseous nerve (PIN)*. The deep branch of the PIN provides sensory input to the posterior of the wrist and carpal bones. The radial innervated muscles include triceps (all heads), brachioradialis, ECRL, ECRB, supinator, EDC, EDM, APL, extensor pollicis longus and brevis, and EI. The last radial innervated muscle is the EI, which becomes important in assessing for recovery following neuropraxia.

INSPECTION

Visual inspection of the elbow requires proper exposure of the extremity from the shoulder to the hand. In the anatomic position, the anterior aspect of the elbow is covered by the biceps muscle and tendon, which are easily visualized. The anterior forearm just distal to the biceps muscle belly and tendon is called the *cubital fossa* or *antecubital fossa*. The cubital vein can be observed and palpated as it passes anterior to the elbow joint just lateral to the biceps tendon. The cephalic vein can be observed on the lateral side of the biceps muscle in the arm. The medial epicondyle of the elbow is the origin of the flexor/pronator muscle mass or the common flexor tendon. On the lateral aspect of the elbow can be seen the muscles that overlie the lateral epicondyle.

The lateral epicondyle is the origin of the extensor muscle mass or the common extensor tendon. On the posterior elbow, the olecranon process of the ulna is noted and is most obvious with the elbow flexed at 90 degrees. The olecranon bursa overlies the posterior elbow. A patient with olecranon bursitis can have a visible swelling with tenderness and warmth over the olecranon.

Observing joint movements through their respective ranges of motion, both actively and passively, is part of inspection. The total joint motion is observed and documented from side to side with quality of movement also noted. The carrying angle in extension and range of motion of the elbow from maximal extension to maximal flexion and from maximal supination to maximal pronation with the elbow flexed to 90 degrees should be documented.

Joint swelling or discoloration and any skin lesions or ecchymosis, hypertrophy, hypotrophy, or frank atrophy of muscles in the arm or forearm should also be documented. Various injuries can be detected immediately through a comprehensive inspection of the extremity. Distally, observation for asymmetry between the hand and wrist in both the supinated and pronated positions, comparing the right with the left sides, is essential. Any tumors, angular deformities, or soft tissue prominence should be noted. Swelling or enlargement of the joints should be noted.

PALPATION

Palpation is a key aspect of the physical examination of any body part and is of critical importance when palpating for potential pathology around the elbow. Palpating the elbow requires pinpointing the exact area of tenderness or pathology.

The medial epicondyle is easily palpable. Just anterior and distal to the medial epicondyle, one can palpate from proximal to distal the muscle origins of the pronator teres, FCR, PL, FDS, and FCU. Just posterior to the medial epicondyle, the ulnar groove can be palpated, as can the ulnar nerve traveling within. On the posterior aspect of the elbow, the olecranon process of the ulna is easily palpable, appreciating the triceps tendon insertion into the olecranon. Midway between the olecranon and the lateral epicondyle, one palpates the anconeus muscle. The lateral epicondyle is covered by a large mass of extensor muscle, called the *extensor bundle* or *wad*. From the lateral supracondylar ridge to the lateral epicondyle, one palpates a number of muscles. The muscles from proximal to distal are the brachioradialis, ECRL, ECRB, and EDC.

Deeper palpation about the lateral elbow can reveal ligamentous and bony abnormalities. The lateral "soft spot" is located between the radial head, lateral epicondyle, and olecranon tip. It should be palpated for fullness, indicating a joint effusion or hemarthrosis, or crepitus, indicating a loose body or fracture. About 2 cm distal to the capitellum, the radial head is palpated with the accompanying annular ligament that encircles the structure. In the face of trauma, crepitus and pain while pronating or supinating the forearm in the region of the radial head area should raise suspicion for a radial head fracture. The lateral collateral ligament is difficult to directly palpate because of the overlying musculature; however, the anterior bundle of the medial collateral ligament is usually palpable with the elbow flexed from 30 to 60 degrees.

EXAMINATION OF NERVE COMPRESSION SYNDROMES

The nerves of the upper extremity all have multiple possible sites of compression and nerve entrapment. In order to be able to diagnose the point of entrapment, an intimate knowledge of both neuroanatomy and potential sites of compression is key. This chapter focuses on nerve compressions that are associated with or can be misdiagnosed as musculoskeletal injuries to the elbow.

MEDIAN NERVE LESIONS

The median nerve innervates a number of important muscles in the upper extremity and hand. Sites of compression include the ligament of Struthers, which is a fibrous band off of an anomalous humeral supracondylar process, between the two heads of the pronator teres, by the lacertus fibrosis extension of the biceps tendon and between the fibrous arch of the FDS.

With compression at a supracondylar process on physical exam, the wrist flexors, PT, and median innervated hand muscles present with weakness. The sensation on the thenar and first three and a half digits can be impaired. Wrist flexion occurs with ulnar deviation, as the FCU remains innervated. Upon being asked to make a fist, the patient will be unable to flex the index finger, and in many cases, the middle finger as well, actively or against resistance. When both the index and middle finger cannot be flexed, the hand forms the "active papal hand" or "benediction sign." Over time, high median nerve injuries may result in "ape hand" deformity, because the radial nerve innervating the APL, EPL, and EPB pull the first metacarpal into the plane of the palm.

PRONATOR SYNDROME

As mentioned, entrapment may also occur under the lacertus fibrosus between the two heads of the PT or through its muscle belly[19,20]; these are collectively referred to as *pronator syndrome*. Pronator muscle function is spared because its innervation is established before the median nerve is compressed. However, all muscles distal to the PT are affected and will result in wrist flexor weakness or lost or impaired sensation over the thenar and lateral three and a half digits.

Symptoms of the pronator teres syndrome mimic carpal tunnel syndrome (CTS). In contrast to CTS, patients will often exhibit pain to palpation over the nerve entrapment site, which is proximal in the volar forearm. Additionally, there are characteristically fewer night symptoms than patients with CTS, and the palmar cutaneous branch of the median nerve that innervates the palm is involved, whereas in CTS, it is spared.[21,22]

Two tests that have been described for pronator syndrome include the resisted elbow flexion with forearm supination (Fig. 5.6) and the resisted elbow extension with forearm pronation (Fig. 5.7). The resisted pronation test is designed to compress the nerve between the two heads of the pronator teres, and the supination test is designed to compress the nerve under the lacertus fibrosus.[22,23]

In this syndrome, repetitive pronation and flexion of the wrist can trigger vague numbness and paresthesias in the

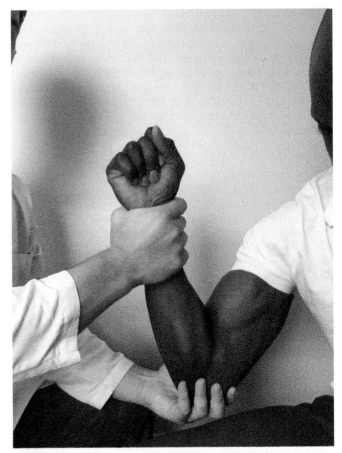

Figure 5.6 Resisted elbow flexion with forearm supination. The test is designed to compress the median nerve under the lacertus fibrosus. Notice the examiner is resisting flexion and supination of the patient.

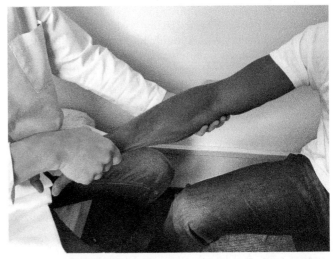

Figure 5.7 Resisted elbow extension with forearm pronation. This test is designed to compress the median nerve between the two heads of the pronator teres. The test is considered positive if the symptoms of forearm pain are reproduced.

forearm. Hartz[24] described tenderness in the proximal part of the PT in 39 subjects with this condition. This finding is supported by Werner's[20] results in nine patients, all of whom had local tenderness over the median nerve and the AIN 4 to 5 cm distal to the elbow. All patients also experienced pain during provocative maneuvering of active forearm pronation against resistance, with the elbow in 30 degrees of flexion. In contrast, resisted active forearm supination with the elbow similarly flexed failed to elicit pain. Additionally, a positive Tinel sign over the entrapment site (tapping the proximal edge of the pronator) was reported in 4 of 9 patients by Werner[20] and 20 of 39 patients by Hartz.[24]

The AIN can be compressed by a fibrous band of either the FDS or FDP muscle bellies. The AIN syndrome results in weakness of the AIN-innervated FPL, FDP to the index and long finger, and the PQ.[22,25] The AIN is purely a motor nerve; therefore, there are no sensory disturbances. Patients will, however, commonly present with a dull forearm ache. On physical exam, lack of flexion of the distal phalanx of the thumb and index finger result in the inability of the patient to make the "okay" sign. When pinching paper between the thumb and index finger, the patient uses the adductor pollicis (ulnar-innervated muscle) to substitute for FPL weakness. Pronator quadratus weakness is tested with the elbow fully flexed placing the PT at a mechanical disadvantage. The most common median nerve entrapment is CTS, which is discussed in another chapter.

ULNAR NERVE LESIONS

The ulnar nerve enters the arm as an extension of the medial cord of the brachial plexus with nerve fibers from the root levels C8 and T1. Sites of compression of the ulnar nerve are multiple and can occur from proximal to distal at the arcade of Struthers, medial triceps head and medial intramuscular septum, cubital tunnel, the aponeurosis of the flexor pronator mass, and Guyon canal at the wrist.

The most common site for ulnar neuropathy in the arm is at the cubital tunnel. The arcade of Struthers is an aponeurotic band from the medial head of the triceps to the intermuscular septum that is present in up to 70% of people.[26,27] Ulnar nerve entrapments at the cubital tunnel can spare the fibers innervating the FCU and FDP to the ring and small fingers. Proximal and distal ulnar nerve lesions have the same effect on all of the hand intrinsics. Proximal lesions that denervate the forearm muscles allow the patient wrist flexion with radial deviation, and wrist flexion strength is usually mildly decreased (Video 5-1). Multiple provocative maneuvers have been developed to diagnose cubital tunnel syndrome, which is discussed in another chapter.

RADIAL NERVE LESIONS

The radial nerve can be injured proximally secondary to axillary crutch use or compression against the back of a chair, a condition referred to as "Saturday night palsy." Proximal injury above the level of tricipital innervation will result in involvement of the triceps along with all other distally innervated muscles and cutaneous nerves. Injury along its course down the spiral groove, on the posterior aspect of the humerus, will result in sparing of the triceps as the branches to the triceps are proximal to the groove. However, the remainder of radial and posterior interosseous nerve–innervated muscles will be weakened, resulting in wrist drop (any flexion of the wrist). Wrist drop places the

wrist and finger flexors at a mechanical disadvantage that leads to weakened grip strength. The posterior interosseous nerve, a branch of the radial nerve, can also be entrapped as it enters the supinator muscle or at the arcade of Frohse, a fibrous arch at the origin of the supinator.[28,29]

Radial tunnel syndrome or PIN syndrome spares the fibers innervating the supinator muscle as well as the radial sensory nerve but affects muscles innervated more distal by the posterior interosseous nerve. On physical exam, patients are able to extend the wrist with radial deviation due to the loss of ulnar extension from the PIN-innervated ECU and unopposed extensor carpi radialis (ECR) firing. On examination, they typically have a point of maximal tenderness 3 to 5 cm distal to the lateral epicondyle. This corresponds to the supinator muscle mass.[30] Provocative physical exam maneuvers that have been described include pain with resisted active forearm extension and pain with extension of the middle finger against resistance (Fig. 5.8).

Diagnostic injections of local anesthesia into the point of maximal tenderness are another diagnostic tool that may help distinguish radial tunnel syndrome from lateral epicondylitis. However, one must be careful to ensure that the local anesthetic does not spread proximally and anesthetize the lateral epicondyle and extensor tendons. Placement of rope or handcuffs at the wrist may reveal more distal involvement of the radial sensory nerve at the wrist, in particular, a condition termed *cheiralgia paresthetica*, which results in sensory loss on the dorsal thumb.

PHYSICAL EXAMINATION OF THE ELBOW

EXAMINATION OF LATERAL EPICONDYLITIS

The term *tennis elbow* developed out of the term used in 1883 by Winkworth, "lawn tennis elbow."[31] Originally, Winkworth described medial epicondylitis; however, today tennis elbow describes lateral epicondylitis, and "golfer's elbow" is commonly used to describe medial epicondylitis.[32] Commonly, patients will have tenderness over the lateral epicondyle that may radiate to the forearm. Palpation 2 to 5 mm distal and anterior to the lateral epicondyle usually isolates the point of maximal tenderness.[33]

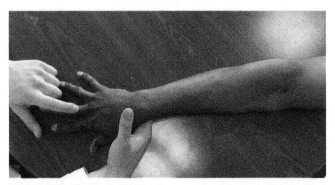

Figure 5.8 Resisted middle finger extension test. The patient attempts to extend the middle finger against resistance. The test result is positive if symptoms are reproduced with pain 3 to 5 cm distal to the lateral epicondyle.

EXTENSOR CARPI RADIALIS BREVIS TEST OR TENNIS ELBOW TEST

The ECRB test should be considered synonymous with the tennis elbow test. The Cozen test has been described to stress this musculotendinous origin (Video 5-2). To perform the test, have the patient hold the elbow extended and the forearm pronated while making a fist and extending the wrist. The patient should hold this position while the examiner applies resistance. Pain at the origin of the ECRB is suggestive of lateral tennis elbow. The test may be repeated with the elbow flexed 90 degrees. The pain is occasionally worse with the elbow in extension than with the elbow in flexion.

It is widely believed that the pain elicited with the tennis elbow test or resisted wrist extension are due primarily to tendinopathy of the ECRB tendon at or near its origin on the lateral humeral condyle.[34] Nirschl and Pettrone discovered pathologic tissue in 86 of 88 (97%) surgically treated patients at the origin of the ECRB tendon.[35]

RESISTED MIDDLE-FINGER EXTENSION TEST

The resisted middle-finger extension test was originally described for diagnosing the radial tunnel syndrome, but it is also useful in evaluating for lateral epicondylitis (see Fig. 5.8; Video 5-3). With the patient's arm extended and the wrist pronated and at neutral flexion, the examiner resists extension of the middle finger. Pain at the area of the lateral epicondyle or 2 to 4 cm distal is indicative of a positive test result. Lister and coworkers reported 19 of 19 cases of resistant tennis elbow relieved by radial tunnel release had positive resisted middle-finger test results.[36] Werner reported a positive resisted middle-finger test result in 67 of 90 cases of resistant lateral elbow pain.[19] Resistant cases of lateral epicondylitis may be secondary to misdiagnosis of PIN entrapment at the radial tunnel.[30,36,37]

MEDIAL EPICONDYLITIS

Although the incidence of medial epicondylitis is less than that of lateral epicondylitis, it is still a cause of significant morbidity. A comprehensive retrospective review by O'Dwyer and Howie found that of individuals with epicondylitis, 91% had lateral epicondylitis, 8% had medial epicondylitis, and both epicondyles were involved in 1% of individuals.[14] Medial epicondylitis has been referred to as *golfer's elbow* because of the wrist flexion performed with the golf swing. This condition is often seen in manual laborers.[38] Other activities implicated include rowing, baseball (pitching), javelin throwing, bricklaying, hammering, tennis (serving), and typing. Commonly, patients present with tenderness at a point 5 to 10 mm distal to the medial epicondyle.[32,38]

RESISTED WRIST FLEXION AND PRONATION

Symptoms of medial epicondylitis may be reproduced by resisted wrist flexion and pronation. With the elbow flexed to 90 degrees and the forearm supinated, the patient makes a fist and flexes the wrist, maintaining that position as the examiner attempts to forcibly extend the wrist (Video 5-4). If resisted wrist flexion elicits pain at the origin of the FCR, the test result is considered positive. This test should be repeated with the elbow fully extended and the amount of pain elicited with the elbow extended and flexed compared. In contradistinction to lateral epicondylitis, medial tennis elbow is usually more painful with the elbow flexed.

Individuals with suspected medial epicondylitis should also be assessed for ulnar neuropathy at or near the elbow. Vangsness and Jobe[39] reported an ulnar nerve involvement in 23% of cases, and Nirschl and Ashman reported an ulnar nerve involvement of 50% in cases of medial epicondylitis.[37] In contrast, a retrospective study by O'Dwyer and Howie reported 0% nerve involvement with medial epicondylitis.[14] One study of medial epicondylitis in occupational settings has found an 84% risk of concomitant ipsilateral upper extremity pathology[32] (Table 5.1).

TESTS FOR BICEPS TENDON RUPTURE

A rupture of the distal tendon of the biceps as it inserts onto the tuberosity of the radius can be a source of significant pain and discomfort. Tears can present traumatically with significant biceps deformity, ecchymosis, and swelling,

Table 5.1   Tests for Epicondylitis

Test	Description	Reliability	Comments
Cozen test aka "Tennis elbow test"	The patient holds the elbow extended and the forearm pronated while making a fist and extending the wrist against resistance. Repeat with the elbow in 90 degrees of flexion.	Pathologic tissue discovered in 86/88 (97%) of patients treated surgically[35]	
Resistant middle-finger extension test	The arm is extended, and with the wrist pronated and at neutral flexion, the examiner resists extension of the middle finger. Pain at the area of the lateral epicondyle or 2–4 cm distal is indicative of a positive test result.	Positive in 19 of 19 (100%) patients with "lateral epicondylitis" treated with radial tunnel release[36]	Also used to diagnose radial tunnel syndrome
Resisted wrist flexion	With the elbow flexed to 90 degrees and the forearm supinated, the patient makes a fist and flexes the wrist, maintaining that position as the examiner attempts to forcibly extend the wrist. If resisted wrist flexion elicits pain at the origin of the flexor carpi radialis, the test result is considered positive.	None reported	Pain usually greater with flexion than with extension for medial epicondylitis

or they may present with a partial tear and chronic pain and weakness with supination and elbow flexion. As the biceps tendon inserts distally onto the radius, it becomes prominent subcutaneously, especially with the forearm supinated. In order to evaluate for a complete tear of the distal biceps, the Hook test is used (Fig. 5.9). With the patient's arm in 90 degrees of abduction and the elbow flexed 90 degrees and the forearm supinated with the thumb pointing up, the examiner attempts to "hook" the tendon from the lateral side. A positive result occurs when there is no palpable cord, which is indicative of a complete tendon rupture (Video 5-5).[40] Another test for complete tear of the distal biceps is the biceps squeeze test (Fig. 5.10). This test is similar to the Thompson test for Achilles tendon tears. The examiner places the patient's forearm in 60 to 80 degrees of flexion and neutral rotation and squeezes the biceps muscle belly. Lack of forearm supination is indicative of a tendon tear (Video 5-6).[41] One study of patients with presumed complete distal biceps tendon ruptures as evidenced by

deformity, found that the test was positive is 25 of 26 tears (96%).[42] In cases of partial tendon tears, the Hook test may be negative, but may elicit pain on palpation of the distal tendon. In these cases, resisted forearm supination is generally painful, as is resisted forearm flexion with the arm maximally extended[23] (Table 5.2).

ELBOW INSTABILITY

As previously mentioned, the elbow has medial and lateral collateral ligaments as the main stabilizers. However, unlike in the knee, there are no cruciate ligaments to offer translational stability of the humerus in relation to the ulna. Elbow stability is offered mainly by the bony congruency between the humerus and ulna, muscles and their tendons, the joint capsule, and the collateral ligaments. Multiple patterns of elbow instability have been described, with the two most common being posterolateral rotatory instability (PLRI) and medial elbow instability.

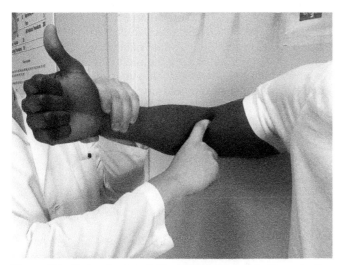

Figure 5.9 Biceps hook test. The test is performed with supination of the forearm and the forearm flexed to 90 degrees. Inability to palpate the tendon indicates a positive test result.

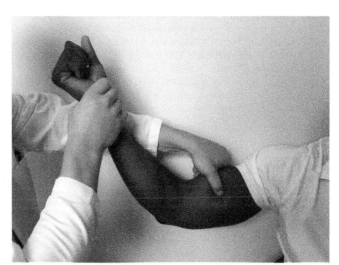

Figure 5.10 Biceps squeeze test. After squeezing the biceps, the forearm should supinate as shown. Lack of supination is indicative of a positive test and a distal tendon tear.

Table 5.2   Tests for Bicep Tendon Tears

Test	Description	Reliability	Comments
Hook test for distal biceps rupture	With the patients arm in 90 degrees of abduction and the elbow flexed 90 degrees and the forearm supinated with the thumb pointing up, the examiner attempts to "hook" the tendon from the lateral side. A positive result occurs when there is no palpable cord, which is indicative of a complete tendon rupture.	None reported	May be falsely negative in partial ruptures
Squeeze test for distal biceps rupture	The examiner places the patients forearm in 60–80 degrees of flexion and neutral rotation and squeezes the biceps muscle belly. Lack of forearm supination is indicative of a tendon tear.	Positive in 25 of 26 cases of presumed complete distal biceps rupture[42]	May be falsely negative in partial ruptures

POSTEROLATERAL ROTATORY INSTABILITY OF THE ELBOW

Posterolateral instability of the elbow can develop following an initially traumatic elbow dislocation or ligament sprain.[12,13,18] The symptoms of recurrent elbow instability are due to disruption of the LUCL. Injury allows for the ulna to have excessive supination or external rotation about the humerus. This leads to a posterior instability of the radiocapitellar joint and can cause the radial head to sublux posteriorly in the radiocapitellar joint with only the annular ligament maintaining its position on the sigmoid notch.[18] Clinically, individuals with posterolateral instability have elbow locking, snapping, and subluxation that occur when the elbow is extended and the forearm supinated.

Lateral Collateral Ligament Complex Examination

The varus stress test is used to assess the radial collateral ligament and is described as follows:

> By placing the patient's arm in 20 degrees of flexion and slight supination beyond neutral, the examiner then places one hand over the medial aspect of the distal humerus and the other hand lateral to the distal forearm. This is followed by a varus stress applied to the forearm with a concomitant counterforce placed upon the humerus. This will create excessive gapping on the lateral aspect of the elbow joint when compared to the contralateral arm (Video 5-7).[10,13]

There are four common tests for PLRI caused by incompetence of the LUCL: the pivot shift test, the rotatory drawer test, the push-up test, and the stand-up test. Tests for PLRI are often difficult to perform and interpret in an awake, alert patient because of the possibility of patient guarding. In order to limit patient apprehension, one of three techniques may be used: (1) intraarticular local anesthetic, (2) fluoroscopy to assess the radiocapitellar subluxation, or (3) the exam can be performed with the patient under sedation.[43]

O'Driscoll and associates[18] described the pivot shift test for the elbow. The PLRI test, or lateral pivot shift test of the elbow, is performed in the supine patient with the arm fully abducted and extended overhead. The examiner applies a valgus stress and axial load with the forearm supinated while the elbow is brought from extension to flexion. Occasionally, the radial head can appear prominent and dimple in extension. As the elbow is flexed, the radial head may reduce with a clunk, often at greater than 40 degrees of flexion, or when awake, the patient feels apprehension as the radial head reduces (Fig. 5.11; Video 5-8).

Another test for PLRI is the posterolateral rotatory drawer test (Fig. 5.12). In this test, the patient is again supine with the arm overhead and the elbow flexed from 40 to 90 degrees. The examiner then, while stabilizing the humerus, applies posteromedial force on the radius attempting to get the radius and ulna to rotate around an intact UCL and the radial head to subluxate posteriorly.

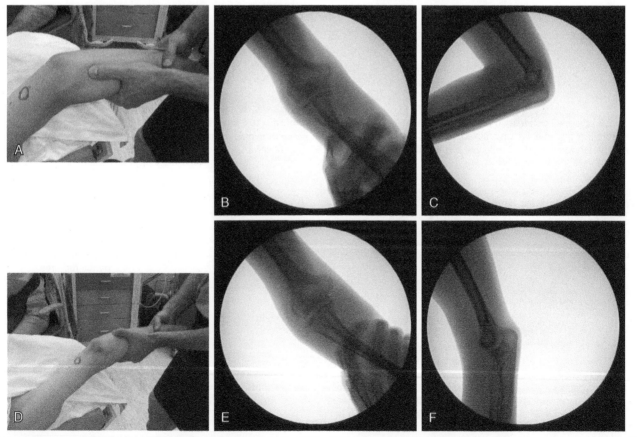

Figure 5.11 Pivot shift test for posterolateral rotatory instability. Notice that this test can be performed under fluoroscopy to evaluate the degree of laxity.

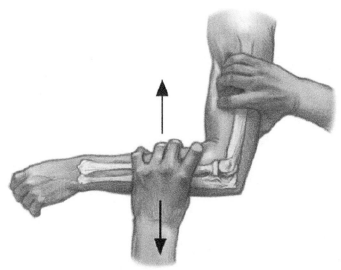

Figure 5.12　Posterolateral drawer test (Video 5-9). (Sanchez-Sotelo J, Morrey BF, O'Driscoll SW. Ligamentous repair and reconstruction for posterolateral rotatory instability of the elbow. *J Bone Joint Surg Br.* 2005;87:54-61.)

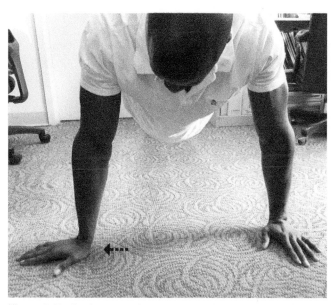

Figure 5.13　Push-up test for posterolateral rotatory instability. The patient performs a push-up with the forearm (right) supinated. If symptoms are re-created with the forearm supinated and disappear with the forearm pronated, then the test result is positive.

The two final tests described for PLRI are the push-up test (Fig. 5.13) and the stand-up test. In the push-up test, the patient starts in a prone position lying on the ground and attempts a push-up with the forearms maximally supinated and repeats a push-up with the forearms maximally pronated. If symptoms occur with the forearms supinated but not pronated, the test has a positive result. In the stand-up test, the patient attempts to get up from a seated position using his or her arms placed behind to push with the forearms maximally supinated. A positive test result will reproduce the patient's symptoms.

In a prospective evaluation by Regan and Lapner[44] of eight patients with PLRI, seven had both positive push-up and chair test results preoperatively, and only three of eight had positive pivot shift or drawer test results while awake. Of note, under anesthesia, all eight patients had a positive drawer test result.

EVALUATION FOR MEDIAL INSTABILITY

The original description by Jobe states that valgus instability can be demonstrated "[by] flexing the elbow 25 degrees to unlock the olecranon from its fossa and gently stressing the medial side of the elbow joint (Video 5-10)."[7] A positive test is produced with pain or laxity. With the arm in supination, there is the possibility for valgus pseudolaxity from subtle PLRI. In order to prevent this, O'Driscoll[13] advocates performing the Jobe test or valgus stress test with the forearm pronated.

The moving valgus stress test and the milking maneuver are two other tests used to assess the competency of the UCL. O'Driscoll and colleagues[13] created the moving valgus stress test in an attempt to recreate the throwing position. The patient's arm is abducted and externally rotated, and the examiner holds the thumb while supporting the elbow and applies a valgus stress throughout flexion and extension (Fig. 5.14). A positive test result occurs when there is pain in the 80- to 120-degree arc of motion at a specific and reproducible point (Video 5-11). The moving valgus stress test, as reported by O'Driscoll and associates, was 100% sensitive and 75% specific for detecting UCL tears when compared with surgical exploration or arthroscopic examination with valgus stress.[13]

The patient, with only observation or support by the examiner, performs the milking maneuver. The patient flexes his or her elbow to 90 degrees and then with the opposite hand passed under the affected arm, pulls the affected thumb in order to stress the medial elbow (Fig. 5.15). The test result is positive if the patient experiences pain, apprehension, or symptoms of instability. The center of the varus–valgus axis is along the center of the trochlea, which is medial to the epicondylar axis. Because of this, even with complete UCL ruptures, the medial joint opening under stress is quite subtle, usually only a few millimeters, and difficult to detect clinically. As a result, pain with stress is an important sign in the diagnosis. Pain with valgus stress testing has been reported to be present in 26% to 53% of patients undergoing surgery for UCL insufficiency, and tenderness has been reported to be present in up to 80% of those undergoing surgery. The subtle degree of valgus laxity may explain why studies noted the ability on physical examination to detect valgus elbow laxity preoperatively of 26% to 82%[5,45] (Table 5-3).

OTHER SPECIAL TESTS FOR THE ELBOW

Tenderness in the posterior aspect of the elbow may indicate an inflammatory condition such as gout or bursitis, a partial or complete triceps rupture, or valgus extension overload (VEO). Bursitis and gout present with warmth and swelling, with the differentiation being distinguished by history and location of swelling. Triceps rupture is an uncommon condition that is often misdiagnosed. It can occur in weightlifters but usually occurs with eccentric contraction associated with bracing a fall. On examination, there is difficulty, inability, or pain with triceps extension overhead, against gravity, or against resistance. Occasionally, a palpable defect in the triceps tendon may be appreciated. A triceps squeeze test,

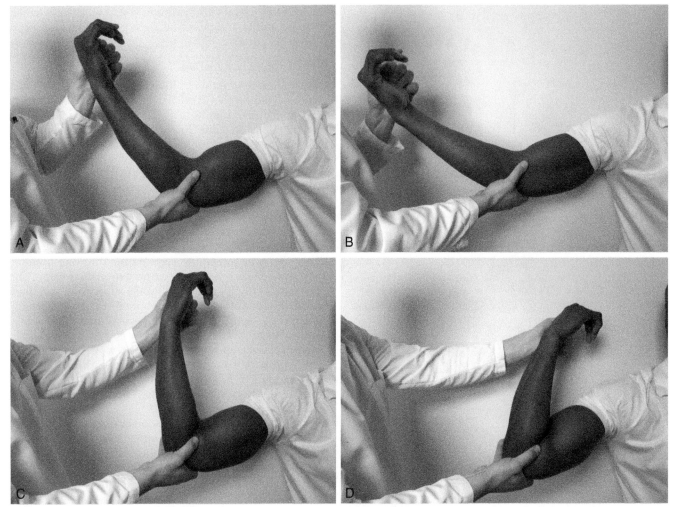

Figure 5.14 Moving valgus stress test. While palpating the medial joint line and ulnar collateral ligament, a valgus stress is applied to the patient's elbow. The test is positive with either pain or the sensation of gapping or instability.

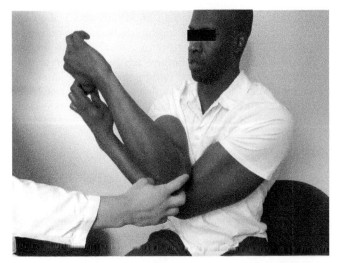

Figure 5.15 Milking maneuver. The patient applies a valgus force on the elbow by grabbing the affected thumb with his opposite hand. Pain over the medial elbow indicates a positive test result.

similar to the Thompson test for the Achilles tendon or biceps squeeze discussed earlier, may also demonstrate no extension with triceps squeeze, indicating a complete rupture. VEO (pitcher's elbow) can occur from repetitive stresses leading to osteophyte formation and pain in the posteromedial olecranon. The patient is frequently tender over the posteromedial elbow, and the arm bar test can be used to reproduce symptoms (Fig. 5-16.) In this test, the patient places the fully extended elbow with the forearm supinated on the examiner's shoulder and, while maintaining extension of the elbow joint, a downward pressure and hyperextension is applied to the elbow. A positive test result occurs when the symptoms are reproduced.

RADIOCAPITELLAR OSTEOCHONDRITIS DISSECANS

Panner disease and radiocapitellar osteochondritis dissecans (OCD) present a spectrum of disease to the cartilage of adolescent and preadolescent athletes that is caused by repetitive lateral compressive trauma. Typically, the patient will present insidiously in the dominant extremity following a period of mild trauma of overuse.[46] In the case of Panner disease, these patients are generally children younger than 10 years of age, while true osteochondritis dissecans occurs

Table 5.3 Tests for Medial and Lateral Elbow Instability

Test	Description	Reliability	Comments
Varus stress test	The patient's arm is placed in 20 degrees of flexion and slight supination beyond neutral. The examiner then places one hand over the medial aspect of the distal humerus and the other hand lateral to the distal forearm. This is followed by a varus stress applied to the forearm with a concomitant counter force placed upon the humerus. This will create excessive gapping on the lateral aspect of the elbow joint when compared with the contralateral arm.	None reported	Tests for radial collateral ligament tear
Pivot shift test	In a supine patient with the arm fully abducted and extended, apply a valgus stress and axial load with the forearm supinated while the elbow is brought from extension to flexion.	3/8 positive when awake[44]	Tests for PLRI in the setting of LUCL tear
Drawer test	The patient is supine with arm overhead and the elbow flexed from 40–90 degrees. While stabilizing the humerus, apply a posteromedial force on the radius attempting to get the radius and ulna to rotate around an intact UCL.	3/8 positive when awake; 8/8 positive when sedated[44]	Tests for PLRI in the setting of LUCL tear
Push-up test	In the push-up test, the patient starts in a prone position lying on the ground and attempts a push-up with the forearms maximally supinated and repeats a push-up with the forearms maximally pronated. Symptoms during supination are indicative of a positive result.	None reported	Tests for PLRI in the setting of LUCL tear
Jobe test	The patient flexes the elbow 25 degrees, and gentle stress is applied to the medial side of the elbow joint.	Laxity detection ranges from 26% to 82% in published studies[5,45]	Tests for UCL tear; result is considered positive with either pain or laxity
Moving valgus stress test	The arm is abducted and externally rotated and the examiner holds the thumb while supporting the elbow and applies a valgus stress throughout flexion and extension. Pain at 80 to 120 degrees arc of motion indicates a positive result.	100% sensitive and 75% specific compared with surgical exploration.[13]	Tests for UCL tear
Milking maneuver	The patient flexes his or her elbow to 90 degrees and then with the opposite hand passed under the affected arm, pulls the affected thumb in order to stress the medial elbow.	None reported	Tests for UCL tear.

LUCL, Lateral ulnar collateral ligament; *PLRI,* posterolateral rotatory instability; *UCL,* ulnar collateral ligament.

in older adolescents and young adults.[47] Mechanical symptoms may also be present such as elbow locking or catching, caused by intraarticular loose bodies. Most patients who present with chondral defects in the radiocapitellar joint will commonly have pain with palpation of the radiocapitellar joint as well as a loss of the terminal 10 to 15 degrees of extension. In the active radiocapitellar compression test,[23,48] the arm is fully extended and the forearm is pronated and supinated while axial compression is applied across the radiocapitellar joint. A positive test result is indicated by pain during forearm rotation. In patients with a suspected radiocapitellar chondromalacia or OCD, hypertrophic synovial plicae have also been reported as a source of pain.[48] In order to evaluate for symptomatic snapping plicae, the plica impingement test may be performed. In this test, the forearm is brought through pronation/supination with elbow flexion and extension while the lateral aspect of the elbow is palpated. A positive test result is indicated by a snapping sensation over the lateral elbow (Table 5-4).

Other causes of elbow "snapping" include unstable ulnar nerve at the cubital tunnel and instability of the triceps tendon. Snapping of the triceps tendon is a rare condition and most commonly occurs on the medial elbow. It may or may not be associated with concomitant ulnar neuritis or

Table 5.4   Other Special Tests for the Elbow

Test	Description	Reliability	Comments
Triceps squeeze test	The arm is abducted to 90 degrees, internally rotated, and the antecubital fossa is supported while the forearm is left to freely hang. The triceps is then squeezed at the distal muscle bulk. Lack of elbow extension indicates a tear.	None reported	May be falsely negative in the setting of partial tears
Arm bar test	The patient places the fully extended elbow with the forearm supinated on the examiner's shoulder, and while maintaining extension of the elbow joint, a downward pressure and hyperextension is applied to the elbow. A positive test result occurs when the symptoms are reproduced.	None reported	

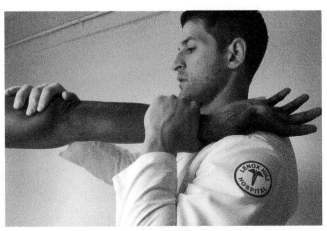

Figure 5.16   Arm bar test. Hyperextension producing pain is indicative of valgus extension overload.

cubital tunnel syndrome. On examination, the snapping can usually be palpated directly over the medial epicondyle as the elbow is brought through flexion and externsion.[49]

SUMMARY

Proper physical examination techniques of the hand, wrist, forearm, and elbow are vital in the correct diagnosis of common traumatic and overuse injuries of the upper extremity. Positive test results may support the use of further diagnostic testing, and negative results may further narrow the differential diagnosis. Understanding both how to perform the tests and how to interpret the results affords the clinician powerful tools in arriving at a correct diagnosis. Additionally, data on the sensitivity, specificity, and reliability of these test maneuvers gives valuable information in how to interpret both positive and negative test results.

Our preferred method of approaching a patient with an elbow or proximal forearm complaint begins with a detailed history in order to categorize the symptoms as being acute or chronic, musculoskeletal or neural, and traumatic or degenerative. Given the patient's profile and history, we then inspect the extremity for signs of trauma, muscle wasting, or other signs of systemic illness. At this point, we then proceed with a thorough physical exam, beginning

with range of motion measurements and following with palpation of common locations of tenderness. This is followed by a complete extremity neurosensory exam to ensure that all major myotomes and dermatomes are functioning appropriately. Only after performing our standard examination do we employ the special tests described in this chapter to provide insight into specific diagnoses and guide our selection of further investigation and management.

REFERENCES

1. Celli A, Celli L, Morrey B. Anatomy and biomechanics of the elbow. In: *Treatment of Elbow Lesions*. Milan: Springer; 2008:1-11.
2. An KN, Zobitz ME, Morrey BF. Biomechanics of the elbow. In: Morrey BF, ed. *The Elbow and its Disorders*. Philadelphia: W.B. Saunders; 1985.
3. Beals RK. The normal carrying angle of the elbow. A radiographic study of 422 patients. *Clin Orthop Relat Res*. 1976;119:194-196.
4. Conway JE, Jobe FW, Glousman RE, et al. Medial instability of the elbow in throwing athletes. Treatment by repair or reconstruction of the ulnar collateral ligament. *J Bone Joint Surg Am*. 1992;74:67-83.
5. Azar FM, Andrews JR, Wilk KE, et al. Operative treatment of ulnar collateral ligament injuries of the elbow in athletes. *Am J Sports Med*. 2000;28:16-23.
6. Davidson PA, Pink M, Perry J, et al. Functional anatomy of the flexor pronator muscle group in relation to the medial collateral ligament of the elbow. *Am J Sports Med*. 1995;23:245-250.
7. Jobe FW, Stark H, Lombardo SJ. Reconstruction of the ulnar collateral ligament in athletes. *J Bone Joint Surg Am*. 1986;68:1158-1163.
8. Kurvers H, Verhaar J. The results of operative treatment of medial epicondylitis. *J Bone Joint Surg Am*. 1995;77:1374-1379.
9. Lee ML, Rosenwasser MP. Chronic elbow instability. *Orthop Clin North Am*. 1999;30:81-89.
10. Morrey BF, An KN. Functional anatomy of the ligaments of the elbow. *Clin Orthop Relat Res*. 1985;201:84-90.
11. Morrey BF, An KN. Articular and ligamentous contributions to the stability of the elbow joint. *Am J Sports Med*. 1983;11:315-319.
12. O'Driscoll SW, Jupiter JB, King GJ, et al. The unstable elbow. *Instr Course Lect*. 2001;50:89-102.
13. O'Driscoll SW, Lawton RL, Smith AM. The "moving valgus stress test" for medial collateral ligament tears of the elbow. *Am J Sports Med*. 2005;33:231-239.
14. O'Dwyer KJ, Howie CR. Medial epicondylitis of the elbow. *Int Orthop*. 1995;19:69-71.
15. Thompson WH, Jobe FW, Yocum LA, et al. Ulnar collateral ligament reconstruction in athletes: muscle-splitting approach without transposition of the ulnar nerve. *J Shoulder Elbow Surg*. 2001;10:152-157.
16. Regan WD, Korinek SL, Morrey BF, et al. Biomechanical study of ligaments around the elbow joint. *Clin Orthop Relat Res*. 1991;271:170-179.

17. O'Driscoll SW, Morrey BF, Carmichael SW. Anatomy of the ulnar part of the lateral collateral ligament of the elbow. *Clin Anat.* 1992;5:296-303.

18. O'Driscoll SW, Bell DF, Morrey BF. Posterolateral rotatory instability of the elbow. *J Bone Joint Surg Am.* 1991;73:440-446.

19. Werner CO, Haeffner F, Rosen I. Direct recording of local pressure in the radial tunnel during passive stretch and active contraction of the supinator muscle. *Arch Orthop Trauma Surg.* 1980;96:299-301.

20. Werner CO, Rosen I, Thorngren KG. Clinical and neurophysiologic characteristics of the pronator syndrome. *Clin Orthop Relat Res.* 1985;197:231-236.

21. Morris HH, Peters BH. Pronator syndrome: clinical and electrophysiological features in seven cases. *J Neurol Neurosurg Psychiatry.* 1976;39:461-464.

22. Rodner CM, Tinsley BA, O'Malley MP. Pronator syndrome and anterior interosseous nerve syndrome. *J Am Acad Orthop Surg.* 2013;21:268-275.

23. Hsu SH, Moen TC, Levine WN, et al. Physical examination of the athlete's elbow. *Am J Sports Med.* 2012;40:699-708.

24. Hartz CR, Linsheid RL, Gramse RR, et al. The pronator teres syndrome: compressive neuropathy of the median nerve. *J Bone Joint Surg Am.* 1981;63:885-890.

25. Nakano KK, Lundergran C, Okihiro MM. Anterior interosseous nerve syndromes. Diagnostic methods and alternative treatments. *Arch Neurol.* 1977;34:477-480.

26. Wadsworth TG, Williams JR. Cubital tunnel external compression syndrome. *Br Med J.* 1973;1:662.

27. Assmus H, Antoniadis G, Bischoff C, et al. Cubital tunnel syndrome-a review and management guidelines. *Cent Eur Neurosurg.* 2011;72:90-98.

28. Goldman S, Honet JC, Sobel R, et al. Posterior interosseous nerve-palsy in the absence of trauma. *Arch Neurol.* 1969;21:435-441.

29. Kaplan PE. Posterior interosseous neuropathies: natural history. *Arch Phys Med Rehabil.* 1984;65:399-400.

30. Mohammad Hosein E, Moradi A, Jupiter JB. Diagnosis and treatment of radial tunnel syndrome. *Arch Bone Joint Surg.* 2015; 3:156–162.

31. Winkworth CE. *Lawn-tennis elbow. Br Med J.* 1883;708.

32. Descatha A, LeClerc A, Chastang JF, et al. Medial epicondylitis in occupational settings: prevalence, incidence and associated risk factors. *J Occup Environ Med.* 2003;45:993-1001.

33. Jobe FW, Ciccotti MG. Lateral and medial epicondylitis of the elbow. *J Am Acad Orthop Surg.* 1994;2:1-8.

34. Ahmad Z, Siddiqui N, Malik SS, et al. Lateral epicondylitis; a review of pathology and management. *Bone Joint J.* 2013;95:1158-1164.

35. Nirschl RP, Pettrone FA. Tennis elbow. The surgical treatment of lateral epicondylitis. *J Bone Joint Surg Am.* 1979;61:832-839.

36. Lister G, Belsole R, Kleinert H. The radial tunnel syndrome. *J Hand Surg.* 1979;4:52-59.

37. Nirschl R, Ashman E. Tennis elbow tendinosis (epicondylitis). *Instruct Course Lect.* 2003;53:587-598.

38. Ciccotti MG, Ramani MN. Medial epicondylitis. *Tech Hand Up Extrem Surg.* 2003;7:190-196.

39. Vangsness C, Jobe F. Surgical treatment of medial epicondylitis. Results in 35 elbows. *J Bone Joint Surg Br.* 1991;73:409-411.

40. O'Driscoll SW, Goncalves LB, Dietz P. The hook test for distal biceps tendon avulsion. *Am J Sports Med.* 2007;35:1865-1869.

41. Ruland RT, Dunbar RP, Bowen JD. The biceps squeeze test for diagnosis of distal biceps tendon ruptures. *Clin Orthop Relat Res.* 2005;437:128-131.

42. Ruland RT, Dunbar RP, Bowen JD. The biceps squeeze test for diagnosis of distal biceps tendon ruptures. *Clin Orthop Relat Res.* 2005;Aug:128-131.

43. Mehta JA, Bain GI. Posterolateral rotatory instability of the elbow. *J Am Acad Orthop Surg.* 2004;12:405-415.

44. Regan W, Lapner PC. Prospective evaluation of two diagnostic apprehension signs for posterolateral instability of the elbow. *J Shoulder Elbow Surg.* 2006;15:344-346.

45. Safran M, Ahmad CS, Elattrache NS. Ulnar collateral ligament of the elbow. *Arthroscopy.* 2005;21:1381-1395.

46. Ahmad CS, Vitale MA, ElAttrache NS. Elbow arthroscopy: capitellar osteochondritis dissecans and radiocapitellar plica. *Instruct Course Lect.* 2011;60:181-190.

47. Kobayashi K, Burton KJ, Rodner C, et al. Lateral compression injuries in the pediatric elbow: Panner's disease and osteochondritis dissecans of the capitellum. *J Am Acad Orthop Surg.* 2004;12: 246-254.

48. Antuna SA, O'Driscoll SW. Snapping plicae associated with radio-capitellar chondromalacia. *Arthroscopy.* 2001;17:491-495.

49. Vanhees MK, Geurts GF, Van Riet RP. Snapping triceps syndrome: a review of the literature. *Shoulder Elbow.* 2010;2:30-33.

6 Examination of the Wrist and Hand

Keith Bengtson, MD

INTRODUCTION

The physical examination of the hand and wrist can be very rewarding because the majority of the anatomy is readily available to the examiner's fingertips. One may palpate, stretch, or stress most of the underlying structures. Therefore, armed with a broad knowledge of the anatomy of the distal upper extremity, one may develop a quick differential for the patient's pathology without the use of expensive imaging or tests.

ANATOMY

BONES, LIGAMENT, AND JOINTS

The bones of the upper extremity increase in number from proximal to distal. The single humerus forms the upper arm and the two bones of the forearm are the radius and ulna. If one considers the pisiform a mere sesamoid bone, then the proximal carpal row has three bones (the scaphoid, lunate, and triquetrum), while the distal carpal row contains four (the trapezium, trapezoid, capitate, and hamate). Finally there are five sets of metacarpals and digits (Fig. 6.1).

DISTAL RADIOULNAR JOINT

In conjunction with the proximal radial-ulnar joint and the interosseous membrane, the distal radioulnar joint (DRUJ) provides for pronation and supination of the forearm. The DRUJ is a synovial pivot joint. The ulnar head articulates with the sigmoid notch of the much larger distal radius. The DRUJ has dorsal and palmar radioulnar ligaments. These ligaments attach the distal radius and ulna offering stability. Nestled between and blended with these two ligaments is the cartilaginous disc of the triangular fibrocartilage forming the triangular fibrocartilage complex (TFCC) (Fig. 6.2).

RADIOCARPAL JOINT

As the name suggests, the radiocarpal joint is the articulation between the distal radial bone and the proximal row of carpal bones.[1-6] There are eight carpal bones in the wrist joint, arranged in a proximal and a distal row (see Fig. 6.1). The proximal-row carpal bones (radial to ulnar) are the scaphoid, lunate, triquetrum, and pisiform. The pisiform bone lies on the palmer aspect of the triquetrum, so

essentially, there are functionally only three carpal bones in the proximal row. The distal-row carpal bones (radial to ulnar) are the trapezium, trapezoid, capitate, and hamate. It follows that the distal radius articulates with the proximal row of carpal bones, the proximal row of carpal bones articulates with the distal row of carpal bones, and the distal row of carpal bones articulates with the metacarpal heads. Each "row" of articulation has a separate compartment and is physically distinct from the next. Therefore, each synovial cavity has its own synovial fluid production and can have its own "effusion."

LIGAMENTS

The wrist has a tremendous number of ligaments.[1-6] The intrinsic ligaments include the palmar, dorsal, and interosseous ligaments, which connect the carpal bones together (Fig. 6.3). The remaining ligaments are the extrinsic ligaments. The ulnar collateral ligament connects the ulnar head with the (proximal carpal row) triquetrum and pisiform. Then the ulnar collateral ligament sends fibers to the (distal carpal row) hamate, and finally fibers extend to the base of the fifth metacarpal. The ulnar head is separated from the trapezium by the TFCC and forms one of the synovial compartments of

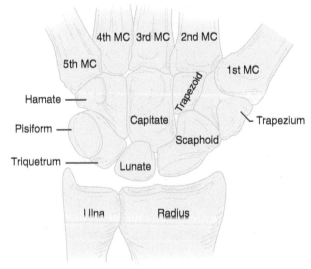

Figure 6.1 Skeletal anatomy of the wrist joint. *MC,* Metacarpal. (Adapted from Steinberg BD, Plancher KD: Clinical anatomy of the wrist and elbow. *Clin Sports Med.* 1995;14:301.)

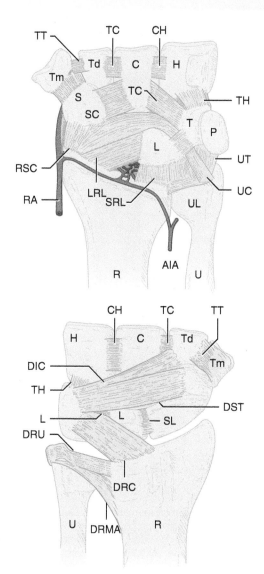

Figure 6.2 Ligaments of the wrist. *AIA,* anterior interosseous artery; *C,* capitate; *CH,* capito-hamate; *DIC,* Dorsal intercarpal; *DRC,* dorsal radiocapitate; *DRMA,* Dorsal radial ulnar ligament; *DRU,* dorsoradio-ulnar; *DST,* dorsal scaphotriquetral; *H,* hamate; *L,* lunate; *LRL,* long radiolunate; *LT,* lunotriquetral; *P,* pisiform; *R,* radius; *RA,* radial artery; *RSC,* radioscaphocapitate; *S,* scaphoid; *SC,* scaphocapitate; *SRL,* short radiolunate; *SL,* scapholunate; *T,* triquetral; *TC,* triquetrocapitate; *Td,* trapezoid; *TH,* triquetrohamate; *Tm,* trapezium; *TT,* trapezio-trapezoid; *U,* ulna; *UC,* ulnocapitate; *UL,* ulnolunate; *UT,* ulnotriquetral. (Adapted from Berger RA. The ligaments of the wrist: a current overview of anatomy with consideration of the potential functions. *Hand Clin.* 1997;13:423.)

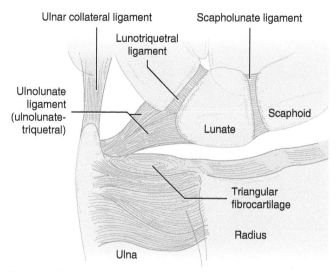

Figure 6.3 The triangular fibrocartilage complex. (Adapted from Steinberg BD, Plancher KD. Clinical anatomy of the wrist and elbow. *Clin Sports Med.* 1995;14:300.)

the wrist (see Fig. 6.2). On the lateral side of the hand, the radial collateral ligament sends fibers from the distal radius to the (proximal carpal row) scaphoid and fibers continue to the (distal carpal row) trapezium.

The radiocarpal joint or the proximal row of articulation is a condyloid joint. The joints between adjacent carpal bones are arthrodial joints. The distal radius articulates with the scaphoid, lunate, and triquetrum. There are interosseous ligaments between the scaphoid and lunate, as well as between the lunate and triquetrum. Therefore, the second synovial cavity of the "wrist" is bounded medially by the ulnar collateral ligament, laterally by the radial collateral,

proximally by the radius, distally by the first row of carpal bones and their interosseous ligaments. This constitutes the radiocarpal joint. The third and largest synovial cavity of the wrist joint is distal to the proximal row of carpal bones and their interosseous ligaments. This synovial cavity includes the distal row of carpal bones and ends at the metacarpal heads and their interosseous ligaments and constitutes the midcarpal joint. The fourth synovial cavity in the wrist region, bounded by carpometacarpal (CMC) ligaments, is between the trapezium and the first metacarpal head (base of the thumb) forming the thumb CMC joint. The fifth and final synovial cavity in the wrist region is between pisiform and the triquetrum bones forming the pisotriquetral joint.

There are multiple ligaments, both palmar and dorsal, interconnecting the carpal bones (see Fig. 6.3).

CARPAL TUNNEL

The carpal tunnel is a semirigid bony and ligamentous structure that is clinically important as the site of pathology in carpal tunnel syndrome and is the most common area of compression of the median nerve. The transverse carpal ligament connects the most volar bony structures of the wrist, which are called the pillars. These are the scaphoid tubercle on the radial side of the wrist and the pisiform and hook of the hamate on the ulnar side of the wrist (Fig. 6.4). This ligament and the carpal bones beneath form the carpal tunnel. Nine tendons (flexor pollicis longus [FPL] and four each from the flexor digitorum superficialis [FDP] and flexor digitorum profundus [FDP]) and one nerve (median) pass beneath the transverse carpal ligament.

GUYON CANAL

Guyon canal is clinically important as the second most common site of ulnar nerve compression. Unlike the carpal tunnel, the borders of Guyon canal are less rigid and more heterogeneous. Guyon canal lies volar to the carpal tunnel on the ulnar side of the wrist, and the transverse carpal ligament, along with the hypothenar muscles, form the floor of Guyon canal. The roof consists of the volar carpal ligament.

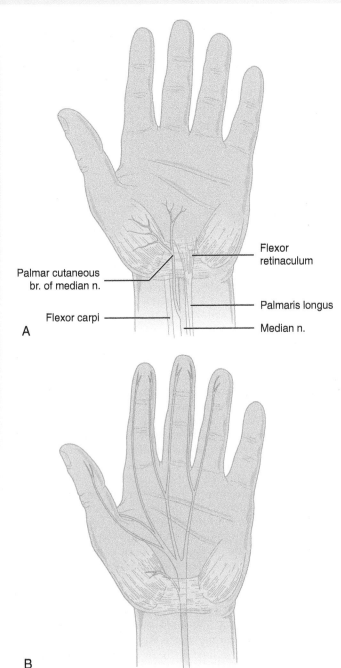

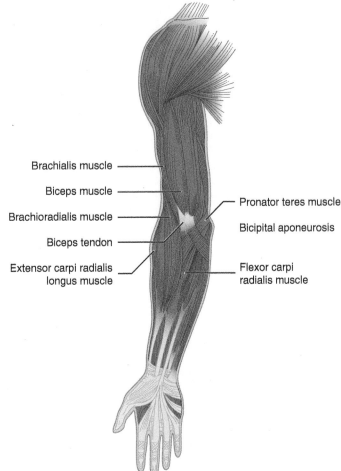

Figure 6.5 Superficial muscles of the anterior elbow region. (Adapted from Anderson TE. Anatomy and physical examination of the elbow. In: Nicholas J, Hershman E, eds. *The Upper Extremity in Sports Medicine.* 2nd ed. St. Louis: Mosby; 1995:262.)

Figure 6.4 The median nerve under the flexor retinaculum. **A,** Flexor retinaculum removed. **B,** Flexor retinaculum intact. (Adapted from Entrapment neuropathy. In: Birch R, Bonney G, Wynn Parry CB, eds. *Surgical Disorders of the Peripheral Nerves.* Edinburgh: Churchill Livingstone; 1998:269.)

MUSCLES

FOREARM BASED (EXTRINSICS)

Our discussion of the extrinsic and intrinsic muscles of the hands focuses on the major action and innervation.[1-6] A full discussion of each and every muscle, including origins and insertions of the muscles, should be sought in an anatomy text.

FLEXOR GROUP

The pronator teres (PT) arises from the medial epicondyle of the humerus and the medial coronoid process of the ulna (Fig. 6.5). It inserts onto the lateral edge of the middle third of the radius. The median nerve innervates the PT, and the root levels are C6 and C7. The major action is forearm pronation with the elbow slightly flexed.

The pronator quadratus (PQ), as the name indicates, is a quadrangular shaped muscle with origin and insertion on the distal ulna and radius, respectively. The PQ assists pronation of the forearm and is the last muscle innervated by the anterior interosseous nerve (AIN), the root level most commonly sited at C7 and C8 (perhaps some T1).

The radial border is the hook of the hamate, and the ulnar border is the pisotriquetral joint, the pisiform, and abductor digiti minimi muscle belly. Smaller ligaments that are clinically important include the pisohamate and pisometacarpal. As their names suggest, these ligaments run from the pisiform bone to the hamate and fifth metacarpal, respectively. The ligament from the pisiform to the hook of the hamate also forms the roof of Guyon canal. Both branches of the ulnar nerve enter this canal already divided into the deep and superficial palmar branches (see Ulnar Nerve).

The palmaris longus (PL) is absent in a certain percentage of the population and does not travel beneath the flexor retinaculum at the wrist. The PL origin is at the medial epicondyle of the humerus from the common flexor tendon, and the insertion is at the palmar aponeurosis of the hand. The major action is assisting wrist flexion. The median nerve innervates the PL and the root levels are C7, C8, and some T1.

The flexor carpi radialis (FCR) is medial to the PT and lateral to the PL and flexor carpi ulnaris. The FCR muscle's origin is at the medial humeral epicondyle from the common flexor tendon, and the insertion is at the second and third metacarpal bones in the hand (see Fig. 6.5). The FCR does not go deep to the flexor retinaculum at the wrist and, therefore, similar to the PL, is not within the carpal tunnel. The major action of the FCR is wrist flexion with a slight pronation component. The major innervation is from the median nerve from the root levels C6 and C7.

The flexor carpi ulnaris (FCU) has two heads of origin: from the medial humeral epicondyle and common flexor tendon and from the proximal posterior surface of the ulna just medial to the origin of the extensor carpi ulnaris. The major action of the FCU is wrist flexion with ulnar deviation. The major innervation is from the ulnar nerve from the root levels C8 and T1.

The FDS has two heads of origin: from the medial to the humeral epicondyle at the common flexor tendon and coronoid process of the ulna and from the lateral radius just distal to the insertion of the supinator. The median nerve and the ulnar artery lie deep to this muscle and pass between the two heads of the FDS. The FDS muscle gives rise to four tendons in the distal forearm. These four tendons pass deep to the flexor retinaculum at the wrist and therefore the FDS lies within the carpal tunnel at the wrist. The four tendons then continue on to each of digits two, three, four, and five. The final insertion of the tendons of the FDS is the middle phalanx of digits two to five. Interestingly, each tendon splits just proximal to the final insertion to allow the tendon of the FDP to pass through. Therefore, the tendons of the FDS insert on both the medial and lateral aspects of the middle phalanx of digits two to five. The major action of the muscle is flexion of the middle phalanx of digits two to five. In addition, this muscle can aid in flexion at the metacarpal phalanges (MCP) and wrist joints. The median nerve innervates the FDS from the root levels C7, C8, and T1.

The FDP has extensive origin from the anterior and medial ulna and adjacent interosseous membrane. The FDP muscle then gives rise to four tendons that pass deep to the flexor retinaculum at the wrist. Therefore, similar to the FDS, the FDP tendons lie within the carpal tunnel. The four tendons of this muscle then divide, and one tendon goes to each of digits two to five. The final insertion is the proximal distal phalanx, after passing through the split tendons of the FDS muscle. The major action of the FDP is flexion of the distal phalanx. The FDP can also secondarily aid more proximal phalangeal flexion and wrist flexion. The lateral portion of the FDP to digits two and three is innervated by the AIN, whereas the medial portion to the fourth and fifth digits is innervated by the ulnar nerve. The root levels innervating the FDP are C7 and C8.

The FPL originates just lateral to the FDP on the interosseous membrane and the adjacent radial bone. In fact, the AIN runs between the two muscles and innervates them both. The insertion of the FPL is at the base of the distal phalanx of the thumb. The FPL tendon passes within the carpal tunnel and is the most laterally situated tendon. The major action of the FPL is flexion of the distal phalanx of the thumb. The FPL can secondarily flex the more proximal phalanx and the wrist with radial deviation. It is innervated by the AIN from root levels C7 and C8.

EXTENSOR GROUP

The extensor carpi radialis longus (ECRL) originates at the lateral supracondylar ridge of the humerus, the adjacent intermuscular septum, and the lateral humeral epicondyle (Fig. 6.6). It inserts at the base of the second metacarpal bone. The major action of the ECRL is extension of the wrist with a lateral or radial deviation. The innervation of the ECRL is from the radial nerve, root levels C7 and C8.

The extensor carpi radialis brevis (ECRB) originates at the lateral humeral epicondyle at the common extensor tendon (see Fig. 6.6). The ECRB and the ECRL share a common tendon sheath and extensor compartment at the wrist. The ECRB inserts at the base of the third metacarpal.

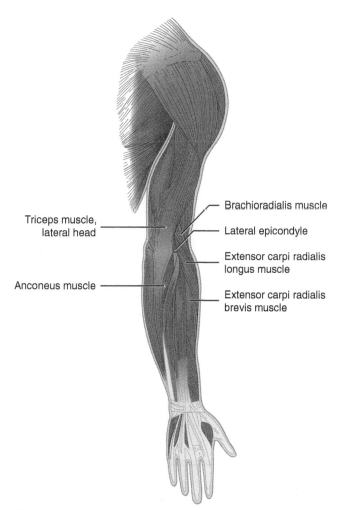

Triceps muscle, lateral head

Anconeus muscle

Brachioradialis muscle

Lateral epicondyle

Extensor carpi radialis longus muscle

Extensor carpi radialis brevis muscle

Figure 6.6 The superficial muscles of the posterior elbow region. (Adapted from Anderson TE: Anatomy and physical examination of the elbow. In: Nicholas J, Hershman E, eds. *The Upper Extremity in Sports Medicine.* 2nd ed. St. Louis: Mosby; 1995:262.)

The major action of the ECRB is wrist extension. The radial nerve innervates the ECRB from the root levels C7 and C8.

The extensor digitorum communis (EDC) originates from the common extensor tendon at the lateral humeral epicondyle and inserts into the middle and distal phalanges of digits two, three, four, and five. The major action is extension of these digits. The radial nerve innervates the EDC from the root levels C7 and C8.

The extensor digiti minimi (EDM) is a small muscle originating at the common extensor tendon of the lateral humeral epicondyle and runs immediately adjacent to the EDC. The EDM has a separate extensor compartment at the wrist from the EDC and is considered a separate muscle from the EDC. It inserts at the middle and distal phalanx of the fifth digit (Fig. 6.7). The major action is to extend the fifth digit. The radial nerve innervates the EDM from root levels C7 and C8.

The extensor carpi ulnaris (ECU) originates from the lateral humeral epicondyle at the common extensor tendon and from the posterior surface of the proximal ulna. The ECU is the most medial muscle in the extensor group. It inserts at the base of the fifth metacarpal bone (see Fig. 6.7). The major action is extension of the wrist with ulnar deviation. The radial nerve innervates the ECU from the root levels C7 and C8.

The abductor pollicis longus (APL) originates on the proximal ulna, adjacent intermuscular septum, and the radius, just distal and posterior to the insertion of the supinator. The insertion of the APL is at the base of the first metacarpal bone. The major action of the APL is abduction of the thumb. The radial nerve innervates the APL from the root levels C7 and C8.

The extensor pollicis longus (EPL) originates distal to the APL on the intermuscular septum and the ulna just lateral to the origin of the extensor carpi ulnaris. The insertion of the EPL is the proximal end of the first distal phalanx (see Fig. 6.7). The major action is extension of the distal phalanx of the thumb. A secondary action of the EPL is wrist extension with radial deviation. The radial nerve innervates the EPL from root levels C7 and C8.

The extensor pollicis brevis (EPB) originates on the posterior surface of the radius and the adjacent intermuscular septum. The insertion is at the base of the proximal phalanx of the thumb. The major action is extension of the proximal phalanx of the thumb. The radial nerve innervates the EPB from root levels C7 and C8.

The extensor indicis (EI) originates on the distal posterior radius and inserts on the extensor surface of the index finger at the middle and distal phalanx (see Fig. 6.7). The major action is extension of the index finger. The EI is the last muscle innervated by the radial nerve from root levels C7 and C8.

HAND BASED (INTRINSICS)

This section discusses the muscles that have their origin and insertion entirely within the hand, distal to the wrist. These are also called the intrinsic muscles.[1-6]

The abductor pollicis brevis (APB) originates from the flexor retinaculum, trapezium, and scaphoid. The APB muscle inserts at the base of the proximal phalanx of the pollicis (thumb), with some fibers inserting on the adjacent extensor expansion (Fig. 6.8). The major action of the APB muscle is abduction of the thumb. In addition, the fibers inserting on the extensor expansion can extend the thumb's interphalangeal joint. The median nerve innervates the APB muscle from root levels C8 and T1.

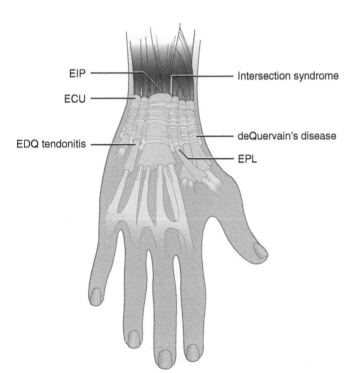

Figure 6.7 Extensor tendons and sites of overuse. *ECU,* Extensor carpi ulnaris; *EDQ,* extensor digiti quinti; *EIP,* extensor indicis proprius; *EPL,* extensor pollicis longus. (Adapted from Kiefhaber TR, Stern PJ. Upper extremity tendinitis and overuse syndromes in athletes. *Clin Sports Med.* 1992;11:39-55.)

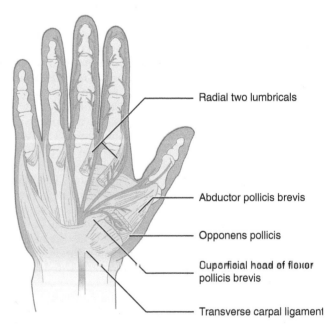

Figure 6.8 Musculature about the thenar eminence. (Adapted from Chase RA. *Atlas of Hand Surgery,* vol. 2. Philadelphia: W.B. Saunders; 1984.)

The flexor pollicis brevis (FPB) has superficial and deep heads. The superficial head originates from the flexor retinaculum and trapezium. The deep head originates from the trapezoid and the capitate. The two heads converge and insert on the base of the proximal phalanx just palmar to the insertion of the APB muscle (see Fig. 6.8). The major action of the FPB is flexion of the first MCP and CMC joints. The FPB can also help in adduction and opposition of the thumb. The FPB has dual innervation with the median nerve innervating the superficial head from root levels C8 and T1. The ulnar nerve innervates the deep head from root levels C8 and T1.

The opponens pollicis (OP) originates from the flexor retinaculum and the adjacent trapezium. The OP inserts along the entire shaft of the first metacarpal on the radial side (see Fig. 6.8). The major action is opposition of the first metacarpal bone toward the other digits. The median nerve innervates the OP from root levels C8 and T1.

The adductor pollicis (AP) has an oblique head and a transverse head. The transverse head originates from the third metacarpal bone, and the oblique head originates from the adjacent carpal bones: capitate, trapezoid, trapezium, and probably a small slip from the base of the second metacarpal. The two heads converge and insert on the base of the first digit's proximal phalanx. The major action of the AP is adduction and flexion of the thumb. The ulnar nerve innervates the AP from root levels C8 and T1.

The lumbrical muscles originate from the four tendons of the FDP and insert on the extensor tendon hood of digits two, three, four, and five (see Fig. 6.8). The major action of lumbricals is extension of the distal interphalangeal joints and flexion of the MCP joints. Lumbricals have dual innervation with the median nerve innervating the lateral two lumbricals (digits 2 and 3), whereas the ulnar nerve innervates the medial two lumbricals (digits 4 and 5).

Three palmar interosseous muscles are numbered 1, 2, and 3. They originate on the volar aspect of the shaft of the second, fourth, and fifth metacarpals. The palmar interosseous muscles insert on the lateral aspect of the base of the corresponding second, fourth, and fifth proximal phalanges and extensor expansion. The first palmar interosseous muscle inserts on the medial (ulnar) side of the second proximal phalanx and extensor expansion (index finger). The second and third insert on the lateral (radial) side of the proximal fourth and fifth phalanx and extensor expansions. It follows that the major action of the palmar interosseous muscles are adduction (bringing the fingers toward midline) of the phalanges. A secondary action is flexion of the metacarpal joints and extension of the interphalangeal joints. The ulnar nerve innervates all interossei muscles from root levels C8 and T1.

Four dorsal interosseous (DI) muscles are numbered 1, 2, 3, and 4. The DI muscles are larger than the palmar interosseous, have two head origins (bipennate), and lie between adjacent metacarpals. The first dorsal interosseous muscle (FDI) originates from both the first (thumb) and second metacarpals (index finger). At the base of the two heads of origin, the FDI has an opening through which the radial artery passes from dorsal to volar. The second DI muscle originates between the second (index) and third (middle) metacarpals. The third DI muscle originates from between the third (middle) and fourth (ring) metacarpals.

The fourth DI muscle originates from between the fourth (ring) and fifth metacarpals. The second, third, and fourth DI muscles all have openings between their two heads through which pass bridging arteries from the dorsal to palmar blood supplies. All the DI muscles insert at the base of the corresponding proximal phalanx and extensor hood, opposite the palmar interosseous insertions. Phalangeal adduction, or movement of the fingers away from the middle finger, is the major action of these muscles. The ulnar nerve innervates the interosseous muscles from root levels C8 and T1.

The abductor digiti minimi (ADM) originates on the pisiform and the tendon of the FCU. The ADM inserts on the medial (ulnar) side of the base of the fifth proximal phalanx and the extensor expansion. The major action is abduction of the fifth digit. Secondarily, the ADM is responsible for flexion of the fifth MCP joint and extension of the fifth interphalangeal joints. The ulnar nerve innervates the ADM from root levels C8 and T1.

The flexor digiti minimi (FDM) originates from the hook of the hamate and the adjacent flexor retinaculum and inserts on the base of the proximal phalanx of the fifth digit. The major action is flexion of the MCP joint of the fifth digit. The ulnar nerve innervates the FDM muscle from root levels C8 and T1.

The opponens digiti minimi (ODM) muscle originates on the flexor retinaculum and the hook of the hamate and inserts along the medial (ulnar) shaft of the fifth metacarpal. The major action is flexion and rotation of the fifth metacarpal bone with respect to the plane of the other metacarpal bones. The ulnar nerve innervates the ODM muscle from root levels C8 and T1.

The palmaris brevis (PB) is a small muscle originating at the medial palmar aponeurosis that runs transversely across the palm and inserts into skin, as well as the pisiform. The palmaris brevis tightens the skin on the palm and may also protect the ulnar nerve and artery. The ulnar nerve innervates this muscle from root levels C8 and T1.

NERVES

MEDIAN NERVE

The median nerve is formed by nerve fibers from the lateral and medial cords of the brachial plexus containing nerve fibers from the cervical root levels C6 to T1 (Fig. 6.9). This nerve enters the arm running with the ulnar nerve and the brachial artery and travels within the forearm just medial to the biceps tendon insertion and anterior to the elbow joint. The median nerve dives deep to the PT, between its two heads, and runs between the FDS and FDP muscles. The median nerve innervates the PT, PL, FDS, and FCR in the forearm. The median nerve gives off the AIN just after crossing the elbow joint. The AIN runs deep to the FDP and innervates the FDP to digits 1 and 2, the FPL, and the PQ. The median nerve continues between the tendons of the FDS and FDP at the wrist, just radial (lateral) to the superficialis tendon, ulnar (medial) to the FCR, and just deep (and lateral) to the PL tendon. The median nerve gives off the palmar cutaneous branch just proximal to the flexor retinaculum. It then passes deep to the flexor retinaculum and supplies the (superficial head) FPB, APB, OP, and lumbricals 1 and 2.

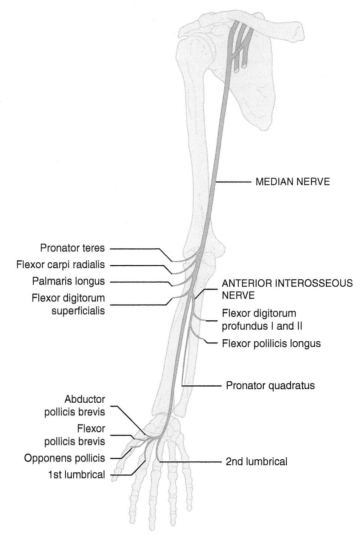

Pronator teres

Flexor carpi radialis

Palmaris longus

Flexor digitorum
superficialis

MEDIAN NERVE

ANTERIOR INTEROSSEOUS
NERVE

Flexor digitorum
profundus I and II

Flexor polilicis longus

Pronator quadratus

Abductor
pollicis brevis

Flexor
pollicis brevis

Opponens pollicis

1st lumbrical

2nd lumbrical

Figure 6.9 The median nerve. (Adapted from Birch R, Bonney G, Wynn Parry CB, eds. *Surgical Disorders of the Peripheral Nerves.* Edinburgh: Churchill Livingstone; 1998:7.)

ULNAR NERVE[7]

The ulnar nerve enters the arm as the extension of the medial cord of the brachial plexus with nerve fibers from the cervical root levels C8 and T1 (Fig. 6.10). The nerve enters the arm slightly posterior to the brachial artery, innervating no muscles in the arm, and passes posterior to the medial humeral condyle in the ulnar groove. In the forearm, the ulnar nerve lies between the FCU and FDP and innervates the FDP to digits 3 and 4 and the FCU. Next, the ulnar nerve crosses the wrist joint medial to the FCU tendon and lateral to the ulnar artery. Once in the hand, the ulnar nerve passes medial to the pisiform bone, splitting into the superficial and deep palmar branches. These two branches enter the canal of Guyon together but exit to different endpoints. The space between the pisiform and the hook of the hamate forms the walls of Guyon canal. The roof of Guyon canal is the distal extension of the FCU tendon, and the floor is the pisohamate ligament. The superficial palmar branch supplies skin sensation to the medial half of the fourth and all of the fifth digits. The deep palmar branch travels (medial side) around the hook of the hamate and

travels laterally to innervate the lumbricals 4 and 5, all interosseous muscles, all hypothenar muscles, the deep head of the FPB, and the AP.

RADIAL NERVE

The radial nerve is the extension of the posterior cord of the brachial plexus with nerve fibers from the root levels C5 to C8 (Fig. 6.11). It enters the upper arm through the quadrangular space (borders teres major, minor, long head of the triceps and the humerus). In general, the radial nerve innervates all extensor muscles of the elbow, wrist, and fingers. The radial nerve has cutaneous innervation to the back of the arm, forearm, and hand. Once in the arm, the radial nerve lies against the humerus traveling distally and laterally in the spiral groove of the humerus, between the lateral and medial heads of the triceps. In the distal arm, the radial nerve lies between the anterior brachialis muscle and the posterior brachioradialis and ECRL muscles. At the elbow, the radial nerve courses anterior to the lateral condyle of the humerus and splits into superficial and deep branches before entering the belly of the supinator. The superficial branch travels under the brachioradialis muscle lateral half of digit 4 are innervated by the digital branches of the median nerve after exiting from the carpal tunnel. The thumb is innervated from the C6 root level and the middle finger (digit 3) from C7. The ulnar nerve cutaneous branches, root level C8, innervate the hypothenar area and the medial dorsum of the hand (proximal to the distal interphalangeal joint). These cutaneous branches leave the ulnar nerve before the wrist. The dorsal ulnar cutaneous nerve leaves the ulnar nerve 8 cm proximal to the wrist and loops around the medial aspect of the distal ulna head to reach the dorsum of the hand. The dorsal ulnar cutaneous nerve innervates the medial one third of the dorsal hand. The medial antebrachial cutaneous nerve innervates the medial forearm from root level T1. This cutaneous nerve originates from the medial cord of the brachial plexus and travels with, but separate from, the ulnar nerve along the entire arm and forearm, providing cutaneous innervation to the medial forearm. The superficial radial nerve provides cutaneous innervation, from root levels C7 and C8, to the lateral dorsal three and a half digits proximal to the distal interphalangeal joints. The posterior cutaneous nerve of the forearm supplying a small strip on the extensor forearm is a branch of the radial nerve.

EXAMINATION

PALPATION

WRIST

The palpation of the surface anatomy of the wrist is particularly helpful because a large portion of the structures of the wrists are quite superficial and directly underneath the skin. Therefore, knowledge of the underlying anatomy allows the examiner to see or feel pathology without special imaging techniques. In general, one can find examination of the hand and wrist quite rewarding because so much information is available to the examiner's fingertips.

Volar/Flexor Surface of the Wrist

The carpal tunnel and the transverse carpal ligament obscure many of the volar structures. However, three tendons and three bony structures are readily palpable. The three tendons on the volar surface that are readily palpable are the FCR, the PL, and the FCU. The FCR and FCU may be stressed by resisted wrist flexion and slight radial deviation for the FCR and slight ulnar deviation of the FCU. The PL is most easily seen (and stressed) by holding the tips of the thumb and small finger together while flexing the wrist.

The three bony prominences that are palpable on the volar surface of the wrist include the scaphoid tubercle, the hook of the hamate, and pisiform. These three structures are known as "the pillars" and are the attachment points for the transverse carpal ligament. More superficially, another landmark is the flexion crease of the wrist, which forms the border between the forearm and the palm and is often referenced in regard to underlying anatomy (Fig. 6.12).

Dorsal/Extensor Surface of the Wrist

As we move the dorsal aspect of the wrist, many more structures are available to the examiner's fingertip. Most superficially are the six dorsal compartments (see Figs. 6.7 and

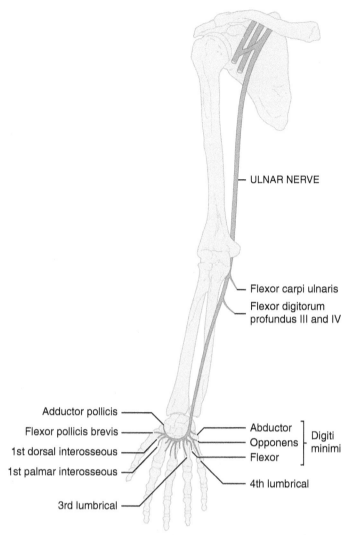

Adductor pollicis
Flexor pollicis brevis
1st dorsal interosseous
1st palmar interosseous
3rd lumbrical

ULNAR NERVE

Flexor carpi ulnaris
Flexor digitorum profundus III and IV

Abductor
Opponens   Digiti
Flexor   minimi
4th lumbrical

Figure 6.10. The ulnar nerve. (Adapted from Birch R, Bonney G, Wynn Parry CB, eds. *Surgical Disorders of the Peripheral Nerves.* Edinburgh: Churchill Livingstone; 1998.7.)

becoming subcutaneous lateral to the tendon in the distal forearm. The superficial branch provides cutaneous innervation to the dorsum of the lateral hand and base of the thumb. The deep branch travels distally between the superficial and the deep extensor muscle groups. After innervating the supinator muscle, the radial nerve is called the posterior interosseous nerve (PIN). The deep branch (PIN) provides sensory input to the posterior of the wrist and carpal bones. The radial innervated muscles include the triceps (all heads), brachioradialis, ECRL, ECRB, supinator, EDC, EDM, APL, EPL, EPB, and EI. The last radial innervated muscle is the EI.

DERMATOMES

The lateral forearm from the elbow to the radial styloid has cutaneous innervation from the lateral antebrachial cutaneous (extension of the musculocutaneous nerve), nerve root level C5. Cutaneous branches of the median nerve innervate the lateral palm (thenar area). These branches from the C6 root leave the median nerve before the nerve enters the carpal tunnel. The rest of the palm, digits 1 to 3, and the

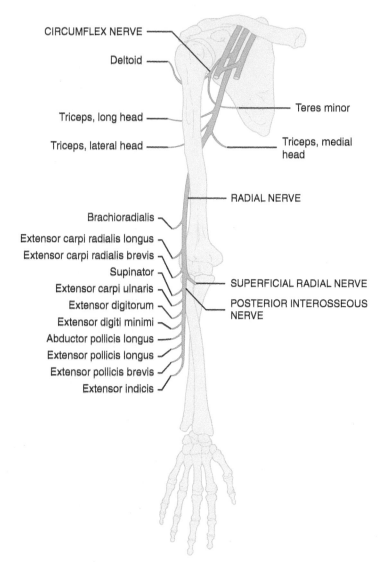

CIRCUMFLEX NERVE

Deltoid

Triceps, long head

Triceps, lateral head

Teres minor

Triceps, medial head

RADIAL NERVE

Brachioradialis

Extensor carpi radialis longus

Extensor carpi radialis brevis

Supinator

Extensor carpi ulnaris

Extensor digitorum

Extensor digiti minimi

Abductor pollicis longus

Extensor pollicis longus

Extensor pollicis brevis

Extensor indicis

SUPERFICIAL RADIAL NERVE

POSTERIOR INTEROSSEOUS NERVE

Figure 6.11 The radial nerve. (Adapted from Birch R, Bonney G, Wynn Parry CB, eds. *Surgical Disorders of the Peripheral Nerves*. Edinburgh: Churchill Livingstone, 1998:8.)

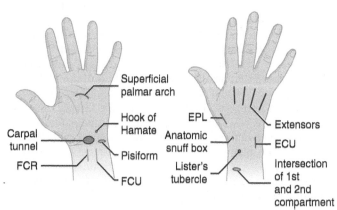

Superficial palmar arch

Hook of Hamate

Carpal tunnel

Pisiform

FCR

FCU

EPL

Anatomic snuff box

Lister's tubercle

Extensors

ECU

Intersection of 1st and 2nd compartment

Figure 6.12 Surface anatomy of the wrist. *ECU*, Extensor carpi ulnaris; *EPL*, extensor pollicis longus; *FCR*, flexor carpi radialis; *FCU*, flexor carpi ulnaris. (Adapted from Nguyen DT, McCue FC, Urch SE. Evaluation of the injured wrist on the field and in the office. *Clin Sports Med*. 1998;17:422.)

6.12). Beginning on the radial side of the wrist, the first and third dorsal compartments form the radial and ulnar borders of the so-called "anatomic snuffbox." The proximal border of the anatomic snuffbox is the distal radius, which includes the radial styloid. The first dorsal compartment contains the adductor pollicis longus (APL) and the EPL. The third dorsal compartment contains the EPL. Both of these structures can be seen by laying the palm flat and having the patient extend their thumb upwards toward the ceiling, with slight extension of the wrist. The structures that are palpable within the snuffbox beginning from the distal end of the snuffbox include the scaphotrapezial trapezoidal (STT) joint, as well as the distal portion of the scaphoid. In order to palpate the most amount of the scaphoid, one can ulnarly deviate the wrist midway so the scaphoid is palpable distal to the radial styloid. Overlying the bony structures is the deep branch of the radial artery, which generally overlies the STT joint. Longitudinally, the superficial radial nerve is also palpable, although it is quite thin at this level and often difficult to palpate. If one follows the EPL into the third dorsal compartment, the bony structure that borders the EPL on the radial aspect is Lister's tubercle. Just distal and ulnar to the EPL is an indentation in the bony structures that is the scapholunate interval. Moving more ulnarly, one can then palpate a broad flat dorsal compartment, which is the fourth dorsal compartment. This contains primarily the EDC and the extensor indicis proprius (EIP), which should be on the radial portion of the fourth dorsal compartment. The EIP is most easily stressed and palpated by having the patient make a fist and extend the index finger because the EDC is most easily palpated and stressed by slightly extending the wrist and extending all of the digits.

As we move farther in the ulnar direction, the fifth dorsal compartment contains only the EDM, and this is most easily palpated and stressed by having the patient make a fist and extend the fifth digit. This rarely is a source of pathology, so it is often neglected during the examination.

Just proximal to the fourth and fifth dorsal compartments, the border between the distal radius and distal ulna can be palpated, and this forms the DRUJ. More ulnarly is a bony prominence, which is the distal ulnar ridge, and one should easily palpate the sixth dorsal compartment, which contains the extensor carpi ulnaris (ECU). The ECU is highly mobile, and when the patient's hand is in the pronated position, the ECU is located more on the ulnar surface of the wrist and primarily acts as an ulnar deviator; however, when the hand is supinated, the ECU is more of a wrist extensor. Because of its mobility, it is prone to snapping and, at times, one can appreciate snapping of the sixth dorsal compartment by palpating it while the patient circumducts the wrist or moves the wrist from radial to ulnar deviation.

The underlying bony structures are then easily palpable, and all of the carpal bones can be palpated dorsally except for the pisiform. The most prominent bony landmarks include Lister's tubercle, which is just radial to the third dorsal compartment and the distal ulna, which is directed underneath the sixth compartment. Distally, the scaphoid can be palpated from the STT joint and the distal end of the anatomic snuffbox to the waist at approximately the end of the anatomic snuffbox with the hand in ulnar deviation. Between the third and fourth dorsal compartments, the scapholunate interval and the radial portion of the lunate are palpable. The lunotriquetral interval lies between the fourth and fifth dorsal compartment, and the triquetrum lies just distal to the prominence of the distal ulna. The triquetrum can be better appreciated by grasping the dorsal aspect of the triquetrum with the examiner's thumb. The examiner's index finger is placed under the pisiform at the base of the hypothenar eminence. In this position, one may toggle the pisotriquetral complex up and down. The dorsal aspect of the hamate is palpable between the triquetrum and the fourth and fifth CMC joints, which form the base of the fourth and fifth metacarpals. Then, moving more radially, one can palpate the capitate just proximal to the third metacarpal or the third CMC joint. Finally, the trapezium is palpated on either side of the distal end of the EPL and into the distal anatomic snuffbox.

HAND

Just like the structures in the wrist, the structures of the hand and fingers are all fairly close to the surface and,

therefore, easily examined by simple palpation and manipulation.

Beginning with the palm, the structures on the surface that are most prominent are those of the thenar and hypothenar muscles, which form the intrinsic muscles to the thumb and small finger, respectively. There is a fairly prominent crease from the ulnar border of the thenar muscle, which is the thenar crease. More distally and transversally are the proximal and distal palmar creases. The proximal crease essentially forms the flexor crease from the second and third MCP, and the distal crease forms the flexor surface for the fourth and fifth MCP. This should not be confused with the more distal palmar digital creases, which are in reality about the level of the midshaft of the proximal phalanx. The flexor tendons are fairly easily palpable beginning at the MCP joints and ending at the distal interphalangeal joints. Many times patients will have flexor tendon nodules at or just distal to the level of the MCP joints. These can be sensitive, and there may be crepitus. In more extreme cases, these are the etiologies for trigger fingers or stenosing flexor tenosynovitis. The flexor tendon nodules are most easily appreciated if one passively flexes and extends the patient's finger while palpating with the opposite hand over the proximal flexor tendon sheath just distal to the MCP joints.

The second and third MCP joints are quite mobile. They not only allow primarily flexion and extension of the digits but also radial and ulnar deviation, and to a lesser extent, rotatory movement and pronation in supination. The metacarpal head is dome shaped, and this allows for this multiplanar movement. The radial and ulnar collateral ligaments are quite lax when the MCP is held in extension. Their origin is just dorsal to the center of rotation of the MCP; therefore, on flexion the collateral ligaments tighten up. Similarly, the bony surface of the metacarpal head when the joint is in extension is quite narrow at the metacarpal head, whereas it widens more volarly and thus provides a tighter bony fit when the joint is brought into flexion. This is important when one is trying to stress the radial and ulnar collateral ligaments such as in the case of examining for a sprained ligament. This means that it is very difficult to stress the ligaments when the joint is held in extension; therefore, the best way to stress these is to hold the MCP at 90 degrees of flexion and then radially and ulnarly deviate. The proximal interphalangeal (PIP) joints and distal interphalangeal (DIP) joints are bicondylar joints and therefore much more of a straightforward hinged joint with very little in the way of radial and ulnar deviation or pronation/supination. The primary movement is almost exclusively flexion and extension. As such, the radial and ulnar collateral ligaments have their origin at the center of motion and therefore do not tighten appreciably in flexion and extension. Nonetheless, one should stress the radial and ulnar collateral ligaments at various degrees of flexion and extension because different portions of the ligaments will be tightened at various levels of flexion and extension.

There are two flexor tendons for each of the second through fifth digits—the FDP and the FDS. The primary action of the FDS is flexion at the PIP joint, whereas the primary action of the FDP is flexion at the DIP joint. The FDP has individual muscle bellies for each digit, whereas the FDS tends to be a single muscle belly for the third through

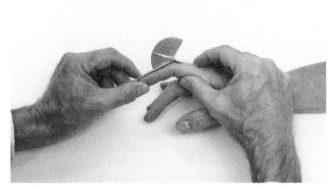

Figure 6.13 Range of motion of the proximal interphalangeal joints measured with a goniometer.

fifth digits. As such, one can press the FDP to all the digits at once, whereas the FDS should be tested with each digit individually. For example, in testing the third finger FDS, one should hold the second, fourth, and fifth digits in extension while having the patient flex the third digit, which the patient will naturally accomplish at the PIP joint.

Range of Motion

Range of motion of the hand and wrist are typically measured with a handheld goniometer. Various sizes of goniometers are available to measure both medium and small joints of the hand and wrist (Fig. 6.13). One could also use electric goniometers to accomplish this task.

Wrist range of motion may be measured in flexion and extension, radial and ulnar deviation, and pronation and supination. Pronation and supination are the most difficult to determine and are really more of an estimation rather than an accurate measurement. A common way of measuring pronation is to have the patient either in a standing or seated position with his or her elbow at the side and flexed at 90 degrees and the palm upward or in a supinated position. One leg of the goniometer is placed at the volar wrist crease, and as the examiner faces the patient, one will align the other leg of the goniometer with the plane of the patient's humerus. This should be an acute angle with zero degrees of neutral being with the patient's volar wrist in line with the humerus. Similarly, pronation is measured in the same general position with the palm facing downward and one leg of the goniometer placed over the dorsal aspect of the wrist at the level of the distal radius and ulna. The other leg of the goniometer is then aligned with the patient's humerus. Again, this should be at an acute angle with zero degrees or neutral indicating that the dorsum of the wrist is aligned with the patient's humerus. Another way to estimate pronation/supination is for the patient to hold a pencil in his or her fist, and the pencil then substitutes for the leg of the goniometer that was otherwise aligned with either the volar wrist crease or the dorsum of the patient's wrist. Again, pronation/supination should measure an acute angle with neutral being in position with the pencil completely vertical or aligned with the patient's humerus.

Wrist flexion is measured with the patient seated and facing the examiner with their elbows on the examination table and at 90 degrees. The wrist is then flexed, one leg of the goniometer is placed on the extensor surface of the forearm, and the other leg is over the dorsum of the third metacarpal or third ray. Neutral or zero degrees would be with the third metacarpal aligned with the surface of the extensor forearm.

Wrist extension is measured with the patient in the same position but with the wrist extended. One leg of the goniometer is then placed along the flexor surface of the forearm, and the other leg is on the palm of the hand and passes between the third and fourth digits; thus, the patient can have slightly flexed digits without affecting the measurement of extension. Again, zero degrees or neutral would be where the palmar surface is aligned with the flexor surface of the forearm.

Radial and ulnar deviations of the wrist are measured with the patient seated with his or her hand palm down on the examination table. One leg of the goniometer is aligned with the third ray, and the other leg of the goniometer is aligned with the extensor surface of the forearm or the underlying radius. The goniometer center should be placed over the lunate. Zero degrees or neutral in radial/ulnar deviation is defined as the position in which the third metacarpal or third ray is in alignment with the radius.

Range of motion measurements of the digits are easiest with a smaller goniometer that is placed on the dorsum of the digits (see Fig. 6.13). The measurement of MCP, PIP, and DIP joints is accomplished in similar fashion. One leg of the goniometer is placed in alignment with the digit, and the other leg of the goniometer is over the dorsum of the corresponding metacarpal. Neutral in this case is when the proximal and distal bones are in alignment. Similarly, the PIP DIP joints are measured over the dorsum of the digit with neutral or zero degrees being the proximal and distal bones in alignment over their distal surfaces.

Many times the multiple measurements of digits are confusing and do not easily bring a picture to mind as far as the overall positioning of the hand. Therefore, a shorthand method has been developed to give a more facile picture of the patient's hand. The flexion and extension lags are single measurements for extremes of flexion and extension of each digit. The definition of the flexion lag is the distance between the tip of the finger and the flexion crease of the palm. For the second and third digits, this is the proximal flexion crease, and for the fourth and fifth digits, this is the distal flexion crease. For the thumb, this is the distance between the tip of the thumb and the base of the fifth finger, roughly at the level of the MCP joint. The extension lags can be measured with the patient's hand flat on the examination table and the palm upward. The second through fifth extension lag is the distance between the tip of the fingernail and the surface of the examination table. The thumb extension lag, however, must be measured with a straight edge held along the thumb metacarpal, and the thumb extension lag is the distance between the tip of the thumbnail and that flat surface.

NEUROLOGIC EXAMINATION

STRENGTH

There are a number of neurologic tests that are specific to the hand and wrist. These are covered in more detail in this chapter. Strength is generally measured through manual muscle testing using the 0- to 5-point scale developed by the British Medical Research Council (BMRC). This is a convenient method and is widely accepted in the medical community. Fortunately, more accurate measures of grip and pinch strength can be obtained using various grip and pinch dynamometers that are available in both analogue and digital formats. Grip dynamometers are generally patterned after the Jebson model, which has five positions. A typical convention is to measure grip strength in position II for women and children and in position III for men. However, one can also measure in all positions depending on the conventions of the particular clinic or area. Typically, one would make three measurements of strength and average the three to get the overall grip strength.

Pinch dynamometers are also available to measure opposition and supposition pinch. Opposition pinch is also known as the 3-point chuck. Opposition pinch is the pinch between the tip of the thumb against the tips of the second and third finger tips. In doing so, the patient must hold the thumb in opposition, hence the name of the pinch. Conversely, the apposition pinch is accomplished by pinching the tip of the thumb against the radial aspect of the flexed index finger. This is also known as the key pinch because this is how one typically grasps a key for a lock. Similar to grip measurements, one usually takes three measurements of each pinch and uses the average for final determination. In general, the opposition and apposition pinch strengths are very similar in each individual. Usually, this is less than a 1-kg difference from side to side. The opposition pinch is thought to be largely a measurement of median nerve function because it uses the thenar muscles and the FDPs of the second and third digits. The apposition pinch is considered more of a test of ulnar innervated muscle because it uses the adductor pollicis and the first dorsal interosseous muscles.

SENSATION

The sensory modalities of light touch, vibration sense, and temperature sense are covered more fully in other parts of this book. These modalities may be used in the hand and wrist in a very similar fashion. Two-point discrimination, however, is a modality that is used almost exclusively in the hand, particularly at the fingertips. This is a measure of neural fiber density and is commonly used as a measure of fingertip sensation. This test is performed using a commercially available wheel, which has points that are measured 2 mm through 8 mm apart. The patient is asked to keep his or her eyes closed while the examiner places the points on their fingertips at various distances apart. The measurement of two-point discrimination then is the closest distance at which the patient can determine two separate points. Normal is considered 3 to 4 mm apart, with 5 mm apart being a borderline measurement.

TINEL SIGN

In 1915 in *La Presse Medicale*, a French medical journal, Dr. J. Tinel originally described the sign that now bears his name.[8] Tinel noted that tapping the proximal stump of an injured axon may create a tingling sensation, or fourmillement as Tinel called it, in the nerve's distal cutaneous distribution. In testing for carpal tunnel syndrome (CTS), this test is performed as follows (Video 5-1):

[Extend] the wrist and [tap] in a proximal to distal direction over the median nerve as it passes through the carpal tunnel, from the area of the distal wrist crease, 2 to 3 cm toward the area between the Thenar and Hypothenar eminences.[8]

The maneuver was not initially used as a diagnostic sign of CTS but rather as a sign of axonal regeneration of peripheral nerves that had been transected.[8,9]

The sensitivity and specificity of Tinel sign varies widely in the literature. Novak and associates[10] contend that, overall, Tinel sign will be positive in only 32% of patients with CTS. The authors offer that a positive Tinel sign is indicative of regenerating nerve fibers, which implies degeneration and then regeneration of nerve fibers. Gellman and coworkers[11] found similar results with a sensitivity and specificity of 44% and 94%, respectively. Gerr and Letz[12] compared the frequency of positive Tinel signs with patients complaining of CTS symptoms who also had confirmed CTS by electrophysiologic testing. They found the sign to be 25% sensitive but 98% specific for CTS. Therefore, a positive result will assure the examiner that CTS is present, but one should not rely on the test as a diagnostic tool. This wide range, which seems to mirror the results noted for other studies noted in the literature, suggests that Tinel sign, when used as a diagnostic tool, is only minimally to moderately useful in detecting the presence of CTS accurately.

ARTERIES

The blood supply to the hand comes from the radial artery on the lateral side of the wrist and the ulnar artery on the medial side of the wrist. In 1929, Allen described a physical exam maneuver testing the patency of the radial or ulnar artery in a paper on thromboangiitis obliterans. The following describes how to perform the Allen test (Fig. 6.14; Video 6-1):

If obstruction of the ulnar artery is suspected, the radial arteries are located by their pulsations; the examiner places one thumb lightly over radial, the four fingers of each hand

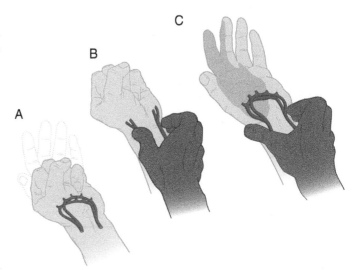

Figure 6.14 Allen Test. (Reproduced with permission from Stokes W: Ulnar neuropathy (elbow). In: Frontera WR, Silver JK, eds. *Essentials of Physical Medicine and Rehabilitation*. Philadelphia: Hanley & Belfus; 2002:165.)

behind the patient's wrist, thus holding the wrist lightly between the thumb and fingers. The patient closes his hands as tightly as possible for a period of one minute in order to squeeze the blood out of the hand; the examiner compresses each wrist between his thumb and fingers, thus occluding the radial arteries; the patient quickly extends his fingers partially while compression of the radial artery is maintained by the examiner. The return of color to the hand and fingers is noted. In individuals with an intact arterial tree, the pallor is quickly replaced by rubor of a higher degree than normal, which gradually fades to normal color. If the ulnar artery is occluded, pallor is maintained for a variable period, due to the obstruction to arterial inflow in the two main channels; the radials are obstructed by the examiner's thumbs, the ulnars by the occlusive lesions (Video 6-1).[13]

This exam can be repeated to test the integrity of the radial arteries. To test the radial arteries, the examiner must compress the ulnar arteries. There are no studies to test the sensitivity, specificity, reliability, or validity of this test. McGregor used fluorescein angiography to evaluate patients with a positive Allen test, and concluded "the Allen test is of no clinical value."[14] However, use of the Allen test is still commonly taught and encouraged to be performed before obtaining blood gases from the radial or ulnar arteries to avoid possible vascular compromise.

SPECIAL TESTS

Distal Radioulnar Joint (DRUJ) instability is assessed clinically in a largely subjective manner by grasping the distal radius and ulna with either hand and manipulating the two bones in a shearing manner back and forth. Kim has attempted to study this maneuver by comparing it to various imaging studies. This stress test for DRUJ instability is described as follows:

> The radius was grasped by the examiner with the forearm in neutral position, and the distal ulna, which was fixed between the examiner's thumb and index finger, was moved in dorsal and palmar directions with respect to the radius. The test was positive if the ulna was conspicuously displaced relative to the contralateral side with the presence of pain or apprehension.[15]

Unfortunately, no clear correlation was found between the physical exam and the imaging studies.

CARPAL TUNNEL SYNDROME

CTS is the most common compressive neuropathy of the upper extremity. It has been studied extensively in regard to diagnosis and treatment. The exact pathophysiology is still somewhat controversial, and therefore the gold standard of diagnosis is not clearly established. As such, the sensitivity and specificity of various diagnostic testing may vary depending on what gold standard is used in studies. In general, the diagnosis is established based on clinical and historical findings plus electromyogram (EMG) and nerve conduction studies, and/or ultrasound imaging of the carpal tunnel.[16]

The physical exam for CTS includes strength testing of the hand as well as sensory testing to look for neurologic

deficits in the median nerve distribution distal to the carpal tunnel. The remainder of the physical examination consists of differing ways of provoking or reproducing the symptoms of CTS. These provocative maneuvers include the Tinel sign (Video 6-2), carpal tunnel compression maneuvers, Phalen's test, and the fist test (Videos 6-3 and 6-4).

MacDermid performed a meta-analysis of the literature on the specificity and sensitivity of various carpal tunnel provocative tests and found that Phalen's test had an estimated sensitivity of 68% and specificity of 73%. Tinel sign had respective estimates of 50% and 77%, and carpal tunnel compression of 64% and 83% (Video 6-5).[17]

Priganc studied the results of various provocative tests and screening tools for CTS and compared them with the severity of CTS as determined by nerve conduction studies alone. In this study only, Phalen's test was correlated with the severity of CTS as determined by nerve conduction studies.[18] A second study by Boland came to the same conclusion.[19] In another study, El Miedany determined that many CTS provocative maneuvers such as Tinel, Phalen's, reverse Palen's, and carpal tunnel compression tests were more specific for the ultrasound-verified diagnosis of wrist flexor tenosynovitis than for CTS.[20]

DE QUERVAIN TENOSYNOVITIS

Tenosynovitis of the first dorsal compartment is termed *de Quervain tenosynovitis*. De Quervain tenosynovitis is commonly seen in those who perform repetitive activities of their thumbs with their wrists held in flexion and/or ulnar deviation. It is particularly common in women directly after pregnancy and has been termed "new mother's tenosynovitis." Tenosynovitis of the wrist is also seen in inflammatory arthritis and can be seen in any of the dorsal compartments.

FINKELSTEIN'S (TABLE 6.1)

Finkelstein first described this well-known test that bears his name as a means to detect the presence of de Quervain tenosynovitis. He describes this as a "pathognomonic objective sign," in which the examiner tugs on the patient's thumb while forcing the wrist into ulnar deviation.[21] A positive test result then reproduces the patient's pain at the region of the first dorsal compartment (Video 6-6). Unfortunately, this test is often confused with a maneuver in which the patient clenches the thumb within the fist and then actively ulnarly deviates the wrist. This is often termed the *Eichhoff maneuver.*[22] In fact, Finkelstein suggested that this maneuver could cause pain even in normal individuals and could cause repeated overstretching of the tendon sheath, resulting in injury to the gliding mechanism. Dawson has suggested a much more gentle form of the test that is done in a careful and progressive manner to better assess the severity of the disease state.[23]

Kutsumi and coworkers studied the biomechanics of Finkelstein's maneuver, finding that the ulnar positioning of the wrist caused significant tethering primarily of the EPB tendon, but not the APB tendon, along with increase in the bulk of the tendon entering the proximal portion of the first dorsal compartment.[24] Accordingly, it appears that the EPB contributes much more to the biomechanics of the disease state than the APL. Alexander hypothesized that patients

Table 6.1   Tests of the Elbow and Wrist

Test	Description	Reliability Validity Test
Finkelstein test	On grasping the patient's thumb and quickly abducting the hand ulnarward, the pain over the styloid tip is excruciating. If one places the thumb within the hand and holds it tightly with the other fingers and then bends the hand severely in ulnar abduction, an intense pain is experienced on the styloid process of the radius, exactly at the place where the tendon sheath takes its course.	Not reported
Ulnar ligaments of the thumb MCP joint	The integrity of the proper collateral ligament is assessed by carrying out valgus stress testing with the MCP joint in 30 degrees of flexion. To avoid a false interpretation, the examiner must prevent MCP rotation by grasping the thumb proximal to the joint. If there is more than 30 degrees of laxity (or 15 degrees more laxity than the noninjured side), rupture of the ligament proper is likely. The thumb is then positioned in extension for repeat valgus testing. If valgus laxity is less than 30 degrees (or 15 degrees less than the noninjured side), the accessory ligament is intact. If the valgus laxity is greater than 30 degrees (or 15 degrees of the noninjured side), the accessory ligament is also ruptured.	Not reported
Thumb basilar joint grind test (Video 6-7)	The basal joint grind test is performed by stabilizing the triquetrum with the thumb and index finger and then dorsally subluxing the thumb metacarpal on the trapezium while providing compressive force with the other hand.	Not reported

MCP, Metacarpal phalanges.

with greater pain on resisted thumb interphalangeal extension (EPL stress) than on resisted thumb abduction (APL stress) would be more likely to have a septum between the two tendons in the first dorsal compartment.[25] Brunelli has suggested an alternative test in which the patient radially deviates the wrist and the examiner resists abduction of the thumb.[26] However, this test has not been studied further.

SCAPHOLUNATE INSTABILITY

In 1978, Kirk Watson described one of the most widely utilized tests for scapholunate instability.[27] Watson test, also known as the scaphoid shift test, was originally used as an assessment tool to identify rotatory subluxation of the scaphoid. Proper performance of this test requires:

> The examiner as if to engage in arm wrestling, [sit] face to face across a table with diagonally opposed hands raised (right to right or left to left) and elbows resting on the surface in between. With the patient's forearm slightly pronated, the examiner grasps the wrist from the radial side, placing his thumb on the palmar prominence of the scaphoid and wrapping his fingers around the distal radius ... The examiner's other hand grasps at the metacarpal level, controlling wrist position. Starting in ulnar deviation and slight extension, the wrist is moved radially and slightly flexed, with constant pressure on the scaphoid (Video 6-8).[28]

As the wrist is brought into radial deviation, the scaphoid is forced to flex. If the lunate is no longer tightly attached to the scaphoid through the scapholunate ligament, then the lunate will suddenly pop into relative extension following the triquetrum to which it is still attached through the lunotriquetral ligament. This is the so-called "catch-up clunk" and signifies a positive test result. It is quite palpable to the examiner and quite painful to the patient. However, as with any

diagnostic exam maneuver, the validity of the result is dependent on the interpretation of the examiner. In fact, Watson himself noted that the scaphoid shift "is not so much a test as a provocative maneuver. It does not offer a simple positive or negative result, but rather a variety of findings."[28]

In 1994, Wolfe and Crisco[29] evaluated the maneuver using an instrumented device to determine degrees of ligamentous laxity noted in asymptomatic individuals with a positive Watson test versus those with a negative scaphoid shift. Interestingly, high degrees of laxity may be associated with a positive scaphoid shift, but this is a result of generalized ligamentous hypermobility, hence giving a false-positive result. This study cautions against making the diagnosis of carpal instability based on a hypermobile scaphoid and reiterates the necessity of concomitant pain for this to be recognized as a positive Watson test result.[29]

The sensitivity of the Watson test has been found to be 69% and the specificity to range between 64% and 68%.[14] Again, based on the modest ability of the test to be both sensitive and specific, the results obtained must be interpreted cautiously, and therefore the test has limited clinical utility.

LUNOTRIQUETRAL INSTABILITY

LUNOTRIQUETRAL BALLOTTEMENT TEST

The lunotriquetral ballottement test has also been called Reagan's test. Reagan and colleagues[30] described the evaluation of lunotriquetral sprains as follows (Fig. 6.15):

> [Fix] the lunate with the thumb and index finger of one hand while, with the other hand, displacing the triquetrum and pisiform first dorsally then palmarly (Video 6-9).

A positive test result is confirmed if pain, crepitus and excessive laxity are elicited. The test is performed with the

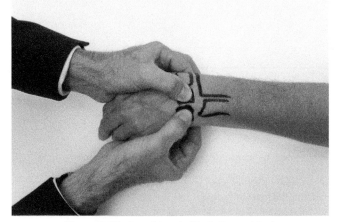

Figure 6.15 Lunotriquetral ballottement test.

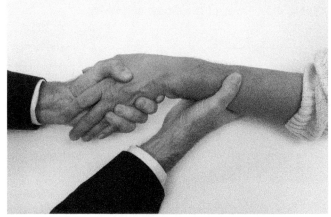

Figure 6.17 Ulnocarpal stress test for triangular fibrocartilage complex tear.

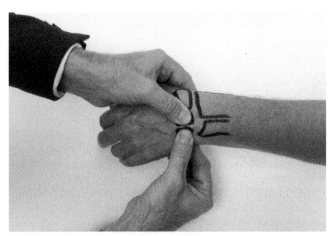

Figure 6.16 Shear test.

Pain that is concordant or similar to the pain or discomfort of the patient is considered a positive test result. Care should be made to compare the right and left wrist exams. There are no studies assessing the specificity or sensitivity of this test.

TRIANGULAR FIBROCARTILAGINOUS COMPLEX

The triangular fibrocartilage complex (TFCC) can be a cause of ulnar-sided wrist pain.[35,36] The TFCC is difficult to test reliably with a physical exam, and radiologic study results are often negative. The use of magnetic resonance imaging (MRI) for evaluating TFCC pathology depends on radiologist experience. Blazar and coworkers[37] compared MRI readings of two different radiologists finding sensitivities of 86% and 80% in detecting TFCC lesions with specificity rates of 96% and 80%.

The complexity of the TFCC increases as we realize the natural degenerative course the TFCC takes with aging. Mikic[38] studied the TFCC in a cadaveric model and found 38.4% had degenerative changes by the third decade of life, and no completely normal discs were found in individuals past their fifth decade. We, therefore, think that examiners should cautiously interpret the results of the physical exam of the TFCC.

ULNOCARPAL STRESS TEST

The ulnocarpal stress test is a provocative test in which the examiner attempts to grind the TFCC between the ulnar-sided carpal bones and distal ulna (Video 6-11). In 1991, Friedman and Palmer first described the ulnocarpal stress test (Fig. 6.17). They found patients generally have chronic or subacute ulnar wrist pain, often exacerbated by activity and relieved by rest. Physical examination reveals swelling and tenderness that is usually localized to the region of the TFCC and lunotriquetral joint. Pronation and supination of the forearm with ulnar deviation of the wrist generally evokes increased symptoms.[39]

Nakamura and coworkers[40] noted "the test is positive when axial stress produces ulnar wrist pain during passive supination–pronation with the wrist in maximum ulnar deviation." When performed correctly, the test compresses

patient's hand palm down, and the examiner is observing the dorsal aspect of the wrist.

The usefulness of this test for determining lunotriquetral instability has been confirmed by others, but its efficacy has not been established.[27,31] Numerous authors have discussed this test, but few have performed controlled studies to determine the sensitivity or specificity of the test. Marx and associates[32] noted the sensitivity of this examination maneuver to be 64% and the specificity to be 44%. As such, it would be difficult at best to base a diagnosis of instability primarily on a positive Reagan's test.

SHEAR TEST FOR LUNOTRIQUETRAL INSTABILITY

The shear test origin could not be determined, but it is used to stress the lunotriquetral ligament (Fig. 6.16). There are multiple sources that describe nearly the same way to perform this test.[33,34]

The shear test is performed with the subject's forearm in neutral rotation and the elbow on the examination table. The examiner's contralateral fingers are placed over the dorsum of the lunate. With the lunate supported, the examiner's ipsilateral thumb loads the pisotriquetral joint from the palmar aspect, creating a shear force at the lunotriquetral joint (Video 6-10).[34]

the TFCC, eliciting clicking and pain in the face of a tear. It is essential to compare the symptomatic side to the uninvolved side, understanding that clicking and snapping may normally be present. There are no studies evaluating sensitivity, specificity, and reliability.

FOVEAL SIGN

The foveal sign test was described by Berger as a means to detect the presence of TFCC tears at the base of the fovea and to detect ulnotriquetral (UT) ligament split tears. This test is performed by "pressing the examiner's thumb distally into the interval between the ulnar styloid process and FCU tendon, between the volar surface of the ulnar head and the pisiform."[41] A positive test result reproduces ulnar-sided wrist pain and should be compared with the unaffected side.

EXTENSOR CARPI ULNARIS INSTABILITY

The ECU tendon and its sheath (the sixth dorsal compartment) are another common source of ulnar sided wrist pain. Because of its high mobility and relatively shallow groove in the dorsal distal ulna, the ECU tendon sheath may become displaced and snap. This is often painful and debilitating to the patient. Ng describes an "ice cream scoop" maneuver in which the patient is asked to simulate the act of scooping ice cream while the examiner resists this movement.[42] The aim of the test is to reproduce the patient's pain and also cause a snap or subluxation of the tendon, which may be palpated and perhaps even seen by the examiner.

THUMB CARPOMETACARPAL ARTHRITIS

The diagnosis of thumb CMC osteoarthritis is largely a clinical diagnosis based on reproduction of the patient's pain with palpation, compression, or manipulation of the CMC joint. Unfortunately, the validity of the physical exam has not been studied. Ideally, the examiner stabilizes the base of the thumb by grasping the scaphoid tubercle and the dorsum of the wrist between her thumb and index finger. With the other hand, the examiner similarly grasps the base of the thumb metacarpal. The examiner is then well positioned to wiggle the joint back and forth, palmarly and dorsally, to assess for both ligamentous laxity and reproduction of the patient's pain.

THUMB METACARPAL PHALANGES INSTABILITY

See Table 6.1.

The thumb MCP joint is a multiaxial diarthrodial hinge joint able to flex, extend, abduct, adduct, and circumduct.[43,44] There are static and dynamic stabilizers of the thumb MCP joint. The main static stabilizers are the radial and ulnar collateral ligaments, as well as the accessory collateral ligament.[44] The ulnar collateral ligament is taut at 30 degrees flexion at the MCP joint, and the ulnar accessory collateral ligament is taut in full extension at the MCP joint.[44] The joint capsule and the dorsal aponeurosis are the other static stabilizers. The dynamic stabilizers are muscles and tendons inserting to this area. Specifically, the AP, APB and the FPL muscles add to the stability about the joint.[43,44]

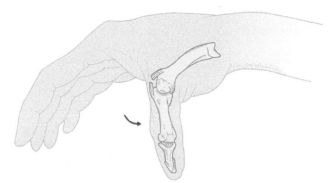

Figure 6.18   Skier's thumb. (Adapted from Mellion MB. *Office Sports Medicine*. 2nd ed. Philadelphia: Hanley & Belfus; 1996.)

In 1955, Campbell described and coined the term gamekeeper's thumb.[45] In his own words:

> The gamekeeper's method of killing a wounded rabbit is to hold the head in one hand and the rear legs in the other. A strong pull is then exerted while the neck is sharply extended … Invariably, a loose grip causes the neck to be stretched against the ulnar side of the thumb. It is the force of the pull, repeated manifold, which stretches the ulnar collateral ligament.

This mechanism of overuse injury is common to rabbit hunters, but traumatic injury is also seen, most commonly in skiers.[46] Therefore, gamekeeper's thumb is anatomically synonymous with skier's thumb. However, the term *gamekeeper's thumb* is usually applied to a repetitive overuse injury, whereas the term *skier's thumb* implies a traumatic injury (Fig. 6.18).[46] The physical exam findings are really an extension of reproducing the valgus force that resulted in the original injury. An original description of testing the ulnar collateral ligament could not be found, but Heyman describes the maneuver as follows:

> The integrity of the proper collateral ligament is assessed by carrying out valgus stress testing with the MCP joint in 30 degrees of flexion. To avoid a false interpretation, the examiner must prevent MCP rotation by grasping the thumb proximal to the joint. If there is more than 30 degrees of laxity (or 15 degrees more laxity than the noninjured side), rupture of the ligament proper is likely. The thumb is then positioned in extension for repeat valgus testing. If valgus laxity is less than 30 degrees (or 15 degrees less than the noninjured side), the accessory ligament is intact. If the valgus laxity is greater than 30 degrees (or 15 degrees of the noninjured side), the accessory ligament is also ruptured (Fig. 6.19).[46]

As with many limb physical exam maneuvers, side-to-side comparison is important. There are no studies to evaluate the specificity and sensitivity of the previously described test. Heyman and others[47] found that individuals with complete collateral ligament tears had greater than 35 degrees of valgus laxity and 15 degrees greater than on the uninjured side. Stener[44] described anatomically the retraction of the collateral ligament in complete lesions that formed a small, palpable nodule; therefore, a palpable mass at the proximal ulnar MCP joint is called a Stener lesion. Heyman and colleagues found a similar palpable mass in 9 of 16 patients

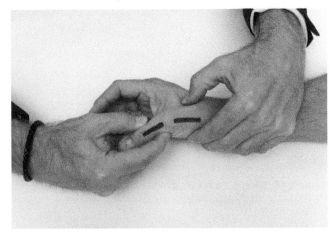

Figure 6.19 Valgus testing for ulnar collateral ligament stability (Video 6-12).

with ligament tears, all of whom had complete ligament tears (proper and accessory ligament tears) at operation. Therefore the specificity of a palpable mass was 100%. On the other hand, there was no palpable mass in 7 patients who had complete tears at operation, making the false-negative rate 46%.

METACARPAL PHALANGEAL JOINTS

The MCP joints of the second through fifth digits are similar to the thumb MCP and highly mobile. The dome-shaped metacarpal head allows for ease of movement, not only in flexion and extension but also for radial and ulnar deviation. There are even some pronation and supination that occur with fine-finger manipulations. As such, the ligaments are difficult not only to injure but also to stress. The origins of the radial and lateral collateral ligaments are dorsal to the center of rotation for flexion and extension about the metacarpal head. Therefore, the ligaments are loosened in extension, allowing ease of radial and ulnar deviation as well as pronation and supination. Only when the joint is flexed will the collateral ligaments be tightened and may be put on stretch. In order to examine the collateral ligaments for injury, the examiner must hold the MCP in 90 degrees of flexion and then radially and ulnarly deviate the digit to stress the ulnar collateral and radial collateral ligaments, respectively. This also mimics the mechanism of injury or the position in which the patient must have acquired such a sprain.

PROXIMAL AND DISTAL INTERPHALANGEAL JOINTS

The PIP and DIP joints have a similar configuration. Both are bicondylar joints that can be thought of as basic hinge joints. Their primary motion is along a flexion extension plane. The radial and ulnar collateral ligaments have their origins near the center of rotation for flexion and extension. Therefore, they remain fairly tight in all angles of flexion and extension and can be stressed at all angles of flexion and extension. As one might expect, they are thus more vulnerable to sprains because of this. The PIP is more vulnerable than the DIP because of the longer lever arm of the digit distal to the joint.

AUTHORS' PREFERRED APPROACH

Each physician develops his or her own routine when examining a patient. I prefer to examine the patient before viewing any of the imaging studies or other tests (and, of course, after taking a thorough history). Many times the tests and imaging have positive findings that are unrelated to the patient's complaint and may lead the physician down many dead-end paths. An exception to this rule is in the case of trauma. Only in context of an appropriate history and examination can one make sense of the subsequent tests.

Typically, I start with a quick view of the active range of motion of the upper extremities and possibly the neck. This may be performed expeditiously by having patients quickly and bimanually:

Close and open their fists.
Oppose and flatten their thumbs.
Extend and flex their elbows.
Flex and extend their wrists.
With their elbows at their side and flexed at 90 degrees, supinate and pronate their forearms.
Raise their hands above their heads.
Externally rotate their shoulders to reach downward behind their backs.
Internally rotate their shoulders to reach upward behind their backs.

This can take as little as 20 seconds to accomplish. Then if any joint movement appears asymmetric or diminished, one can measure this in a more formal manner.

After range of motion, I generally palpate the hand and fingers, feeling the flexor tendons with one hand while flexing and extending the digits passively with the other. I then palpate the muscles of the forearms and finally focus in on the symptomatic area. I then measure grip and pinch strengths followed by two-point discrimination at the finger tips. The remainder of the exam is customized to the patient's complaint and subsequent findings.

CONCLUSION

When examining the hand and wrist, one must acquire a firm grasp of the underlying anatomy. With such knowledge and modicum of practice, the examiner may diagnose most hand and wrist problems with proficiency and without the use of advanced imaging. Of course, knowing the common pathologies and how they may present further refines the accuracy of one's diagnoses.

The author of this chapter would like to acknowledge and thank Drs. Thomas Agesen, Scott F. Nadler, John Wrightson and Jeffrey Miller for their previous contributions to this chapter.

REFERENCES

1. Clemente C. *Anatomy: A Regional Atlas of the Human Body.* 4th ed. Baltimore: Williams and Wilkins; 1997.
2. Gray H, Pick TP, Howden R, eds. *Gray's Anatomy.* New York: Bounty Books; 1978.

3. Hollinshead WH, Rosse C. *Textbook of Anatomy*. 4th ed. Philadelphia: Harper & Row; 1985.
4. Jenkins DB. *Hollinshead's Functional Anatomy of the Limbs and Back*. 7th ed. Philadelphia: W.B. Saunders; 1998.
5. Kendall FP, McCreary EK, Provance PG. *Muscle Testing and Function*. 4th ed. Baltimore: Williams & Wilkins; 1993.
6. Netter FH. *Atlas of Human Anatomy*. East Hanover: Novartis; 1989.
7. Sapira JD. The neurologic examination. The extremities. In: Sapira JD, Sapira JD, eds. *The art and science of bedside diagnosis*. Baltimore: Williams & Wilkins; 1990.
8. Tinel J. Le signe "fourmillement" dans les lesions des neffs periupheriques. *Presse Med*. 1915;23:388-389.
9. Moldaver J. Brief note: Tinel's sign. *J Bone Joint Surg Am*. 1978;60:412-414.
10. Novak CB, Mackinnon SE, Brownlee R, et al. Provocative sensory testing in carpal tunnel syndrome. *J Hand Surg [Br]*. 1992;17:204-208.
11. Gellman H, Gelberman RH, Tan AM, et al. Carpal tunnel syndrome. An evaluation of the provocative diagnostic tests. *J Bone Joint Surg Am*. 1986;68:735-737.
12. Gerr F, Letz R. The sensitivity and specificity of tests for carpal tunnel syndrome vary with the comparison subjects. *J Hand Surg [Br]*. 1998;23:151-155.
13. Allen EV. Thromboangiitis obliterans: methods of diagnosis of chronic occlusive arterial lesions distal to the wrist with illustrative cases. *Am J Med Sci*. 1929;178:237-244.
14. McGregor AD. The Allen test–an investigation of its accuracy by fluorescein angiography. *J Hand Surg [Br]*. 1987;12:82-85.
15. Kim JP, Park MJ. Assessment of distal radioulnar joint instability after distal radius fracture: comparison of computed tomography and clinical examination results. *J Hand Surg Am*. 2008;33:1486-1492.
16. Descatha A, Dale A-M, Franzblau A, et al. Diagnostic strategies using physical examination are minimally useful in defining carpal tunnel syndrome in population-based research studies. *Occup Environ Med*. 2010;67:133-135.
17. MacDermid JC, Wessel J. Clinical diagnosis of carpal tunnel syndrome: a systematic review. *J Hand Ther*. 2004;17:309-319.
18. Priganc VW, Henry SM. The relationship among five common carpal tunnel syndrome tests and the severity of carpal tunnel syndrome. *J Hand Ther*. 2003;16:225-236.
19. Boland RA, Kiernan MC. Assessing the accuracy of a combination of clinical tests for identifying carpal tunnel syndrome. *J Clin Neurosci*. 2009;16:929-933.
20. El Miedany Y, Ashour S, Youssef S, et al. Clinical diagnosis of carpal tunnel syndrome: old tests-new concepts. *Joint Bone Spine*. 2008;75:451-457.
21. Finkelstein H. Stenosing tendovaginitis at the radial styloid process. *J Bone Joint Surg*. 1939;12:509-540.
22. Eichoff E. Zur pathogenese der Tendovainitis stenosans. *Bruns' Beitrage Zur Klinischen*. 1927;746-755.
23. Dawson C, Mudgal CS. Staged description of the Finkelstein test. *J Hand Surg Am*. 2010;35:1513-1515.
24. Kutsumi K, Amadio PC, Zhao C, et al. Finkelstein's test: a biomechanical analysis. *J Hand Surg Am*. 2005;30:130-135.
25. Alexander RD, Catalano LW, Barron OA, et al. The extensor pollicis brevis entrapment test in the treatment of de Quervain's disease. *J Hand Surg Am*. 2002;27:813-816.
26. Brunelli G. Finkelstein's versus Brunelli's test in De Quervain tenosynovitis. *Chir Main*. 2003;22:43-45.
27. Watson HK, Weinzweig J. Physical examination of the wrist [review]. *Hand Clin* [Review]. 1997;13:17-34.
28. Watson HK, Ashmead Dt, Makhlouf MV. Examination of the scaphoid. *J Hand Surg Am*. 1988;13:657-660.
29. Wolfe SW, Crisco JJ. Mechanical evaluation of the scaphoid shift test. *J Hand Surg Am*. 1994;19:762-768.
30. Reagan DS, Linscheid RL, Dobyns JH. Lunotriquetral sprains. *J Hand Surg Am*. 1984;9:502-514.
31. Alexander CE, Lichtman DM. Ulnar carpal instabilities. *Orthop Clin North Am*. 1984;15:307-320.
32. Marx RG, Bombardier C, Wright JG. What we know about the reliability and validity of physical examination tests used to examine the upper extremity. *J Hand Surg Am*. 1999;24:185-192.
33. Ambrose L, Posner MA. Lunate-triquetral and midcarpal joint instability. *Hand Clin*. 1992;8:653-668.
34. Shin AY, Battaglia MJ, Bishop AT. Lunotriquetral instability: diagnosis and treatment. *J Am Acad Orthop Surg*. 2000;8:170-179.
35. Palmer AK, Werner FW. The triangular fibrocartilage complex of the wrist–anatomy and function. *J Hand Surg Am*. 1981;6:153-162.
36. Palmer AK. Triangular fibrocartilage disorders: injury patterns and treatment. *Arthroscopy*. 1990;6:125-132.
37. Blazar PE, Chan PS, Kneeland JB, et al. The effect of observer experience on magnetic resonance imaging interpretation and localization of triangular fibrocartilage complex lesions. *J Hand Surg Am*. 2001;26:742-748.
38. Mikic ZD. Age changes in the triangular fibrocartilage of the wrist joint. *J Anat*. 1978;126:367-384.
39. Friedman SL, Palmer AK. The ulnar impaction syndrome. *Hand Clin*. 1991;7:295-310.
40. Nakamura R, Horii E, Imaeda T, et al. The ulnocarpal stress test in the diagnosis of ulnar-sided wrist pain. *J Hand Surg [Br]*. 1997;22:719-723.
41. Tay SC, Tomita K, Berger RA. The "ulnar fovea sign" for defining ulnar wrist pain: an analysis of sensitivity and specificity. *J Hand Surg Am*. 2007;32:438-444.
42. Ng CY, Hayton MJ. Ice cream scoop test: a novel clinical test to diagnose extensor carpi ulnaris instability. *J Hand Surg Eur*. 2013;38:569-570.
43. Coonrad RW, Goldner JL. A study of the pathological findings and treatment in soft-tissue injury of the thumb metacarpophalangeal joint. With a clinical study of the normal range of motion in one thousand thumbs and a study of post mortem findings of ligamentous structures in relation to function. *J Bone Joint Surg Am*. 1968;50:439-451.
44. Stener B. Displacement of the ruptured ulnar collateral ligament of the metacarpo-phalangeal joint of the thumb. *J Bone Joint Surg*. 1962;44:869-879.
45. Campbell CS. Gamekeeper's thumb. *J Bone Joint Surg Br*. 1955;37-B:148-149.
46. Heyman P. Injuries to the ulnar collateral ligament of the thumb metacarpophalangeal joint. *J Am Acad Orthop Surg*. 1997;5:224-229.
47. Heyman P, Gelberman RH, Duncan K, et al. Injuries of the ulnar collateral ligament of the thumb metacarpophalangeal joint. Biomechanical and prospective clinical studies on the usefulness of valgus stress testing. *Clin Orthop Relat Res*. 1993;292:165-171.

7

Physical Examination of the Lumbar Spine and Sacroiliac Joint

David N. Woznica, MS, MD | Joel M. Press, MD

INTRODUCTION

Because of the multifactorial nature of the complaint of low back pain (LBP), patients presenting with LBP necessitate a detailed history and physical examination. Nonspecific or incorrect diagnoses can lead to ineffective treatment plans that prolong morbidity and result in suboptimal utilization of community health resources. History collection should include traumatic events, personal and family histories of cancer diagnoses, rheumatologic disorders, bowel inflammatory disorders, and skin disorders, and the review of systems should be sensitive enough to identify potential systemic symptoms. Pain-relieving and pain-exacerbating activities should be identified through history because they may provide clues toward potential mechanical relief of the back pain with physical therapy and/or increased general physical activity. The examiner must also keep in mind the importance of the sacroiliac joint (SIJ) and the hip joint within the differential diagnosis of LBP; the description of hip joint pain and examination is addressed in Chapter 8.

ANATOMY AND BIOMECHANICS

The joints of the pelvis are intrinsically stable, and proper functioning is essential for normal biomechanics about the pelvis. High forces and repetitive loads can lead to ligamentous, muscle, and bone injuries or overuse syndromes. The pelvis also adapts to injuries of the spine and the lower extremities, which may lead to maladaptive syndromes.[1] SIJ dysfunction occurs when there is an alteration of the structural or positional relationship of the sacrum on the ilium. This dysfunction commonly originates through asymmetric force transmission, as well as degenerative changes.[1] Despite these well-known biomechanical changes, it is still unclear whether altered motion at the SIJ is the source of pain.

The pelvis serves as the central base through which forces are transmitted both directly and indirectly (Fig. 7.1). In contrast to the lumbar spine, the joints of the pelvis are relatively stable; however, repetitive load, trauma, or maladaptive compensatory gait patterns from spine or lower extremity injury can result in SIJ dysfunction. The natural degenerative changes that take place must be recognized as well. The SIJ can be affected in rheumatologic disorders such as seronegative spondyloarthropathies including reactive arthritis, psoriasis, juvenile chronic arthritis, ulcerative colitis, and Crohn disease. It can also be affected by autoimmune and infectious diseases and malignancy with and without metastasis. Radiographic changes about the SIJ have been well documented in ankylosing spondylitis (AS), including joint space narrowing, subchondral sclerosis, and osteophytosis.[2-5]

Bodyweight and postural changes may create or inhibit motion at the SIJ, while the majority of indirect motion occurs secondary to the muscle groups surrounding the joint. These include the gluteals, hamstrings, hip external rotators, iliopsoas, abdominals, latissimus dorsi, quadratus lumborum, and erector spinae (Fig. 7.2). Restriction of any of these muscle groups may subsequently alter mechanics about the SIJ. Acquired hyper- or hypomobility about the SIJ results in altered load transmission, which may have an impact on the other components of the lower extremity kinetic chain. Studies have shown various ranges of motion about the SIJ, but most agree that approximately 4 degrees of rotation and 1.6 mm of translation occur.[6,7] The amount of joint motion decreases with age. Women develop degenerative changes that restrict motion at age 50 years, and men develop them around age 40 years.[6,7] At the present time, the clinical impact of age-related degeneration about the SIJ is unclear.

The presentation of SIJ dysfunction can be similar to other forms of LBP, which may make clinical diagnosis more challenging.[8] SIJ-mediated pain can also be confounding in the appearance of lumbosacral radicular pain, with a prevalence between 15% and 30% and an unknown incidence.[9-12] Ebraheim et al.[13] via a cadaveric dissection study, determined that the fifth lumbar nerve root and lumbosacral trunk coursed across the sacroiliac at a level 2.0 ± 0.2 cm below the pelvic brim and were relatively fixed to the sacral ala with fibrous connective tissue. Bernard and Kirkaldy-Willis[14] reported that of 1293 patients with LBP, SIJ dysfunction was thought to be the pain generator in 22.5% based on history and physical exam, with a referral pattern mainly involving the buttock and posterolateral calf, although SIJ syndrome occurred in isolation in only 61% of this subgroup. SIJ pain referral patterns have been documented after provocative SIJ injection, and show extension to the medial/lateral buttocks, greater trochanter, and the superior-lateral thigh.[8,12,15-18] Pain or tenderness over the region of the posterior superior

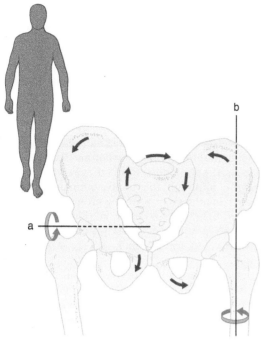

Figure 7.1 Biomechanics of the sacroiliac joints during walking: *a,* rotation of the iliac bone at the non–weight-bearing side around a frontal horizontal axis; *b,* rotation of the iliac bone at the weight-bearing side around a vertical axis. (Adapted with permission from Ombregt L, Bisschop P, Ter Veer HJ, et al. Applied anatomy of the sacroiliac joint. In: Ombregt L, Bisschop P, Ter Veer HJ, et al, eds. *A System of Orthopedic Medicine.* London: W.B. Saunders; 1995:694.)

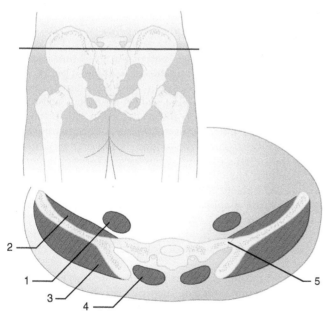

Figure 7.2 Musculature about the sacroiliac joints: *1,* psoas; *2, iliacus; 3,* gluteus; *4,* erector spinae; *5,* sacroiliac joint. (Adapted with permission from Ombregt L, Bisschop P, Ter Veer HJ, et al. Applied anatomy of the sacroiliac joint. In: Ombregt L, Bisschop P, Ter Veer HJ, et al, eds. *A System of Orthopedic Medicine.* London: W.B. Saunders; 1995:690.)

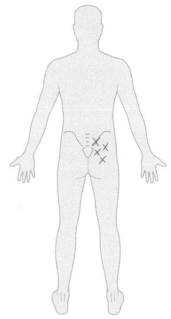

Figure 7.3 Typical pain location for sacroiliac joint dysfunction. (Adapted with permission from George SZ, Delitto A. Management of the athlete with low back pain. *Clin Sports Med.* 2002;21:112.)

iliac spine is the most common symptom in patients with SIJ pain.[19-21] The area of maximal pain has been defined from the medial buttock extending approximately 10 cm caudally and 3 cm laterally from the posterior superior iliac spine (PSIS) (Fig. 7.3).[20,21]

With these diagnostic challenges in mind, frequently used factors on history and physical examination include the determination of exacerbating activities, location pattern of the pain (midline vs paramidline), and presence or absence of the centralization/peripheralization phenomenon. On history, SIJ pain is frequently aggravated after prolonged sitting or standing and with loading of the leg of the affected side while the hip is in flexion. Transitional pain may also be a feature, such as during sit-to-stand motions.[1]

To evaluate the utility of the location pattern of LBP as a predictor of the pain's source, Delpalma and coworkers[22] performed a retrospective chart review of 170 cases with definitive diagnoses of the LBP origin. A significantly greater percentage of patients with internal disc disruption reported midline LBP (95.8%) compared with facet-mediated (15.4%) or SIJ-mediated pain (12.9%). A significantly lower percentage of patients (67.3%) with internal disc disruption reported paramidline pain compared with facet-mediated (95%) or SIJ-mediated pain (96%). The specificity of midline LBP for internal disc disruption was 74.8% compared with 28.0% for facet-mediated pain and 36.0% for SIJ-mediated pain. They concluded that the presence of midline LBP increased the probability of internal disc disruption and decreased the probability of symptomatic facet or sacroiliac dysfunction, while isolated paramidline LBP increased the probability of symptomatic facet or SIJ pain and mildly reduced the likelihood of internal disc disruption.

The centralization/peripheralization phenomenon is noted clinically as the movement of pain centrally toward the lumbar spine or peripherally toward the extremities in response to repeated lumbar movements. This phenomenon has been associated with pain from discogenic rather than sacroiliac sources and has shown high sensitivity but low specificity in patients with chronic LBP.[23,24]

A comprehensive physical examination of LBP patients includes evaluation of the neurologic, vascular and musculoskeletal system. Physical examination of this region should flow through a specific sequence repeatedly by an examiner in order to avoid missing key elements. A commonly performed sequence includes: inspection, palpation, range of motion (ROM), flexibility, functional and neurologic assessments, and provocative maneuvers. Motion testing and provocative maneuvers should be performed for both the low back and for the sacroiliac and hip joints. The following sections separate physical exam of the lumbar spine from that of the SIJ.

PHYSICAL EXAM OF THE LUMBAR SPINE

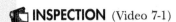 **INSPECTION** (Video 7-1)

Examination of the low back begins with the initial observation of the patient, noting the patient's preferred position while awaiting the physician. Patients with uncomfortable discogenic and radicular pain may be noted to be standing or moving as opposed to being seated while they wait. At other times, patients with LBP will maintain rigid postures, and motions will be noted to be hesitant to avoid bending or twisting, which may exacerbate their pain. An antalgic or listing posture should be noted if present. Patients should disrobe to either an examination gown or disposable examination shorts with an easily removed top to allow complete visualization.

Bony landmarks are useful in determining site of pain in the lumbar spine. Important landmarks include the anterior superior iliac spine (ASIS) at the level of the sacral promontory and the PSIS at the level of the spinous process of the second sacral vertebra.[25] A commonly used reference line is created by passing a horizontal line connecting the highest points of both iliac crests, which crosses the vertebral column at the level of the L4 to L5 intervertebral space or the L4 vertebra. Notably, Duniec and coworkers[26a] performed a recent study comparing palpation guided identification of this line by an anesthetist with ultrasound evaluation before lumbar puncture and found that in 36% of cases, the palpatory exam was off by a mean of one level. This study corroborated similar results found by Locks et al.[27] in 2010, who found that the L3 to L4 space determined anatomically in the seated position in obese and nonobese women undergoing elective cesarean section was only 49% and 53% accurate, respectively, when confirmed with ultrasound evaluation.

Forming a line through the tubercles of the iliac crests creates the intertubercular plane, which cuts the body of the fifth lumbar vertebra. The upper margin of the greater sciatic notch is opposite the spinous process of the third sacral vertebra, and slightly below this level is the posterior inferior iliac spine (PIIS). The surface markings of the posterior inferior iliac spine and the ischial spine are both situated in a line that joins the posterior superior iliac spine to the outer part of the ischial tuberosity; the posterior inferior spine is 5 cm and the ischial spine 10 cm below the posterior superior spine; the ischial spine is opposite the first portion of the coccyx. With the body erect, the line joining the pubic tubercle to the top of the greater trochanter is practically horizontal; the middle of this line overlies the acetabulum and the head of the femur.

Patients should be observed from the front, side, and rear. Anterior observation should assess head position, height symmetries of the shoulders and iliac crests, patellar directionality, and lower limb positioning. The head should sit straight on the shoulders, which themselves should be of equal height, although the hand-dominant side may be slightly lower in athletic or sporting individuals. (Fig. 7.4A). The iliac crest height should be equal (Fig. 7.4B). The patellae should be pointing anteriorly and the lower limbs straight, with any deformity such as valgus–varus misalignment noted.

Posterior observation involves inspection of spinal, bone, and soft tissue alignment. Shifting of the pelvis or shoulders may be noted in the face of nerve root injury or gluteus medius weakness, similar to a Trendelenburg sign.[25] With a disc herniation lateral to the nerve roots, the patient may list away from the side of the irritated nerve root in an attempt to draw the nerve root away from the disc; this is termed a *lateral shift*. When the herniation is medial to the nerve root, the patient may list toward the side of the lesion. The reliability of lateral shift judgments was examined by Clare and others[28] in different levels of physical therapists with training in the McKenzie method using stable photographic slides of 45 patients with LBP, and it was found that lateral shift judgments had only moderate reliability (intraclass coefficient [ICC] range of 0.48 to 0.64).

Scoliotic curves may be evaluated by inspection of the height of the shoulders, scapula, and iliac crests. The spines of the scapulae begin at the level of the third thoracic vertebra (T3) and should be at the same angle. The inferior angles of the scapula (T8) should be equidistant from the spine. Any curve in the spine should be noted, as well as muscular asymmetry. A rib hump deformity can be noted with trunk forward flexion or may be seen through apparent scapular winging. The waist angles should be equal. Comparing the heights of the iliac crests or posterior superior iliac spines for any differences may identify pelvic obliquity, which could indicate a functional leg length discrepancy, or may stem from a spinal deformity such as scoliosis or an anomalous vertebrae.[29] The relationship between the PSIS and the ASIS should be noted to assess for level of pelvic tilt. In addition, the gluteal folds and popliteal creases should be level.

Upon examining a patient from the side, the ear should drop a plumb line even with the tip of the shoulder and the peak of the iliac crest. A gentle lumbar lordotic curve is normal. Any exaggerated or increased curve should be noted. Exaggerated lordosis may be associated with a hip flexor contracture, weak hip extensors, or spondylolisthesis. The alignment of the lower extremities should also be observed from the side in neutral stance.

The skin may reveal ecchymosis after blunt trauma, erythema with infection or inflammation, or rashes with shingles or infection. Atrophy of the tissues may be noted with the presence of nerve root or peripheral nerve injury.

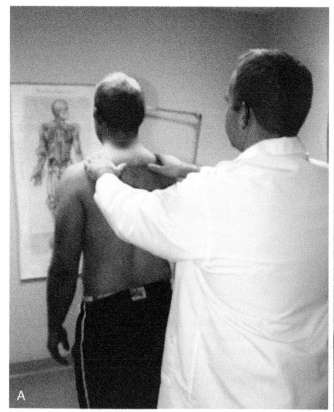
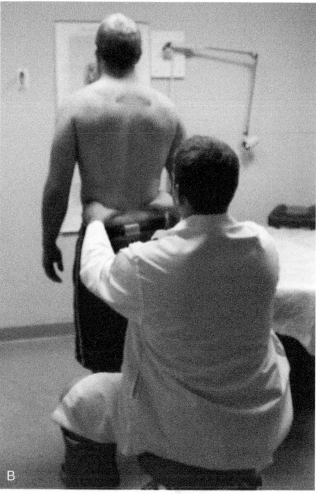

Figure 7.4   Inspection. **A,** Assessment of shoulder height. **B,** Assessment of iliac crest height.

PALPATION

Palpatory examination in ambulatory patients begins in the standing position, usually with the examiner placing their fingers along the tops of the iliac crests with thumbs directed toward the midline L4 to L5 interspinous level. Palpation as such will allow further assessment of iliac crest height and symmetry in patients with obese body habitus that obscures visual examination. While the patient is standing, the spinous processes are palpated sequentially, not only to evaluate for pain but also for the presence of a possible step-off deformity from one level to the next, which may be indicative of spondylolisthesis. Palpation of the paraspinal musculature is performed to identify tender or trigger points as well as regions of muscle spasm; tenderness may be found in regions of referred pain such as the gluteal musculature. Midline palpation may elicit pain with symptomatic intervertebral disc disorders. Tenderness to palpation or percussion of the vertebrae should be noted because it may be suggestive of metastasis, compression fractures, or osteomyelitis and should be correlated with the patient's history. Deyo and others[30] described palpation of soft tissue and bony tenderness as having both poor reproducibility (kappa coefficient [κ] = 0.40) and specificity; however, it is essential to perform. To complete the examination, palpation of the posterior superior iliac spines, iliac crests, the greater trochanters, and ischial tuberosities are all important in localizing the etiology of the patient's symptoms.

RANGE OF MOTION

Lumbar ROM is used to measure impairment and identify restrictions in patients with LBP. The literature supports greater accuracy of passive range assessment over active range assessment.[31] Motion must be assessed in all planes, document any side-to-side differences. ROM may be affected by age and sex.[32] Total sagittal ROM, flexion angle, and extension angle decline as age increases.[33] A comprehensive normative database of lumbar ROM indices was determined by Troke and associates,[34] who examined 405 asymptomatic subjects (Table 7.1).

Mellor and colleagues[35] found greater variations in proportional motion between lumbar vertebrae in subjects with LBP versus controls using quantitative fluoroscopy. In a systematic review and meta-analysis, Laird and associates[36] found that on average, persons with LBP have reduced lumbar ROM and proprioception and move more slowly than healthy counterparts.

Table 7.1   Maximum and Minimum Median Ranges of Lumbar Spinal Motion Across All Subjects (Overall Age Range of Subjects, 16 to 90 Years)

Movement	Male		Female	
	Max	Min	Max	Min
	(Median of Values) (Deg)		(Median of Values) (Deg)	
Flexion	73	40	68	40
Extension	29	7	28	6
Right lateral flexion	28	15	27	14
Left lateral flexion	28	16	28	18
Right axial rotation	7	7	8	8
Left axial rotation	7	7	6	6

Reproduced with permission from Troke M, Moore AP, Maillardet FJ, et al. A normative database of lumbar spine ranges of motion. Man Ther 2005;10:198-206.

Table 7.2   Segmental Range of Motion (in Degrees)

Level	Flexion	Extension	Lateral Bending	Axial Twist
L1/L2	8	5	6	2
L2/L3	10	3	6	2
L3/L4	12	1	8	2
L4/L5	13	2	6	2
L5/S1	9	5	3	5

Reproduced with permission from McGill SM. Low Back Disorders: Evidence-based Prevention and Rehabilitation. Champaign, IL: Human Kinetics; 2002.

Studies have measured lateral flexion from different reference points, which has led to differing normative data. Using T12–L1 to L5–S1 as the reference points for measuring lateral flexion, the range on both sides was 49 to 77 degrees,[37] and Pearcy and associates[38,39] measured the segmental ROM of the spine (Table 7.2).

A common starting measurement is forward flexion, which is composed of both lumbar and pelvic movement.[40,41] It is generally considered that the first 60 degrees takes place in the lumbar spine, while any further motion takes place in the hips; however, strict measurements validating this have not been performed.[42] Torso flexion is accomplished with a combination of hip and lumbar spine motion.[42] Caillet[43] has demonstrated that the initial 45 degrees of trunk flexion is essentially the reversal of lumbar lordosis and that the remainder of the motion is a result of pelvic rotation.

Radiographic analysis is considered the gold standard for determining ROM; there is no physical examination gold standard to measure ROM of the lumbar spine in the peer-reviewed literature.[44] Studies have used external measurements with comparison with plain radiographs with inconsistent findings.[45,46] Mayer and coworkers[47] and Saur and associates[48] have found good correlation between these measurements. Mayer and coworkers[47] found no significant differences between radiographic ROM measurements and noninvasive inclinometer techniques. Saur and associates[48] found a very close correlation ($R = 0.93$) of ROM taken with and without radiologic evaluation using an inclinometer. A systematic review by Littlewood and May[44] indicated limited positive evidence that the double inclinometer method is valid for measuring total lumbar ROM, conflicting evidence for double inclinometer measurement of flexion range, and limited evidence that the modified–modified Schober test is not valid for measurement of lumbar flexion range.

FINGERTIPS-TO-FLOOR

The finger-to-floor distance integrates lumbar spine and hip ROM. Patients stand with their knees extended and bend forward towards the floor. The distance between the fully extended middle finger and floor can be measured or visually estimated. When used quantitatively, the intratester reliability has been shown to be 76% and the intertester reliability 83% for using this method.[49] The specificity of this method has been shown to be 88.8% with a sensitivity of 45.3%.[50,51] Robinson and Mengshoel[52] obtained a smallest detectable change of 9.8 cm at which an examiner can be certain a change has occurred. In a study evaluating 111 adolescents aged 12 to 14 years, finger-to-floor distance achieved an acceptable intrarater and interrater agreement (ICC ≥ 0.75), although the study was limited to comparison between two experienced chiropractors.[52a] Observation of the maneuver can expose limitations in pelvic mobility if the motion is noted to initiate and maintain primarily in the lumbar spine, potentially secondary to tight hamstring musculature.

Right and left lateral flexion of the lumbar spine is assessed similarly. Thomas et al.[53] evaluated 344 patients with new-onset LBP and 118 individuals without LBP. Lateral flexion was measured as the distance covered by the fingertips on the lateral thigh. Right lateral flexion had a sensitivity of 23% and a specificity of 94%, while left lateral flexion had a sensitivity of 26% and a specificity of 92%.

SCHOBER TEST AND MODIFICATIONS THEREOF

In 1937, Schober first described a test to measure segmental motion of the lumbar spine.[54] It is described as follows:

> The first sacral spinous process is marked, and a mark is made about 10 cm above this mark. The patient then flexes forward, and the increased distance is measured. If there is normal motion of the lumbar spine with absence of disease, there should be an increase of 4–5 cm.

This test is used only to measure flexion, with intratester variation reported to be just 4.8%.[55] The Schober test has been criticized because of the difficulty in isolating surface landmarks through different depths of subcutaneous tissue.[56] A smallest detectable change of 1.8 cm was determined by Robinson and Mengshoel.[52] In a study comparing subjects with ankylosing spondylitis with healthy control participants, Rezvani and colleagues[57] found excellent intrarater reliability but only a weak correlation between the Schober test and radiographically analyzed spinal motion.

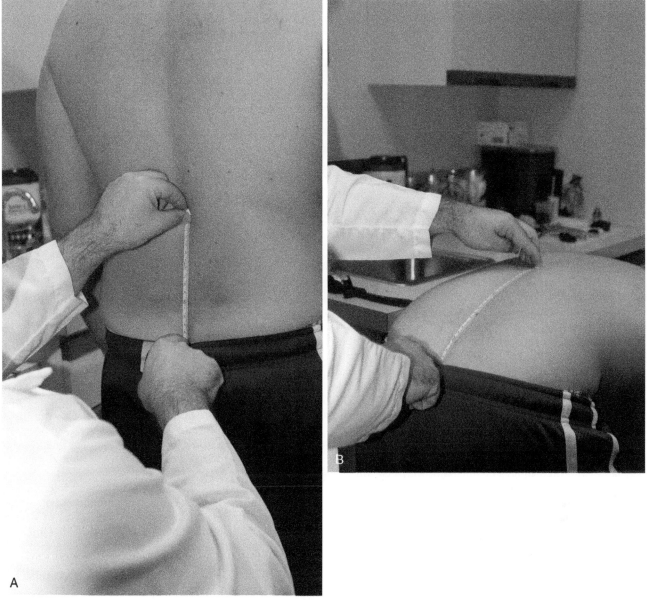

Figure 7.5 A, Modified Schober technique (neutral standing). **B,** Modified Schober technique (full flexion).

MODIFIED SCHOBER TEST

In 1969, Moll and Wright[58] modified the Schober technique for the assessment of patients with ankylosing spondylitis and others, with the addition of a mark 5 cm below S1. It is described as follows:

> With the subject standing erect but relaxed, a point is drawn with a skin marker at the spinal intersection of a line joining the dimples of Venus (S1). Additional marks are made 10 cm above and 5 cm below S1. Subjects are asked to bend forward. The distance between the marks 10 cm above and 5 cm below S1 is measured.

The rationale for this modification was an observation that, on forward flexion, both the lumbosacral junction and superiorly placed 10-cm skin marks tended to move less relative to the spinous processes and the skin than the previously used mark 5 cm inferior to the sacrum (Fig. 7.5).[59]

Reynolds[60] found this measurement of motion to have good reliability in flexion and extension, with reasonable variation in flexion. Fitzgerald and others[61] reported a Pearson correlation coefficient of 1.0 for lumbar flexion and 0.88 for lumbar extension in a study of young healthy subjects. Rezvani and associates[57] found that the modified Schober test reflected spinal mobility better than the original Schober test.

Gill and colleagues[62] concluded that the modified Schober method was the most reproducible method of measurement. The coefficient of variation (CV) was excellent, ranging from 0.9% for flexion and 2.8% for extension.

Miller and associates[63] noted overall good interrater reliability ($R = 0.71$) of the modified Schober method. Potential errors that affect the reliability of this clinical test were (1) the presence or absence of dimples of Venus, (2) anatomic location of the dimples of Venus, (3) anatomic variability of the 10 cm line, (4) problems introduced by skin distraction, and (5) problems in developing a normative database. Stankovic and coworkers[64] noted an intrarater correlation coefficient of 0.95 and an interrater correlation coefficient of 0.94 utilizing the modified Schober test. Thomas and others[51] determined the specificity to be 95% and sensitivity to be 25% when comparing patients with and without LBP.

Viitanen and associates[65] compared the modified Schober test with the thoracolumbar flexion measure using a simple tape method and correlated the results with radiologic changes in patients with ankylosing spondylitis (AS). The Schober test and tape methods correlated fairly highly (modified Schober $R = 0.71$, 0.62; tape method $R = 0.49$, 0.42) with radiologic changes. Macrae and Wright[25] found the validity of modified Schober against radiographs was strong ($r = 0.97$) while Rahali-Khachlouf[66] found it to be moderate ($r = 0.59$).

In conclusion, the modified Schober test has been found to be moderately reproducible and specific but not sensitive when examining patients with and without LBP, and at least moderately reflects lumbar spine motion compared to radiographs.[57,67]

MODIFIED–MODIFIED SCHOBER TEST

The modified–modified Schober technique was first described by Van Adrichem and Van der Korst in 1973.[68] Williams and associates[59] reported interrater reliability, with Pearson correlation coefficients from 0.72 for flexion and 0.76 for extension, using the further modified Schober technique.

Tousignant and colleagues[69] examined 31 subjects with LBP and found moderate validity with the gold standard of radiography, with a Pearson correlation coefficient of 0.67. This is in contrast to Rezvani and coworkers[57] who found it reflected spinal motion poorly in subjects with ankylosing spondylitis. Therefore, the modified–modified Schober (MMS) test may be more a valid ROM measurement in patients with LBP of nonspondylarthritic origin.

INCLINOMETER

An inclinometer is a handheld, circular, fluid-filled disc with a weighted gravity pendulum that remains vertically oriented. The inclinometer technique has been described using single and dual techniques, with dual inclinometry demonstrating superior results. Dual inclinometry requires one inclinometer to be placed on the sacrum to measure hip motion and the other placed on the first lumbar vertebra to measure hip and lumbar ROM. Loebl[70] described a method of measuring four spinal segments with one inclinometer placed on the T12 spinous process and the other at a point 15 cm above the S1 spinal level. This test was based on the assumption that the curvature of the spine can be determined by the angle formed by the tangent of one point on the curve with the tangent of another point on the curve.[49] ROM is then measured by calculating the differences between angles measured while the back is in neutral, flexed, and extended positions.

The AMA Guides to the Evaluation of Permanent Impairment, 5th edition[70a], recommends the use of dual inclinometry for measuring lumbar ROM with techniques as described by Loebl. Nattrass[71] evaluated the validity of spinal ROM methods as outlined in the second and fourth editions of the AMA Guidelines for Impairment and Disability. Comparing goniometry and dual inclinometry, interrater and intrarater reliability were found to be poor (Pearson correlation coefficient ranges from −0.38 to 0.54) with measurement error for thoracolumbar and lumbar movements as large as ± 30 degrees, with the smallest error being 9 degrees. Reliability measures have varied greatly in the literature (Table 7.3).[71]

With the development and use of computerized digital inclinometers (CDIs), their reliability and validity have been studied. MacDermid and coworkers[79] measured sagittal plane ROM in 20 subjects with LBP and 20 without, comparing CDIs with the MMS test. They found high to very high intratrial reliability for both methods (ICC 0.85 to 0.96 for CDI and 0.84 to 0.98 for MMS); however, intertrial reliability of the CDI was poor to moderate, and poor correlations were found between the CDI and MMS for flexion measurements. Bedekar and associates[80] found moderate to high reliability of an iPod with goniometer software, but they did not compare it with standard measurement devices. Kolber and colleagues[81] compared an iPhone inclinometer with dual bubble inclinometry in 30 asymptomatic subjects and found good intrarater and interrater reliability with nearly equivalent ICCs for bubble inclinometry (≥0.81) and the iPhone application (≥0.80). Validity between the two devices was good with an ICC ≥ 0.86, but it was noted that individual differences of up to 18 degrees may exist when devices were used interchangeably.

The inclinometer can be used to measure lateral flexion, which is determined by subtracting measurements between the T12 and sacral inclinometers, with good to excellent intrarater reliability (0.60 to 0.96).[56,71,73,77] Ohlen and others[82] measured 82 degrees of lateral flexion with a COV of 19%.

In conclusion, the inclinometer is moderately reliable but is not consistent in patients with LBP.

NEUROLOGIC EXAMINATION

MANUAL MOTOR TESTING (Video 7-2)

Strength assessment is typically performed in a sequential manner, evaluating muscle groups innervated by different peripheral nerves and nerve roots. Lumbar radiculopathy is usually characterized by weaknesses affecting two or more muscles from the same spinal segment but different peripheral nerves. For example, an L5 radiculopathy may affect both the dorsiflexors of the foot and toes (peroneal nerve) and abduction of the hip (superior gluteal nerve). The strength examination should include the assessment of the hip flexors (L1–L3), quadriceps (L2–L4), tibialis anterior (L4–L5), extensor hallucis longus (L5), and gastrocnemius-soleus (S1). The latter muscle may be assessed via the performance of 10 toe raises (unilaterally) or the ability to ambulate on toes.[40,41] Functional testing of the hip abductors should be performed with the patient

Table 7.3 Tests of Lumbar Spine Motion

Test	Description	Reliability/Validity Tests	Comments
Fingertips to floor	The subject is asked to stand erect with knees extended and bend forward as far as possible. The distance between the middle finger and the floor is measured with a measuring tape.	Merrit et al. 1986[49] Intratester reliability: 76% Intertester reliability: 83% The specificity of this method has been shown to be 88.8% with a sensitivity of 45.3%.[51,53]	Not specific for lumbar spine because it assesses both lumbar and hip motion Smallest detectable change of 9.8 cm at which an examiner can be certain a change has occurred[52]
	Lateral flexion of lumbar spine can be measured in a similar manner.		

		Thomas et al. 1998[53]
		Right lateral flexion:
		  Sensitivity: 23%
		  Specificity: 94%
		Left lateral flexion:
		  Sensitivity: 26%
		  Specificity: 92%
			Compared spinal ROM in 344 patients with new-onset LBP with 118 without LBP. The subject stood with head and buttocks pressed against the wall with no knee flexion, and was asked to bend sideways.[53]

Schober test	The first sacral spinous process is marked, and a mark is made about 10 cm above this mark. The patient then flexes forward, and the increased distance between marks is measured.[56]	Biering-Sorensen 1984[55]
		Intratester variation reported to be only 4.8%.
		
		Rahali-Khachlouf et al. 2001[66]
		Reliability:
		  Strong intrarater: (r = 0.96)
		  Strong interrater: (r = 0.90)
		Robinson and Mengshoel 2014[52]
		Smallest detectable change of 1.8 cm
		Validity correlation with radiographic data:
		Macrae and Wright 1969[25]
		Strong (r = 0.90)
		Rahali-Khachlouf et al. 2001[66]
		Moderate (r = 0.68)
			Schober test is only used to measure flexion
			Criticized for difficulty in isolating surface landmarks with different tissue depths

Modified Schober test	With the subject standing erect but relaxed, a point is drawn with a skin marker at the spinal intersection of a line joining the dimples of Venus (S1). Additional marks are made 10 cm above and 5 cm below S1. Subjects are asked to bend forward. The distance between the marks 10 cm above and 5 cm below S1 is measured.[25]	Reynolds 1975[60]
		Pearson correlation coefficients:
		  0.59 for lumbar flexion
		  0.75 for extension
		COV:
		  11.65% for flexion
		  21.57% for extension
		
		Fitzgerald et al. 1983[61]
		Pearson correlation coefficients:
		  1.00 for lumbar flexion
		  0.88 for lumbar extension
		
		Gill et al. 1988[62]
		COV:
		  0.9% for flexion
		  2.8% for extension	

			Study performed on young healthy subjects, may not translate to older individuals
			Concluded that modified Schober method was most reproducible method of measurement as compared to fingertip-to-floor, modified–modified Schober, inclinometer, and photometric techniques
		Miller et al. 1992[63] Interrater reliability: 0.71	Potential errors: (1) Presence or absence of dimples of Venus (2) Anatomic location of the dimples of Venus (3) Anatomic variability of the 10-cm line (4) Problems introduced by skin distraction (5) Problems in developing a normative database

Continued on following page

Table 7.3   Tests of Lumbar Spine Motion (Continued)

Test	Description	Reliability/Validity Tests	Comments
		Rahali-Khachlouf et al. 2001[66] Interrater reliability: 0.92 Intra-rater reliabilitiy: 0.96	
		Stankovic et al. 1999[64] Intrarater CC: 0.95 Interrater CC: 0.94	
		Thomas et al. 1998[53] Specificity: 95% Sensitivity: 25%	Comparing patients with and without LBP
		Validity correlation with radiographic data:	In patients with AS

		Viitanen et al. 1999[65]
		    Moderate to strong
		    (r = 0.71, 0.62)
		    Macrae and Wright 1969[25]
		    Strong (r = 0.97)
		    Rahali-Khachlouf et al. 2001[66]
		    Moderate (r = 0.59)	

Modified–modified Schober test	The PSISs are identified and a mark is made on the midline of the lumbar spines horizontal to the PSIS. Another mark is placed on the spinous processes 15 cm superior to the PSIS line. A tape measure is aligned between the two marks, and the patient is asked to bend forward or backward depending on the motion being measured. The new distance between the markings is measured. The difference between the two measurements is recorded.[68]	Van Adrichmem and Van der Korst[68]
		Pearson correlation coefficients:
		    Lumbar flexion: 0.78 and 0.89
		    Lumbar extension: 0.69 and 0.91
		Interrater reliability:
		    Flexion: 0.72
		    Extension 0.76
		
		Williams et al. 1993[59]
		Interrater reliability:
		    Flexion: 0.72
		    Extension: 0.76
		Rezvani et al. 2012[57]
		Intrarater reliability:
		    Flexion: 0.97
		
		Validity correlation with radiographic data:
		
		Tousignant et al. 2005[69]
		Moderately valid
		Pearson correlation coefficient 0.67
		
		Rezvani et al. 2012[57]
		No validity established	

Inclinometer	Dual inclinometry requires one inclinometer to be placed on the sacrum to measure hip motion and the other placed on the first lumbar vertebra to measure hip and lumbar range of motion. ROM is then measured by calculating the differences between angles measured while the back is in neutral, flexed, and extended positions.	Nattrass et al. 1999[71] Pearson correlation coefficient ranged from −0.38 to 0.54 Measurement error for thoracolumbar and lumbar movements as large as ±30 degrees, with the smallest error being 9 degrees.	Evaluated the validity of spinal ROM methods as outlined in the second and fourth editions of the *AMA Guidelines for Impairment and Disability*; compared goniometry and dual inclinometer

		Reynolds 1975[60]
		Intertester reliability:
		    Flexion, R = 0.76
		    Extension, R = 0.87
			Standard inclinometer

Table 7.3   Tests of Lumbar Spine Motion (Continued)

Test	Description	Reliability/Validity Tests	Comments
		Burdett et al. 1986[45] Intertester reliability: 　Flexion, R = 0.73 　Extension R = 0.15	Gravity inclinometer
		Merrit et al. 1986[49] Intertester reliability: 　CV flexion: 9.6 　CV extension: 65.4 Intratester reliability: 　CV flexion: 13.4 　CV extension: 50.7	Standard inclinometer
		Dillard et al. 1991[72] Intertester reliability: 　Flexion, $R = 0.78$ 　Extension, $R = 0.27$ Intratester reliability: 　Lateral flexion, $R = 0.66$	Dual inclinometer
		Saur et al. 1996[48] Intertester reliability: 　Flexion, $R = 0.88$ 　Extension, $R = 0.94$	Standard inclinometer
		Ng et al. 2001[73] Intratester reliability: 　Flexion, $R = 0.87$ 　Extension, $R = 0.92$ 　Right lateral flexion, $R = 0.96$ 　Left lateral flexion, $R = 0.94$ 　Right axial rotation, $R = 0.96$ 　Left axial rotation, $R = 0.94$	Modified inclinometer with pelvic restraint
		Dopf et al. 1994[74] Intratester reliability: 　$R = 0.93$	
		Nattrass et al. 1999[71] Intratester reliability 　Flexion, $R = 0.90$ 　Extension, $R = 0.70$ 　Lateral flexion, $R = 0.89$–0.90	Dual inclinometer
		Williams et al. 1993[59] Intratester reliability: 　Flexion, $R = 0.13$–0.87 　Extension, $R = 0.28$–0.66	
		Keeley et al. 1986[75] Intratester reliability: 　Extension, $R = 0.90$–0.96	Dual inclinometer
		Portek et al. 1983[46] Intratester reliability: 　Flexion, $R = 0.86$	Standard inclinometer
		Mellin 1986,1987[76-78] Intratester reliability: 　Flexion, $R = 0.86$ 　Extension, $R = 0.93$ 　Lateral flexion, $R = 0.6$–0.85	Dual inclinometer
		Gill et al. 1994[62] Intratester reliability: 　CV flexion: 9.3–33.9 　CV extension: 3.6–4.7	Dual inclinometer

AS, Ankylosing spondylitis; *CC,* correlation coefficient; *CV,* coefficient of variation; *LBP,* low back pain; *PSIS,* posterior superior iliac spine; *ROM,* range of motion.

standing on one leg to evaluate for the presence of a Trendelenburg sign, noted as a sagging of the iliac crest on the unloaded side.

Several studies have looked at the sensitivity and specificity of muscle strength testing in patients with lumbar radiculopathy (Table 7.4). Kerr and coworkers[85] demonstrated reduced ankle dorsiflexion in 54% and plantar flexion in 13% of those with lumbar disc protrusions from L4 to S1 with an overall specificity of 89%. Weakness of the extensor hallucis longus had a sensitivity of 12% to 51% with a specificity of 72% to 91% for detecting L5 radiculopathy, whereas weak ankle plantar flexors had an overall specificity between 26% and 99% in detecting S1 radiculopathy. In a cross-sectional study, Ortiz-Corredor[89] correlated physical exam findings to abnormal electromyogram (EMG) findings in LBP patients and found weak plantar flexors were highly specific (97.5%), but weak quadriceps were poorly sensitive (35.67%). In a small retrospective chart review of 28 patients, Iizuka and colleagues[92] found that the most common condition causing a foot drop (manual muscle testing grade of 0 to 3) was compression of two nerve roots. A systematic review and meta-analysis by Al Nezari and others[93] in 2013 determined that motor testing for paresis showed low pooled sensitivities (22% to 40%) and moderate specificities (62% to 79%) for surgically and radiologically determined disc herniations, while motor testing in muscle atrophy exhibited a pooled sensitivity of 32% and a specificity of 76% for surgically determined disc herniations.

SENSORY EXAMINATION (Video 7-3)

The sensory exam should cover the bilateral lower extremities to evaluate for true dermatomal or more diffuse sensory loss as seen in peripheral neuropathies with a "stocking" distribution of loss. Dermatomes define the area of skin innervated by a single nerve root or peripheral nerve (Fig. 7.6). Sensation can be evaluated using many different modalities, including vibration, proprioception, temperature, light touch, and pinprick. The latter two are more commonly used in the neurologic evaluation, although vibration may be more sensitive for injury to large-diameter sensory nerves and proprioception loss may be indicative of posterior column dysfunction such as vitamin B_{12} deficiency and syphilis.[68] The sensitivity and specificity of the sensory examination in the diagnosis of lumbar disc herniation has been described in the literature (see Table 7.4). Suri and

Table 7.4   Neurologic Exam as a Test for Lumbar Disc Herniation

Test	Description	Reliability/Validity Tests	Comments
Muscle strength testing	Assessment of strength must be performed in a sequential manner, evaluating muscle groups innervated by different peripheral nerves and nerve roots. Radiculopathy is characterized by weaknesses affecting two or more muscles from the same spinal segment but different peripheral nerves.	Spangfort 1971[33] Ankle dorsiflexor weakness: Sensitivity: 49% Specificity: 54% Hakelius and Hindmarsh 1970[83] and Hakelius 1972[84] Ankle dorsiflexor weakness: Sensitivity: 20% Specificity: 82% Ankle plantar flexor weakness: Sensitivity: 6% Specificity: 95%	Tested ankle dorsiflexor in 2504 patients; 70–90% of patients with weakness had HNP at L4/L5 level
	The examination should include hip flexors (L1–L3), quadriceps (L2–L4), tibialis anterior (L4–L5), extensor hallucis longus (L5), and the gastrocnemius/soleus complex (S1).	Great-toe extensor weakness: Sensitivity: 37% Specificity: 71% Quadriceps weakness: Sensitivity: <1% Specificity: 99% Kerr et al. 1988[85] Ankle dorsiflexor weakness: Sensitivity: 54% Specificity: 89% Ankle plantar flexor weakness: Sensitivity: 13% Specificity: 100%	
		Kortelainen et al. 1985[86] Ankle dorsiflexor weakness: Sensitivity: 57%	32% HNP at L4/L5 57% HNP at L5/S1
		Knutsson 1961[87] Ankle dorsiflexor weakness: Sensitivity: 63% Specificity: 52%	For L5 root specifically, the sensitivity was 76%, and the specificity was 52%.

Table 7.4   Neurologic Exam as a Test for Lumbar Disc Herniation (Continued)

Test	Description	Reliability/Validity Tests	Comments

		Lauder 2002[88]
		Great-toe extensor weakness:
		    Sensitivity: 61%
		    Specificity: 55%
		Quadriceps weakness:
		    Sensitivity: 40%
		    Specificity: 89%
		Ankle plantar flexor weakness:
		    Sensitivity: 47%
		    Specificity: 76%	

		Ortiz-Corredor 2003[89]
		Ankle plantar flexor weakness:
		    Specificity: 97%
		Quadriceps weakness:
		    Sensitivity 35.67%
			Compared EMG with physical exam

Muscle stretch reflex	Tapping the test tendon stretches the spindle and activates its fibers. Afferent projections from these fibers synapse with the alpha motor neurons, which in turn send impulses to the skeletal muscles, resulting in a brief contraction. This contraction is graded on a standard scale.	Spangfort 1971[33]
		Ankle:
		    Sensitivity: 50%
		    Specificity: 62%
		Patella:
		    Sensitivity: 4%
		    Specificity: 97%
			Ankle: HNP at L5/S1 level in 80%–90% for ages 20–45 years and 60% older than 50 years
			Patella: Sensitivity of 50% in L3/L4 HNP. In 67% of cases of impairment, HNP is at L4/L5 and L5/S1 levels.

		Hakelius and Hindmarsh 1970[83] and Hakelius 1972[84]
		Ankle:
		    Sensitivity: 52%
		    Specificity: 63%
		Patella:
		    Sensitivity: 7%
		    Specificity: 93%	

		Knutsson 1961[87]
		Ankle:
		    Sensitivity: 56%
		    Specificity: 57%
		Patella:
		    Sensitivity: 15%
		    Specificity: 67%
			For S1, the sensitivity was 79%, and the specificity was 62%.

		Kerr et al. 1988[85]
		    Sensitivity: 48%
		    Specificity: 89%
			For L3–L4, the sensitivity was 10%, and the specificity was 85%.

		Lauder 2002[88]
		Ankle:
		    Sensitivity: 47%
		    Specificity: 90%
		Patella:
		    Sensitivity: 50%
		    Specificity: 93%
			For L5–S1, the sensitivity was 78%, and the specificity was 88%.

		Kortelainen et al. 1985[86] Sensitivity: 7%	

		Suri et al. 2011[90]
		Ankle:
		    Sensitivity: 33%
		    Specificity: 91%
		    Likelihood ratio: 3.9
			In 85% of cases of impairment, HNP is at L4–L5 and L5/S1.

		Patella:
		    Sensitivity: 39%
		    Specificity: 95%
		    Likelihood ratio: 7.7
			For L5 impingement

Continued on following page

Table 7.4   Neurologic Exam as a Test for Lumbar Disc Herniation (Continued)

Test	Description	Reliability/Validity Tests	Comments

		Iversen et al. 2013[95a]
		Ankle:
		  Sensitivity: 44%
		  Specificity: 61%
		Patella:
		  Sensitivity: 67%
		  Specificity: 83%
			For L4 impingement
			For L4 impingement
			
			For S1 impingement

Sensory Exam	The sensory examination should cover the bilateral lower extremities to evaluate for dermatomal or diffuse sensory loss. Sensation is evaluated using different modalities, including vibration, proprioception, temperature, light touch, and pinprick.	Kerr et al. 1988[85]
		  Sensitivity: 16%
		  Specificity: 86%
		
		Knutsson 1961[87]
		  Sensitivity: 29%
		  Specificity: 67%
		
		Kosteljanetz et al. 1984[91]
		  Sensitivity: 66%
		  Specificity: 51%
		
		Kortelainen et al. 1985[86]
		  Sensitivity: 38%
		
		Lauder 2002[88]
		  Sensitivity: 50%
		  Specificity: 62%
		
		Suri et al. 2011[90]
		Anterior thigh pinprick:
		  Sensitivity: 50%
		  Specificity: 96%
		  Positive likelihood ratio: 13
		
		Medial ankle pinprick:
		  Sensitivity: 31%
		  Specificity: 100%
		  Positive likelihood ratio:
		    infinity
			
			For L2 impingement
			
			For L4 impingement

EMG, Electromyogram; *HNP,* herniated nucleus pulposus.

coworkers[90] examined pinprick testing at the anterior thigh, medial knee, medial ankle, great toe, and lateral foot for sensitivity and specificity for mid lumbar and low lumbar nerve root impingement as well as level-specific nerve root impingement. For mid lumbar and low lumbar impingement, sensitivities ranged from 0% to 21%, though specificities ranged from 79% to 100%, with the highest specificities and significant likelihood ratios observed for the medial knee and medial ankle in mid lumbar nerve root impingement. For level-specific impingement, anterior thigh pinprick sensation was 50% sensitive and 96% specific and had a positive likelihood ratio (LR) of 13 for L2 impingement, while medial ankle pinprick was 31% sensitive and 100% specific and had an LR approaching infinity for L4 nerve root impingement.

REFLEX EXAMINATION (Video 7-4)

A reflex is the involuntary contraction of muscles induced by a specific stimulus. Tendon reflex activity depends on the status of the alpha motor neurons, the muscle spindles and their afferent fibers, and the gamma neurons whose axons terminate on intrafusal muscle fibers within the spindles. Rapid distension of the tendon stretches the spindle and activates its fibers. Afferent projections form these fiber synapses with the alpha motor neurons, which in turn send impulses to the skeletal muscles resulting in the familiar brief muscle contraction or monophasic stretch reflex.

The reflex is usually named after the muscle being tested. Common stretch reflexes include the quadriceps or patellar reflex involving the L2 to L4 spinal levels, medial hamstring reflex at the L5 level, and Achilles reflex involving the S1 level (Fig. 7.7). A 5-point grading system recommended by the National Institute of Neurological Disorders and Stroke is the most commonly used scale (Table 7.5).[68] Eliciting reflexes may be difficult in the patient who is unable to relax. In 1885, Jendrassik described a technique to elicit reflexes by having the patient "hook together the flexed fingers of his right and left hands and pull them apart as

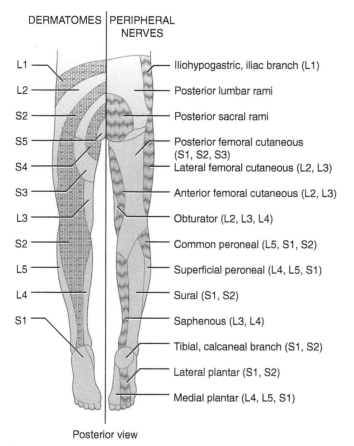

Posterior view

Figure 7.6 Dermatomes and peripheral nerve distribution of the lower extremities. (Adapted with permission from Borenstein, Wiesel, and Boden; Low Back and Neck Pain: comprehensive diagnosis and management. 3rd edition (2004). Chapter 5, Figure 5-14, page 123.)

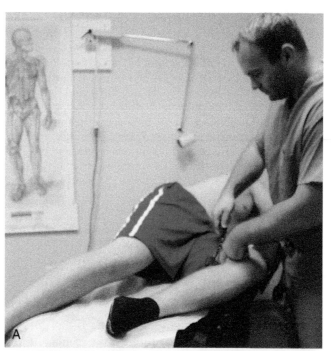

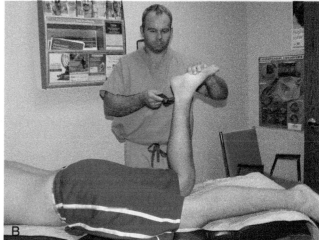

Figure 7.7   A, Medial hamstring reflex. **B,** Prone technique for eliciting Achilles reflex.

strongly as possible" while the clinician taps on the tendon; this enhances the reflexes of patients.

Absent or exaggerated reflexes by themselves do not signify neurologic disease. In older adults, up to 50% without neurologic disease lack an Achilles reflex bilaterally.[68] Small percentages (3% to 5%) of normal individuals have generalized hyperreflexia.[94]

Absent or exaggerated reflex is significant only when it is associated with one of the following clinical settings:

1. The absent reflex is associated with other findings of lower motor neuron disease.
2. The exaggerated reflex is associated with other findings of upper motor neuron disease.
3. The reflex amplitude is asymmetric.
4. The reflex is unusually brisk compared with reflexes from a higher spinal level.[68]

Deyo and others[30] reviewed the relevance of the physical examination in patients with LBP (see Table 7.4). Andersson and Deyo[95] noted a specificity of 0.60 and a sensitivity of 0.50 for the Achilles reflex in diagnosing lumbar disc injury. In patients with a high probability (> 60%) of a herniated disc (which is based on the clinicians' patient population and

Table 7.5	Classification of Muscle Stretch Reflexes
0	Absent
+	Present but reduced
++	Normal
+++	Increased, possibly normal
++++	Greatly increased, often associated with clonus

Reproduced with permission from Nicholas J. Talley and Simon O'Connor. Clinical examination: A systematic guide to physical diagnosis, 7e. Churchill Livingstone, 2014.

the prevalence of LBP), the positive predictive value for an impaired Achilles reflex was 0.65 with a negative predictive value of 0.44. However, in patients with a low probability of a herniated disc, the positive predictive value was 0.04 with a negative predictive value of 0.98. Suri and associates[90] determined a 39% sensitivity, 95% specificity, and significant LR of 7.7 for L4 impingement if the patellar reflex was affected, and a 33% sensitivity, 91% specificity, and LR of 3.9 for L5 impingement if the ankle reflex was affected. Iversen and coworkers[95a] found the knee reflex to be 67% sensitive and 83% specific for L4 impingement and the ankle reflex to be 44% sensitive and 61% specific for S1 impingement.

PROVOCATIVE LUMBAR SPINE MANEUVERS

STRAIGHT-LEG RAISE TEST (Video 7-5)

Lasègue's sign, or straight-leg raise (SLR) test, was initially described by J. J. Frost, a student of Charles Lasègue in 1881, who memorialized his mentor through the naming of this test. In the described test, pain was induced in the distribution of the sciatic nerve upon lifting the leg while maintaining it extended via pressure on the knee. Frost suspected that the activation of pain during this maneuver was the result of pressure from the hamstring on the nerve.[85] Lazarevic described this test in 1880, 1 year earlier than Frost, after he observed six patients to have increased pain during stretching of the sciatic nerve.[96]

Lazarevic described a three-step approach to the test[97]:

In the first step, the patient was asked to flex forward, maintaining his knees straight. In step 2, the patient was asked to lie supine and his trunk was slowly brought into flexion, maintaining his knees extended. In step 3, the supine patient had his leg raised with the knee extended. Elevation of the leg was stopped when the patient began to feel pain, and the angle of elevation and amount of pelvic movement was recorded. The patient was then asked to indicate the distribution of pain. All three maneuvers were noted to reproduce discomfort in the sciatic nerve distribution.

In 1884, Lucien de Beurmann concluded that during the lifting of a stretched leg, pain is evoked by stretching of the nerve rather than from the compression of the muscle.[98] Inman and Saunders[99] noted a 2- to 7-mm distal migration of the spinal nerve roots during performance of straight-leg raising. Falconer and coworkers[100] described a 2- to 6-mm downward migration of the nerve roots through their respective foramen during the test. Goddard and Reid[101] noted the L5 nerve root to move 3 mm and the S1 nerve root to move 4 to 5 mm during performance of SLR. In a recent controlled in vivo radiologic study, Rade and colleagues[102] scanned 16 asymptomatic subjects with a 1.5 T magnetic resonance imaging (MRI) scanner; the displacement of the medullar cone during the SLR was quantified and noted to displace caudally in the spinal canal by 2.31 ± 1.2 mm with right SLR and 2.35 ± 1.2 mm with left SLR, which was speculated to be directly proportional to the sliding of the L5 and S1 nerve roots.

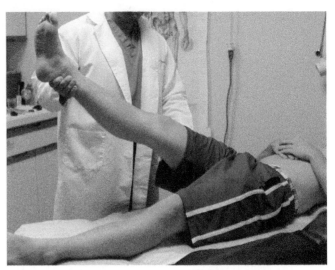

Figure 7.8   Straight-leg raise (SLR) test.

The classic SLR test is considered positive when the supine leg is elevated to between 30 and 70 degrees and pain is reproduced down to the posterior thigh below the knee.[25] Pain below 30 degrees is not considered to be related to nerve root irritation.[103] Kosteljanetz and others[91] noted prolapsed discs in 45 of 52 individuals diagnosed during surgery with a positive SLR on physical examination. In addition, no "typical" Lasègue's sign with pain into the leg was noted beyond 70 degrees of leg elevation. SLRs with pain induced beyond 70 degrees of leg elevation is not believed to be due to nerve root tension. Rather, it is thought likely to be related to tightness within the hamstrings or gluteal muscles (Fig. 7.8).[104]

Several studies have looked at the sensitivity and specificity of the SLR test on physical examination and have compared preoperative results with confirmation at surgery. Spangfort[33] studied 2504 lumbar disc herniation operations and related the incidence of Lasègue's sign to the findings at surgery. He noted that 96.8% of patients with surgically confirmed disc herniations had a positive straight-leg test on physical examination. In patients with herniations from L4 to S1, positive SLR was noted in 96% to 98% of cases, while in those with herniations from L1–L2 to L3–L4, it was positive in only 73%. Of note, 88% of those patients with negative exploration had a positive SLR on examination.

Thomas and associates[51,53] found that SLR testing did not predict the likelihood of disc herniation at operation, although a positive SLR was present in 87% of those with prolapsed discs. The specificity of SLR was 87% with a sensitivity of only 33%. Shiqing and coworkers[104] noted that 98.2% of patients with a positive SLR test had a disc protrusion at a lower lumbar level. In this study, the combination of SLR with ankle dorsiflexion, compression of the peroneal nerve, and flexion of the neck were positive in 70.8%, 73.5%, and 54.8% of subjects, respectively (Fig. 7.9). Kosteljanetz and associates[91,105] found the positive SLR to be present in 49 of 55 patients with unilateral sciatica, 43 of whom had disc pathology at surgery, although the absence of positive SLR did not preclude the presence of a herniated lumbar disc.

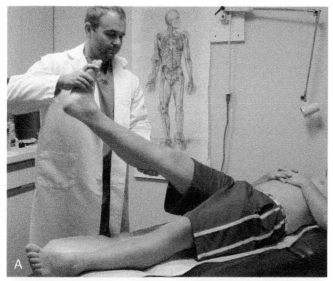

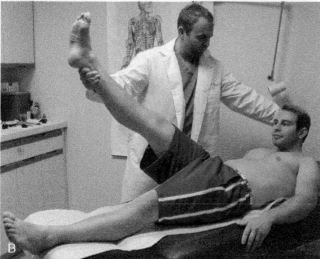

Figure 7.9 Straight-leg raising provocation with ankle dorsiflexion (**A**) and head flexion (**B**).

Andersson and Deyo[95] reported the positive predictive value of the straight-leg test in individuals with a great probability of having a disc herniation to be 67%, whereas the negative predictive value was determined to be 57%. The positive predictive value in patients with a low probability—including patients with no sciatica or neurologic signs or symptoms—was determined to be 4% with a negative predictive value of 99%.

Iglesias-Casarrubios and others[106] found that in 243 patients who underwent hemilaminectomy for herniated lumbar disc, the Lasègue sign assessed 3 months after surgery was predictive for poor functional status at 2 and 3 years, lower return to work, and frequency of reoperation.

Deville and others[107] determined that the pooled sensitivity for the SLR test was 91% (95% confidence interval [CI]: 0.82–0.94), and the pooled specificity was 26% (95% CI: 0.16–0.38). The mean predictive value of a positive test result was 89%, and the negative predictive value was 33%. Deville and colleagues[107] concluded that the studies

evaluated were not representative of the general population, with high prevalence resulting in consequentially higher positive predictive values for SLR. It was also suggested that these studies were prone to verification bias because nearly all studies were retrospective and based on data obtained on surgical patients. Flaws in the design of these studies—including independency of interpretation, verification bias, and retrospective design—were also noted.

Supik and Broom[50] compared the results of the SLR test, Lasègue's sign, ankle dorsiflexion, and crossed SLR (see below) with their patients' postoperative findings. The straight-leg lift was considered positive if hip, buttock, and leg pain were elicited, while Lasègue's sign was performed by raising the leg until pain was elicited then lowering the leg 10 to 15 degrees to reduce discomfort, with subsequent ankle dorsiflexion intensifying the pain. The straight-leg lift was positive in 96% of patients, and Lasègue's sign was positive 71% of the time. In this study of patients, the straight-leg sign was more sensitive than the other maneuvers, independent of level or location of the disc.

Jönsson and Strömqvist[108,109] graded the SLR depending on whether it was positive at 0 to 30 degrees, positive at 30 to 60 degrees, positive at greater than 60 degrees, or negative. In this study, 86% of patients had a positive SLR preoperatively; 42% occurred below 30 degrees, 26% between 30 and 60 degrees, and 18% above 60 degrees. The authors found an almost linear correlation between a positive SLR and pain at rest, pain at night, pain upon coughing, and reduction of walking capacity.

Capra and others[110] performed a retrospective review of 2352 patients with sciatic pain, finding the SLR had a sensitivity of 36% and specificity of 74%; they noted that the discriminative power of the SLR seemed to decrease as age increased, concluding that it may be less conclusive in older patients. In a prospective blinded study, Suri and colleagues[90] found that SLR was 73% sensitive and 63% specific for S1 impingement, while being 69% sensitive and 84% specific for composite lower lumbar impingement (L5 or S1). In a 2010 Cochrane systematic review, van der Windt and colleagues[111] found the SLR to have high sensitivity (pooled estimate, 0.92) with widely varying specificity (0.10 to 1.00; pooled estimate, 0.28) in surgical populations characterized by a high prevalence of disc herniation, although imaging-based studies showed poorer sensitivity. Table 7.6 outlines clinical studies that have examined the prevalence, sensitivity, and specificity of the SLR in lumbar disc herniations. The literature has shown that a positive ipsilateral SLR test is sensitive (72% to 97%) but nonspecific (11% to 66%).[95]

CROSSED STRAIGHT-LEG RAISE TEST (Video 7-6)

In 1901, Fajersztajn first described the crossed straight-leg raise (CSLR) test after noting on cadaveric study that SLR not only stretched the ipsilateral root but also pulled laterally on the dural sac, stretching the opposite root.[129] Woodhall and Hayes[130] demonstrated the CSLR to be strongly predictive for a disc herniation, noting its presence in 92 of 95 subjects with large disc herniations. Hudgins[119] evaluated 351 patients thought to have a herniated disc on physical exam and found the CSLR test result to be positive in 97% of those with a herniated disc; only 64% of subjects with SLR alone had a herniated disc.

Table 7.6 Provocative Maneuvers for Diagnosis of Lumbar Disc Herniation

Test	Description	Reliability/Validity Tests	Comments
Straight-leg raise	The supine patient has his/her leg raised with the knee extended. Elevation of the leg is stopped when the patient begins to feel pain, and the type and distribution of the pain as well as the angle of elevation is recorded.	Charnley 1951[112] Sensitivity: 72% Specificity: 66% Prevalence: 84%	N = 88
		Spangfort 1971[33] Sensitivity: 97% Specificity: 11% Prevalence: 88%	N = 2504 Criteria: leg pain N = 1986 Criteria: leg pain
	The test result is positive when the angle is between 30 and 70 degrees and pain is reproduced down to the posterior thigh below the knee.[113]	Hakelius and Hindmarsh 1970[83] and Hakelius 1972[84] Sensitivity: 96% Specificity: 14% Prevalence: 75%	N = 100
		Kosteljanetz et al. 1988[105] (Leg pain, leg or back pain) Sensitivity: 76%, 91% Specificity: 45%, 21% Prevalence: 58%, 58%	N = 52
		Kosteljanetz et al. 1984[91] (Leg pain, leg or back pain) Sensitivity: 89%, 95% Specificity: 17%, 14% Prevalence: 86%, 86%	Data compiled from the following: Edgar and Park,[114] Kosteljanetz et al.,[91,105] Gurdjian et al.,[115] Jönsson and Strömqvist,[108] Shiqing et al.,[104] Spangfort,[33] Kerr et al.,[85] Knuttson,[87] Aronson et al.,[116] Kortelainen,[86] Albeck,[117] Charnley,[112] Hakelius and Hindmarsh,[83] Hirsch and Nachemson[118]
		Deville et al. 2000[107] Pooled data Sensitivity: 91% Specificity: 26%	
		Capra et al. 2011[110] Sensitivity: 36% Specificity: 74%	N = 2352, retrospective. Felt discriminative power decreases with increased age.
		Suri et al. 2011[90] For S-1 impingement: Sensitivity: 73% Specificity: 63% For lower lumbar impingement: Sensitivity: 69% Specificity: 84%	Prospective, blinded study.
		van der Windt et al. 2010[111] Pooled data Sensitivity: 92% Specificity: 28%	Cochrane Systematic Review
Crossed straight-leg raise	Same technique as straight leg raise, but pain elicited with raising contralateral leg.	Spangfort 1972[33a] Sensitivity: 23% Specificity: 88% Prevalence: 86%	N = 2504 straight-leg Criteria: contralateral leg pain
		Hakelius and Hindmarsh 1972[88] Sensitivity: 27% Specificity: 88% Prevalence: 85%	N = 1986 Criteria: contralateral leg pain
		Hudgins 1979[119] Sensitivity: 24% Specificity: 96% Prevalence: 83%	N = 274 Criteria: contralateral leg pain

Table 7.6   Provocative Maneuvers for Diagnosis of Lumbar Disc Herniation (Continued)

Test	Description	Reliability/Validity Tests	Comments
		Kosteljanetz et al. 1984[91] (Contralateral leg pain, contralateral leg or back pain) Sensitivity: 24%, 42% Specificity: 100%, 85% Prevalence: 86%, 86%	N = 52
		Deville et al. 2000[107] Pooled data Sensitivity: 29% Specificity: 88%	Data compiled from the following: Edgar and Park,[114] Kosteljanetz et al.,[91] Jönsson and Strömqvist,[108] Shiqing et al.,[104] Spangfort,[33] Kerr et al.,[85] Knuttson,[87] Hakelius and Hindmarsh[83]
		Poiraudeau et al. 2001[120] Sensitivity: 29% Specificity: 83%	Imaging reference standard
		Suri et al. 2011[90] Sensitivity: 4–7% Midlumbar specificity: 93% Low lumbar specificity: 96%	
		van der Windt et al. 2010[111] Pooled data Sensitivity: 28% Specificity: 90%	Cochrane Systematic Review
Bowstring sign	After a positive straight-leg raise, slightly flex the knee and apply pressure to the tibial nerve in the popliteal fossa. Compression of the sciatic nerve reproduces the leg pain.[121]	Supik and Broom 1994[50] Positive in 71% of patients with known lumbar disc herniation	
Slump test	The patient is seated with legs together and knees against the examining table. The patient slumps forward as far as possible, and the examiner applies firm pressure to bow the subject's back while keeping sacrum vertical. The patient is then asked to flex the head, and pressure is added to the neck flexion. Lastly the examiner asks the subject to extend the knee and dorsiflexion at the ankle is added.[121]	Stankovic et al. 1999[64] Sensitivity for HNP: 82.6% Specificity for HNP: 54.7% Walsh and Hall 2009[122] Substantial agreement with SLR test: κ = 0.69	N = 105 45 subjects with unilateral leg pain
Ankle dorsiflexion test (Braggard sign)	Elevate the leg as in SLR to the point of pain provocation. Drop the leg to a nonpainful range, and dorsiflex the ipsilateral ankle.[113]	No data	Meant to differentiate neural tension from hamstring pain
Femoral nerve stretch test	With the patient prone, the examiner places a palm at the popliteal fossa as the knee is dorsiflexed. Pain is produced in the anterior aspect of the thigh and/or back. A positive test result should produce pain in the distribution of the patient's complaints.	Positive in 84%–95% of patients with a high lumbar disc[123-125] Suri et al. 2011[90] For midlumbar impingement: Sensitivity: 50% Specificity: 100% For L3 impingement on MRI: Sensitivity: 70% Specificity: 88%	Possibly best test for clinical diagnosis of high lumbar disc herniation

Continued on following page

Table 7.6   Provocative Maneuvers for Diagnosis of Lumbar Disc Herniation (Continued)

Test	Description	Reliability/Validity Tests	Comments
Crossed femoral nerve stretch test	With the patient prone, the examiner places a palm at the popliteal fossa as the asymptomatic side's knee is dorsiflexed. Pain is produced in the anterior aspect of the thigh and/or back. A positive test result should produce pain in the distribution of the patient's complaints.	Suri et al. 2011[90] Found no added sensitivity over femoral nerve stretch test	May support diagnosis of high lumbar radiculopathy, but more research needed

Waddell signs	*Distraction tests*: Once a positive physical finding is demonstrated, this finding is then checked with the patient distracted. Findings that are present only on formal examination and not at other times may have a nonorganic component.	McCombe et al. 1989[32]
		Reliability data, κ coefficients:
		  Distraction: −0.16 to 0.40
		  Overreaction: 0.29 to 0.46
		  Abnormal sensory/motor: −0.03 to 0.26
			Kappa agreement coefficients in which a score of 1 signified complete agreement, 0 signified no agreement, and −1 signified complete disagreement of several physical examination signs
			A coefficient of 0.4 was selected for the "cutoff" point for reliability.

	Overreaction: May take the form of extremes of verbalization, facial expression, muscle tension and tremor, collapsing, or sweating.	Simulation: 0.25 to 0.48 Superficial tenderness: 0.17 to 0.29	Kummel[126] assessed limitation of shoulder motion with production of low back pain and low back pain resulting from active cervical motion in addition to Waddell signs.
	Regional disturbances: Involving a widespread region of neighboring parts such as the leg below the knee, entire leg, or quarter or half of the body. The essential feature is divergence from the accepted neuroanatomy.	Carleton et al. 2009[127] If ≥2 Waddell signs: Great depressive symptoms, pain-related anxiety, fear, catastrophizing, and pain intensity	Prognosis for return to work was poor in subjects with positive Waddell signs: 52.9% did not return to work.
	Simulation tests: On formal exam, a particular movement causes the patient to report pain. The movement is then simulated without being performed. If pain is reported, a nonorganic influence is suggested.		
	Tenderness: Nonorganic tenderness may be either superficial or nonanatomic. Superficial: The skin is tender to light pinch over a wide area of lumbar skin. Nonanatomic: Deep tenderness is felt over a wide area; is not localized to one structure; and often extends to the thoracic spine, sacrum, or pelvis.[128]		
Hoover test	Performed to assess the patient's voluntary effort. The patient's heels are cupped by the clinician and the patient is instructed to individually raise his or her legs. Increased pressure should be felt on the untested cupped heel if true volitional effort is provided.	No study has been performed to formally evaluate the sensitivity, specificity, and reliability.	

Kosteljanetz and others[105] also noted a significant propensity for the CSLR test to be positive because 19 of 20 patients with this finding were noted to have disc herniations at surgery. The CSLR has also been correlated with outcome of treatment. Woodall and Hayes[130] and Edgar and Park[114] noted 32% and 44% of patients with positive findings, respectively, required surgical intervention.

Khuffash and Porter[131] examined the prognostic significance of the CSLR in 113 patients who had root tension signs from a lumbar disc lesion. A positive CSLR sign was found to be associated with poor prognosis for conservative management. Thirty percent of patients who presented with asymptomatic disc protrusion and 59% of those requiring surgery had positive crossed-leg pain, with 58% of patients with crossed-leg pain ultimately requiring discectomy. Certainly, there may have been some selection bias involved in choosing those who would require operative treatment.

Several studies have looked at the specificity and sensitivity of the CSLR. Thomas and coworkers[51,53] determined that the crossed Lasègue's sign had a specificity of 100% with a low sensitivity.

Andersson and Deyo[95] examined the prevalence, sensitivity, and specificity of the CSLR. They showed that the CSLR is less sensitive (23% to 42%), but much more specific (85% to 100%) compared with the SLR, with a positive predictive value of 79% and a negative predictive value of 44%. The positive predictive value in patients with a low probability including patients with no sciatica or neurologic signs or symptoms was determined to be 7%, with a negative predictive value of 98%.

Deville and associates[107] determined that the pooled sensitivity of CSLR was 29% (95% CI: 0.24–0.34), and the pooled specificity was 88% (95% CI: 0.86–0.90) with a positive predictive value of 92% at a prevalence of 0.82 and a negative predictive value of 22%. Poiraudeau and coworkers[120] used an imaging reference standard and found a sensitivity of 29% and specificity of 83%. Suri and others[90] found the CSLR to be only between 4% to 7% sensitive for lumbar root impingement but 93% specific for mid lumbar root impingement and 96% specific for lower lumbar root impingement. Vucetic and associates[132] found the crossed Lasègue's sign to have predictive ability in regard to determining the severity of disc injury, correctly classifying 74% of uncontained herniations and 68% of contained herniations. A 2010 Cochrane systematic review found the CSLR showed high specificity (pooled estimate 0.90, 95%) with low sensitivity (pooled estimate 0.28).[111]

BOWSTRING SIGN (Video 7-7)

In 1888, Cram described the bowstring sign or posterior tibial nerve sign (Fig. 7.10)[133]:

> In this test, when a positive straight leg raising test was noted, the leg was slightly flexed and pressure was applied to the tibial nerve in the popliteal fossa. Popliteal space compression was noted to be anatomically correlated with stretch of the sciatic nerve.

Supik and Broom[50] examined the sensitivity of several diagnostic signs of lower lumbar nerve root compression

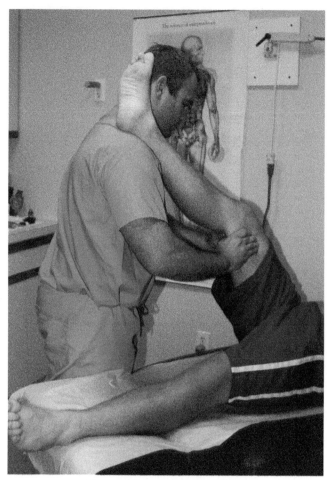

Figure 7.10 The bowstring sign.

associated with disc herniation and found the bowstring test to be positive 71% of the time (Table 7.7).

THE SLUMP TEST (Video 7-8)

The slump test appears to have been initially described by Cyriax in 1942, who noted that sciatic pain was reproduced in the seated individual with the knee of the painful leg extended with the addition of cervical spine and trunk flexion.[121] It is described as follows (Fig. 7.11):

> The subject sits straight with arms behind back, legs together, and posterior aspect of knees against the edge of the couch. The subject slumps as far as possible, producing full trunk flexion; the examiner applies firm pressure to bow the subject's back, and being careful to keep sacrum vertical. The subject is asked to flex his or her head, and over-pressure is then added to the neck flexion. While maintaining full spinal and neck flexion with over-pressure, the examiner asks the subject to extend the knee. Dorsiflexion is then added to knees extension. Neck flexion is then released, and the subject is asked to further extend the knee.

Walsh and Hall[122] performed an observational cross-sectional study of 45 subjects with unilateral leg pain and found substantial agreement between the SLR and slump test ($\kappa = 0.69$). Stankovic and associates[64] noted that 94.2%

Table 7.7 Interrater Reliability for Low Back Examination

Sign	Kappa Coefficient
Bowstring sign	0.11–0.49
Femoral stretch sign	0.27–0.77
CSLR test	0.02–0.74
SLR test reproducing patient symptoms	0.36–0.81
SLR test reproducing back and leg pain	0.44–0.81
MMT	0.04–1.0
Waddell signs: superficial tenderness	0.17–0.29
Waddell signs: simulation	0.25–0.48
Waddell signs: distraction	−0.16–0.40
Waddell signs: overreaction	0.29–0.46
Waddell signs: abnormal sensory/motor	−0.03–0.26
ROM—flexion	0.78–0.91
Movement—rotation pain	0.10–0.58
Movement—extension pain	0.31–0.57
Movement—flexion pain	0.52–0.56
Tenderness on palpation	0.28–0.50

CSLR, Crossed straight-leg raise; MMT, manual muscle testing; ROM, range of motion; SLR, straight-leg raise.

Reproduced with permission from McCombe PF, Fairbank JC, Cockersole BC, et al. Volvo Award in Clinical Sciences. Reproducibility of physical signs in low-back. Spine 1989;14:908-918.

of patients with frank disc herniation had pain reproduction with slump testing compared with 78% of those with bulging discs and 75% with no positive imaging findings on CT or MRI.

THE ANKLE DORSIFLEXION TEST (BRAGGARD SIGN) (Video 7-9)

Straight-leg raising can be further enhanced by different variations, including the ankle dorsiflexion test (see Fig. 7.9A). In 1884, Fajersztajn added the foot dorsiflexion test and neck flexion test, two provocative maneuvers that exacerbate leg pain by further increasing the pressure on the dura around the nerve root.[129] The ankle dorsiflexion test, or Braggard sign, involves elevating the leg to the point of pain provocation, dropping the leg down to a nonpainful range, and subsequent dorsiflexion of the ipsilateral ankle, increasing tension in the sciatic nerve distribution.[25]

FEMORAL NERVE STRETCH TEST (Video 7-10)

In 1918, Wassermann described the femoral stretching test after a systematic search for an objective physical sign in soldiers who complained of pain in the anterior thigh and shin when Lasègue's sign was absent[134]:

> With the patient prone, the examiner places a palm at the popliteal fossa as the knee is strongly dorsiflexed. Excruciating pain is produced in the anterior aspect of the thigh and/or back. Pain was apparent by facial grimacing, loud outcries,

and reflex reaching for the groin area. For the results to be positive, the test should produce pain, usually very severe, in the distribution of the patient's complaints.

The pathophysiologic response is incompletely understood, but the pain is assumed to be caused by stretching of an irritable femoral nerve when there is compression of the L2, L3, or L4 nerve roots.[135] It has been observed that these traction forces result in a 2-mm movement of the L4 root.[136] Overall, high lumbar disc herniations affecting these upper nerve roots are more challenging to diagnose owing to their unusual clinical presentation and overall rarity in comparison to those affecting the L4–L5 and L5–S1 levels.[123-125]

The femoral nerve stretch test is probably the single best screening test to evaluate lumbar radiculopathy secondary to an upper lumbar disc herniation. It has been shown to be positive in 84% to 95% of patients with a high lumbar disc.[123-125] Suri and colleagues[90] found it to be 50% sensitive and 100% specific for mid lumbar root impingement and 70% sensitive and 88% specific for L3 impingement on MRI. Estridge and coworkers[136] demonstrated a strong correlation with L3/L4 disc herniation and a positive femoral stretch test, and Christodoulides[124] noted lateral L4–L5 disc protrusions causing L4 nerve root involvement in 95% of patients with a positive femoral nerve stretch test.

Geraci and Alleva[137] reported increased sensitivity with the addition of hip extension to the femoral nerve stretch test, though no specific research protocol was utilized to support this assertion (Fig. 7.12). Penning and Wilmink[138] showed that, with extension of the spine, the anterior dural surface at the L3–L4 and L4–L5 levels was indented by posterior bulging of the discs, which may lend support to the added benefit of extension during the femoral nerve stretch test.

Trainor and Pinnington[139] investigated the slump knee bend (femoral slump test) as a test for upper or mid lumbar root compression in a study with 16 subjects with radicular leg pain. Sensitivity was 100% and specificity 83%, with good intertester reliability; of note, only 4 subjects had MRI evidence of mid lumbar nerve root compression, and the femoral slump test was falsely positive in 2 subjects without the condition.

The femoral stretching test is not pathognomonic for an upper lumbar disc herniation. The test result is likely to be positive in several conditions, including all forms of femoral neuropathy, tight iliopsoas or rectus femoris muscles, or pathology in or about the hip joint.[40]

THE CROSSED FEMORAL NERVE TEST (Video 7-11)

The crossed femoral stretch test (CFST) was first described by Cyriax in 1947 (the original description is unavailable).[140] Crossed femoral stretch testing has received very little attention in the literature. Dyck[135] suggested that stretching of the psoas and quadriceps femoris muscles puts traction on the third and fourth lumbar nerve roots. Kreitz and others[140] reported a case in which the CFST was positive in a patient with an L3–L4 lateral disc herniation. Nadler and coworkers[41] reported the presence of the crossed femoral nerve stretch test in two cases of high lumbar radiculopathies who presented with a positive femoral nerve stretch test result

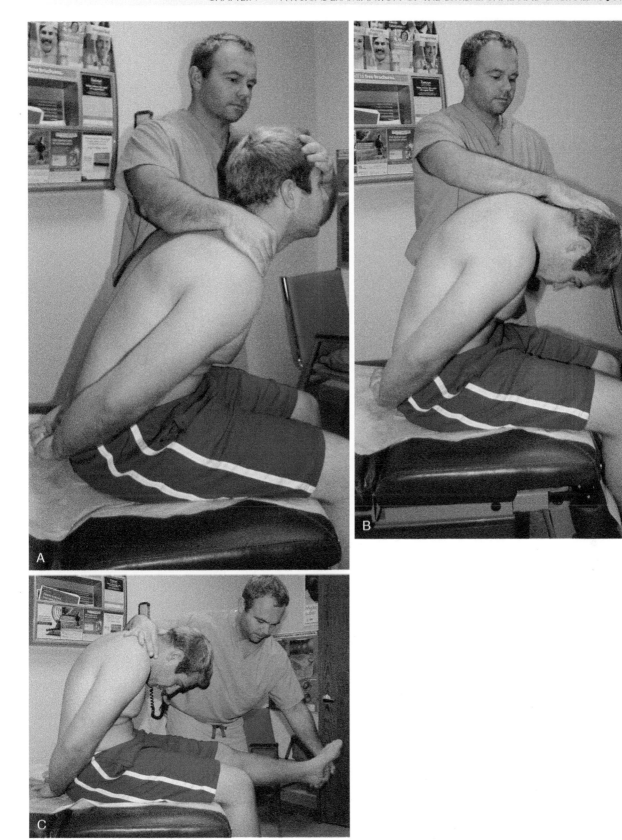

Figure 7.11 Slump test. **A,** Stage I. **B,** Stage II. **C,** Stage III.

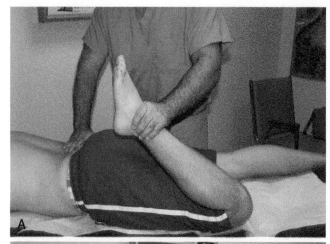

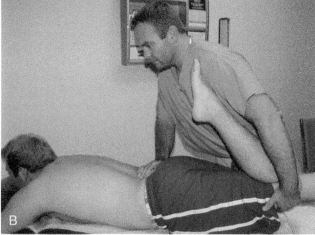

Figure 7.12 **A,** Femoral nerve stretch test (FNST). **B,** Enhancement of FNST with hip extension.

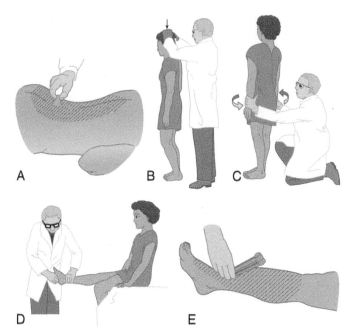

Figure 7.13 Waddell signs. **A,** Superficial sensitivity to light pinch. **B,** Axial loading causing low back pain. **C,** Passive rotation of the shoulders and pelvis in the same plane causing back pain. **D,** Straight-leg raising test in the seated position. **E,** Stocking distribution of sensory deficit. (Adapted with permission from Waddell et al. Nonorganic Physical Signs in Low-Back Pain. Spine. 5(2):117-125.)

along with a CFST; however, unlike the previous cases described in the literature, both patients responded well to conservative treatment.

A CFST may further support the diagnosis of a high lumbar radiculopathy and possibly enhance the specificity of the femoral nerve stretch test.[41] Suri and associates,[90] however, found that the FST was so sensitive that the CFST added no value, and furthermore, the CFST result was positive in only a single subject. Further study is needed to identify the prevalence of the CSFT in patients with upper to mid lumbar radiculopathies and in patients with confirmed herniated lumbar intervertebral discs.

WADDELL SIGNS (Video 7-12)

In 1980, Waddell and colleagues[128] described a standardized group of five types of physical signs: tenderness, simulation, distraction, regional, and overreaction (Fig. 7.13). In scoring, any individual sign counts as a positive sign for that group type, and a finding of three or more of the five types of signs was considered clinically significant. The signs were initially described as discussed in the subsequent sections.

TENDERNESS

Superficial: The skin is tender to light pinch over a wide area of lumbar skin. A localized band in a posterior primary ramus distribution may be caused by nerve irritation and should be discounted.

Nonanatomic: Deep tenderness is felt over a wide area; is not localized to one structure; and often extends to the thoracic spine, sacrum, or pelvis.

SIMULATION TESTS

Axial Loading: LBP is reported on vertical loading over the standing patient's skull by the examiner's hands. Neck pain is common and should be discounted.

Rotation: Back pain is reported when shoulders and pelvis are passively rotated in the same plane as the patient stands relaxed with the feet together. In the presence of root irritation, leg pain may be produced and should be discounted.

DISTRACTION TESTS

A positive physical finding is demonstrated in the routine manner; this finding is then checked while the patient's attention is distracted. The distraction must be nonpainful, nonemotional, and nonsurprising. During examination, parts of the body other than the particular part being overtly tested should be observed. Any finding that is consistently present is likely to be physically based. Findings that are present only on formal examination and disappear at other times may have a nonorganic component. Straight-leg raising is the most useful distraction test. The patient whose back pain has a nonorganic component shows marked improvement in straight-leg raising on distraction as compared with formal testing.

REGIONAL DISTURBANCES

Regional disturbances involve a widespread region of neighboring parts such as the leg below the knee, the entire leg, or a quarter or half the body. The essential feature is divergence from accepted neuroanatomy.

Weakness: Weakness is demonstrated on formal testing by a partial cogwheel "giving way" of many muscle groups that cannot be explained on a localized neurologic basis.
Sensory: Sensory disturbances include diminished sensation to light touch, pinprick, and sometimes other modalities fitting a "stocking" rather than a dermatomal pattern. "Giving way" and sensory changes commonly affect the same area, and there may be associated nonanatomic regional tenderness.

OVERREACTION

Overreaction during examination may take the form of disproportionate verbalization; facial expression; muscle tension; and tremor, collapsing, or sweating.

These provocative maneuvers aid in the identification of individuals who have physical findings without anatomic cause.[40] Three or more of the five types is considered clinically significant and is correlated with a significant psychological overlay consisting of hypochondriasis, hysteria, and depression using the Minnesota Multiphasic Personality Inventory (MMPI) psychological screening tool.[128,132,141] These signs were found to be more than 80% reproducible with a κ coefficient between 0.55 and 0.71. Multiple positive signs should be considered a "yellow flag" and suggest that the patient does not have a straightforward physical problem, and psychological factors need to be considered.[113] Multiple positive signs should not be used to indicate that a subject is malingering. Repeated testing and numerous questions in combination with the results of the entire physical examination will improve reliability.[95]

THE HOOVER TEST (Video 7-13)

The Hoover test may be performed to assess the patient's voluntary effort. The patient lies supine, and his or her heels are cupped by the clinician. The patient is instructed to individually raise his or her legs. Increased pressure should be felt on the untested cupped heel if true volitional effort is provided. No study has been performed to formally evaluate the sensitivity, specificity, and reliability of the Hoover test.

OTHER TESTS

Kummel[126] assessed the prognostic value of the limitation of shoulder motion with production of LBP, as well as LBP resulting from active cervical motion in addition to Waddell signs. Prognosis for return to work was poor in subjects with positive Waddell signs—52.9% did not return to work. However, with the additional finding of limitation of shoulder motion resulting in LBP, the prognosis was worse—

69.6% did not return to work. If cervical motion additionally produced LBP, the outlook was even poorer, with no return to work in 73.1%.

THE SACROILIAC JOINT

Proper evaluation and treatment of patients with SIJ pain can be difficult. No gold standard for diagnosis by physical examination exists, and evidence is often accrued clinically through a combination of maneuvers and observations. The complex biomechanics of the SIJ involve interactions with the hip, pubic symphysis, and spine, requiring the clinician to keep the SIJ within the differential diagnosis of LBP with radicular symptoms.

PHYSICAL EXAM OF THE SACROILIAC JOINT

In general, tests for SIJ dysfunction are divided into tests of motion or provocation. The gold standard for mobility tests needs to be further delineated because reliability is not well established and a significant percentage of asymptomatic individuals may have positive tests.[142,143] In vivo studies or the use of three-dimensional recording systems have been used; however, the conclusions are mixed.[142] Colachis and associates[144] embedded pins into the iliac spines of medical students, and movement was measured in sitting, standing, trunk flexion, and extension. Movement varied significantly among individuals, with differences of 5 mm recorded between iliac spines. Frigerio[145] demonstrated movement in cadavers and living subjects using radiographic techniques. In living specimens, it was observed that movement between the sacrum and iliac crests varied up to 26 mm with torsional and flexion motions.

Provocative maneuvers for the SIJ are likewise difficult to interpret in isolation. Gemmell and Jacobson,[146] Miraeu and colleagues,[147] and Dreyfuss and colleagues[148] have shown positive provocative maneuvers in 26%, 33%, and 16% of asymptomatic populations.

SACROILIAC MOTION TESTS (Video 7-14)

Standing Flexion Test

The standing flexion test was initially described by Henry Fryette in 1918, although he did not specifically call it a standing flexion test. Mitchell and others[149] described the standing flexion test as follows (Fig. 7.14):

> This test is performed with the patient standing, facing away from the examiner, with his feet approximately 12 inches apart so that the patient's feet are parallel and approximately acetabular distance apart. The examiner then places his thumbs on the inferior aspect of each PSIS. The patient is asked to bend forward with both knees extended. The extent of the cephalad movement of each PSIS is monitored. Normally, the PSIS should move equally. If one PSIS moves superiorly and anteriorly to the other, this is the side of restriction and hypomobility.

There are varied suggestions for the distance the feet should be apart.[150] Bourdillon and coworkers[151] stated that the heels should be spaced about 6 inches. Schwarzer and associates[11]

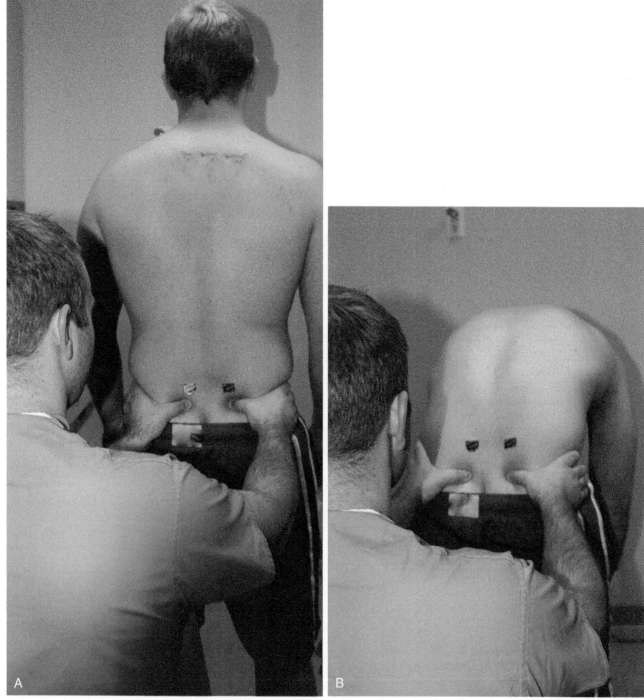

Figure 7.14   A and **B,** Standing flexion test.

found no association between this test and those patients who had a positive fluoroscopically guided injection of lidocaine into the SIJ.

Potter and Rothstein[152] found a 44% interexaminer reliability for this test. Riddle and Freburger[153] reported 55% interexaminer reliability with a κ coefficient of 0.32, indicating fair agreement. Vincent-Smith and Gibbons[150] reported an interexaminer reliability of 42% and a κ coefficient of 0.052, demonstrating poor reliability.

Levangie[154] assessed the association between innominate torsion and four clinical tests of the SIJ, including the standing forward flexion test in 150 patients with LBP and 138 without. This study found the standing flexion test to have a sensitivity of 17%, specificity of 79%, a positive predictive value of 61%, and negative predictive value of 35%.

Dreyfuss and others[148] determined the incidence of false-positive screening tests for SIJ dysfunction. Subjects were all asymptomatic and had no back pain for the past 6 months.

The control group consisted of subjects with active LBP, but SIJ was not the confirmed source of the subject's pain. For all 101 subjects, the incidence of false-positive results on either side for the standing flexion test was 13%.

This test only indicates asymmetry in motion or loss of lumbopelvic rhythm. A standing flexion test can be positive with an ipsilateral tight quadratus lumborum, contralateral tight hamstrings, SIJ arthritis, or hip joint restriction.[155] At best, it appears that this test is useful in assessing symmetry of motion.

Seated Flexion Test (Video 7-15)

This is a test of the sacroiliac mobility that is used to differentiate sacroiliac from iliosacral dysfunction. Mitchell and colleagues[149] described the seated flexion as follows (Fig. 7.15):

> This test is performed with the patient seated; both feet are flat on the floor facing away from the examiner and are firmly supported. The lower extremities should be abducted slightly to allow the patient's shoulders to descend between them.

The examiner stands or sits behind the patient with the eyes at the level of the iliac crests and then the examiner should place his thumbs on each PSIS. The patient should be instructed to forward flex until his/her hands touch the floor as the examiner maintains contact with the PSISs. The test is positive if one PSIS moves unequally cephalad with respect to the other PSIS. The side with the greatest cephalad excursion implies articular restriction and hypomobility. While the patient is seated, the innominates are fixed in place, thus isolating out iliac motion.

A seated flexion test result may be positive for reasons other than SIJ pain including a tight ipsilateral quadratus lumborum.[156-158] Beal[159] reported poor interexaminer reliability of this test. Potter and Rothstein[152] examined the interexaminer reliability of the 13 tests including the seated flexion test for SIJ dysfunction and reported a 50% interexaminer reliability. Dreyfuss and others[160] concluded that this test has a low specificity as a result of the false-positive rate of 13.3%. Levangie[154] determined the sensitivity to be 9%, the specificity to be 93%, the positive predictive value to be

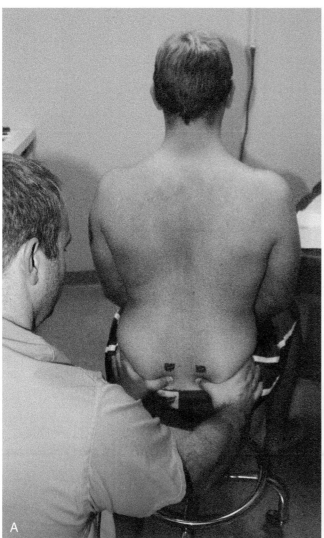
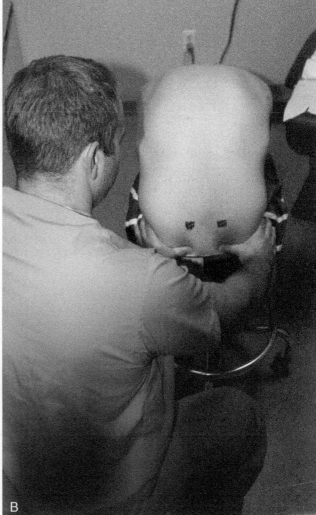

Figure 7.15 A and **B,** Seated flexion test.

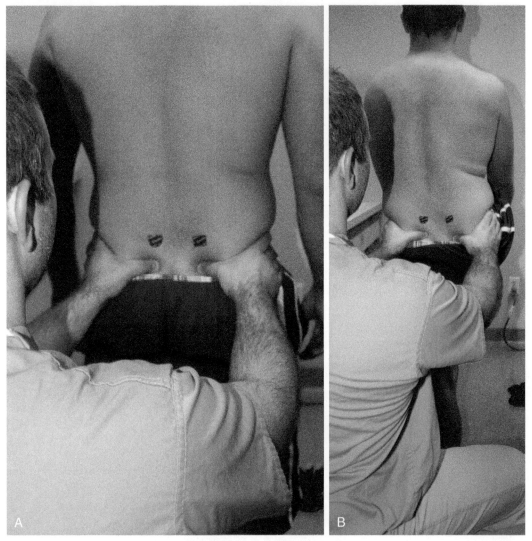

Figure 7.16   A and **B,** Gillet test.

78%, and the negative predictive value to be 28%. There is great disparity in the studies of reliability, specificity, and sensitivity of the seated flexion test.

Gillet Test (One-Leg Stork Test) (Video 7-16)

The Gillet test was described by Gillet and Liekens in 1981 to be a sensitive procedure to detect so-called partial iliosacral and SIJ dysfunction.[161] It is performed as follows (Fig. 7.16)[162]:

> This test is performed with the patient standing, facing away from the examiner, with his feet approximately 12 inches apart. Once each PSIS is localized by the examiner's thumbs, the patient is asked to stand on one leg while flexing the contralateral hip and flexing his knee to his chest.

Another method, the modified Gillet–Liekens test, has been described throughout the literature[146,152]:

> The examiner places one thumb directly under one PSIS and the other thumb at the S2 tubercle. The patient then stands on one leg and flexes the other hip toward the chest. The test

is positive if the PSIS on the side of hip flexion fails to move posterior and inferior with respect to the other PSIS.

There are mixed results regarding the intertester reliability of this test. Three studies found high interexaminer reliability for this maneuver. Wiles[163] evaluated 46 young asymptomatic patients and found an interrater reliability of 78%. Herzog[164] evaluated 11 patients examined by 10 chiropractors and determined the interexaminer reliability to be between 54% and 78%. Carmichael and others[165] looked at 53 healthy college students and determined the interexaminer reliability for the Gillet test to be 85%, and intraexaminer reliability to be 89.2%. Carmichael modified the original Gillet test by having the patient raise the leg as high as possible without bending the knee.

Several studies question the utility of the Gillet test.[161,166] Potter and Rothstein[152] found a 46% interexaminer reliability among 8 therapists who evaluated 17 patients with lateral buttock pain. Meijne and others[162] found the intraexaminer to have a κ coefficient of 0.03 to 0.08 in all subjects (poor correlation) and an agreement of 70% to 83%. The interexaminer reliability had a κ coefficient of –0.05 to 0.00 and 76% to 77% agreement. The authors concluded that this test has a very low level of reliability.

Dreyfuss and associates[148] found this test to have nearly 20% false-positive value, with females having more false positives (26%) than males (12.5%). In a follow-up study, Dreyfuss and coworkers[160] evaluated 85 patients with SIJ-mediated LBP. Patients were diagnosed with SIJ dysfunction based on a 90% reduction in pain after fluoroscopically guided injection of lidocaine and steroid. Twelve clinical examinations were evaluated on patients with pain reduction after fluoroscopy. The Gillet test was performed on 45 patients and was found to have a sensitivity of 43% and a specificity of 68%. The interexaminer reliability was found to be poor with a κ coefficient of 0.22 and agreement 45% of the time.

Levangie[154] assessed the association between innominate torsion and several physical examination tests, including the Gillet test. This study looked at 150 patients with LBP and compared them to 138 patients without LBP. The Gillet test was found to have a sensitivity of 8%, a specificity of 93%, a positive predictive value of 67%, and a negative predictive value of 35%.

Sturesson and others[142,143] studied the Gillet test with an invasive radiostereometric method looking at 22 patients with a positive Gillet test result and presumptive SIJ dysfunction. No significant difference was noted between the left and right SIJ using the Gillet test, and it was concluded that this test was of no value.

McCombe and colleagues[32] examined the reproducibility among observers of physical exam maneuvers in patients with LBP. A total of 88 patients were examined, and the interexaminer reliability for the Gillet test was found to have a poor κ coefficient of 0.16 to 0.09.

Maigne[167] concluded that there was no statistically significant association between the Gillet test and patients who responded to fluoroscopically guided anesthetic injections.

Sturesson and associates[142,143] additionally evaluated the standing flexion test by using radiostereometric analysis. Only very small movements were registered in the SIJs, and the authors indicated that the standing flexion test could not be supported as a diagnostic test for SIJ motion.

On a practical note, despite controversy regarding its ability to detect motion abnormalities, the Gillet test can assess standing tolerance and balance.

OTHER TESTS

PALPATION

O'Haire and associates[24] tested the interexaminer and intraexaminer reliability of 10 senior osteopathic students using static palpation on 10 asymptomatic subjects. Four assessments including the palpation of the PSIS, sacral sulcus (SS), and the sacral inferior lateral angle (SILA) were performed on every subject by all examiners. Intraexaminer reliability ranged between κ = 0.21 (poor) to 0.33 (poor to fair) for palpation of the SILA, κ = 0.33 (poor to fair) for palpation of the PSIS, and κ = 0.24 (poor) for the SS. Interexaminer reliability was poor for all palpation measurements, with κ scores ranging from 0.04 to 0.08.

Potter and Rothstein[152] determined that palpation in standing of iliac crest and PSIS levels had an interexaminer reliability of only 35% for each assessment individually. The poor reliability of clinical tests involving palpation may be partially explained by error in landmark location.

Dreyfuss and coworkers[148,160] found sacral sulcus tenderness to be 90% sensitive and 15% specific when comparing the results to a diagnostic SIJ block. Interexaminer reliability demonstrated a κ coefficient of 0.41 (fair). In a study of 56 women and five men, Robinson and Mengshoel found the palpation test to have poor interexaminer reliability with a κ coefficient of –0.06.

FORTIN FINGER TEST

Fortin described this test in 1991, as a simple diagnostic aid to clinicians to consider SIJ dysfunction[20,21]:

> The subject is asked to point to the region of pain with one finger. Positive sign was if the patient can localize the pain with one finger, the area pointed to was immediately inferomedial to the PSIS within 1 cm, and the patient consistently pointed to the same area over at least two trials.

Fortin and Falco[21] used provocation-positive SIJ injections to identify patients with SIJ dysfunction. Sixteen subjects were chosen from 54 consecutive patients by using the Fortin finger test. All 16 patients subsequently had provocation-positive joint injections validating SIJ abnormalities. A subset of 10 individuals underwent additional evaluation to exclude the possibility of confounding discogenic or posterior joint pains. All 10 patients had no indication of either discogenic or zygapophyseal joint pain generators. These results prompted the authors to conclude that a positive finding of the Fortin finger test successfully identified patients with SIJ dysfunction.

A study in 2008 by Murakami and coworkers[168] examined 38 patients who could reproducibly localize their pain with a single finger; 25 of the 38 indicated pain at the PSIS or within 2 cm of the PSIS, confirmed by fluoroscopy. Eighteen of these patients showed positive response to periarticular SIJ block, leading the authors to concur that if patients point to within 2 cm of the PSIS as their pain site, the SIJ should be considered the origin of their pain.

SACROILIAC PROVOCATIVE MANEUVERS

COMPRESSION TEST (Video 7-17)

The history and description of the compression test are limited in the literature. However, the value of the compression test was debated in 1927 by F. J. Gaenslen, though the test was not fully described. In 1957, Newton[169] illustrated the SI compression test as performed in the supine position as follows (Fig. 7.17):

> The examiner places both hands on the patient's ASIS and exerts a medial force bilaterally to implement the test. The compression test is more frequently performed with the patient in the side-lying position. The examiner stands behind the patient with their elbows locked in extension and palms interlocked over the anterolateral or upper part of the patient's iliac crest. The examiner exerts a medial or downward force towards the floor.

This test is reported to stretch the posterior ligaments and capsule dorsally over the reference and compresses the

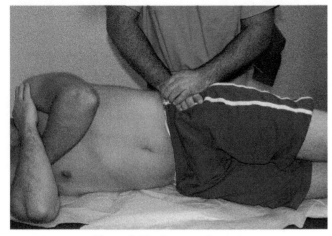

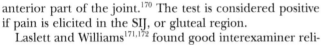

Figure 7.17 Compression test.

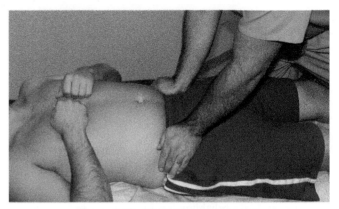

Figure 7.18 Distraction/gapping test.

anterior part of the joint.[170] The test is considered positive if pain is elicited in the SIJ, or gluteal region.

Laslett and Williams[171,172] found good interexaminer reliability using seven pain provocation tests for SIJ dysfunction in 51 patients with LBP. The interexaminer agreement was over 90% with a κ coefficient of 0.73 (good reliability). However, the majority of published studies indicate significant variability of the interexaminer reliability for this test. Potter and Rothstein[152] found a 76% intertester agreement, while Strender and others[173] noted a poor κ coefficient (0.26) for this test. However, neither of these studies addressed sensitivity or specificity, controls were not evaluated, and subjects did not have validated SIJ pathology.

With regard to the validity of SIJ tests, van der Wurff[166,174] calculated the sensitivity of the compression test to be 19% based on a study done by Rantanen and Airaksinen,[175] 0% based on a study by Blower and Griffin,[176] and 7% based on a study by Russel and others.[177] The specificity was calculated from Blower and Griffin's study to be 100% specific and 90% specific based on the study by Russel and coworkers.[177]

In a study of SIJ arthropathy pain confirmed by injection, Werner and coworkers[178] found the pelvic compression test to be poorly sensitive (<35%) but with good specificity (>90%). In a 2009 systematic review, Szadek and others[179] found the compression test to have discriminative power for diagnosing SIJ pain, with an odds ratio of 3.88. In 2007, Stuber[180] reviewed six studies and found the compression test to have greater than 60% specificity and sensitivity in at least one study. These studies contrast with a 2002 review by Cattley and associates[181] who concluded the compression test is invalid and unreliable.

GAPPING TEST (DISTRACTION) (Video 7-18)

The history and description of the gapping (distraction) test are also limited in the literature (Fig. 7.18). In 1957, Newton[169] described the SI gapping test as follows:

> The gapping test, also known as the distraction test, is performed with the patient in a supine position. The examiner places the heel of both hands at the same time on each ASIS, pressing downward and laterally.

This procedure is reported to stretch the anterior ligaments and capsule ventrally and compress the posterior part of the joint.[170] If lumbar pain is elicited, support is placed at the low back to rule out lumbar involvement. The test result is positive if pain is described in the gluteal or posterior crural areas.

Potter and Rothstein[152] and Laslett and Williams[171,172] showed more than 94% and 88% interexaminer agreement, respectively, when the gapping test was used to diagnose SIJ dysfunction. Laslett and Williams[171,172] demonstrated a κ coefficient of 0.69 (good reliability), while a κcoefficient of 0.36 (poor reliability) was previously demonstrated by McCombe and coworkers[170] who concluded it to be unreliable. The sensitivity for the gapping test has been documented to range only between 11% and 21%, whereas the specificity ranges from 90% to 100%.[166,174-177] However, in a 2005 study, Laslett[182] obtained a sensitivity of 60% and a specificity of 81% and found the gapping test to have the single highest positive predictive value for diagnosing SIJ dysfunction.

Maigne[167] found no statistically significant association between the gapping test and patients who had 75% or greater pain relief from fluoroscopically guided SIJ injections with lidocaine and steroid.

PATRICK (FABERE) TEST (Video 7-19)

In 1917, Hugh Patrick described the FABERE test originally for patients with hip arthritis.[183] This examination maneuver later became known as the FABERE sign, an acronym for flexion, abduction, external rotation, and extension (Fig. 7.19). It is described as follows:

> With the patient supine on a level surface, the thigh is flexed and the ankle is placed above the patella of the opposite extended leg. With the knee depressed and the ankle maintaining its position above the opposite knee, the patient will complain of pain before the knee reaches the level obtained in normal persons.

Kenna and Murtagh[184] in 1989 described the Patrick test for use in those with hip or SIJ dysfunction as follows:

> The patient lies supine on the table and the foot of the involved side is externally placed on the opposite knee. The hip joint is

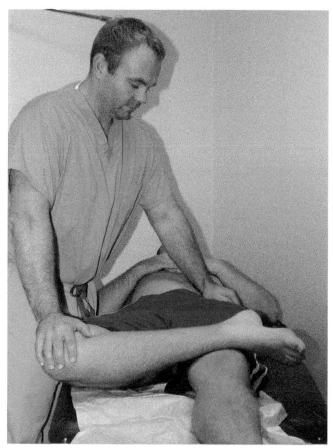

Figure 7.19.   FABERE test.

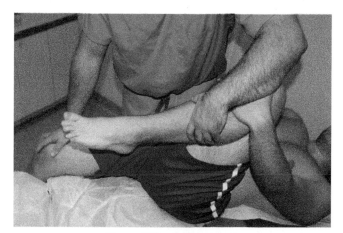

Figure 7.20   Gaenslen test.

GAENSLEN TEST (Video 7-20)

In 1929, F. J. Gaenslen described a diagnostic maneuver to differentiate between lumbosacral and sacroiliac lesions (Fig. 7.20).[187] He described the following:

> The patient lies supine, flexes the ipsilateral knee and hip with the thigh crowded against the abdomen with the aid of both the patient's hands clasped about the flexed knee. This brings the lumbar spine firmly in contact with the table and fixes both the pelvis and lumbar spine. The patient is then brought well to the side of the table, and the opposite thigh is slowly hyperextended with gradually increasing force by pressure of the examiner's hand on the top of the knee. With the opposite hand, the examiner assists the patient in fixing the lumbar spine and pelvis by pressure over the patient's clasped hands. The hyperextension of the hip exerts a rotating force on the corresponding half of the pelvis in the sagittal plane through the transverse axis of the sacroiliac joint. The rotating force causes abnormal mobility accompanied by pain, either local or referred on the side of the lesion.

now flexed, externally rotated and abducted. This position stresses the hip joint so that the inguinal pain on that side is a pointer to a defect in the hip joint or surrounding soft tissue. The range of motion for the hip joint in this position can be taken to the end point by pressing the knee downwards and simultaneously pressing on the region of the ASIS of the opposite side. This stresses the hip point as well as the SIJ on that side. If low back pain is reproduced, the cause is likely to be due to a disorder of the SIJ.

Strender and associates[173] examined 71 patients with LBP and evaluated the interexaminer reliability of clinical tests used in the physical exam of patients with LBP. Patrick's test was found unreliable in this study ($\kappa = 0.50$ with 95% agreement). Deursen and colleagues[185] also found this test to be unreliable ($\kappa = 0.38$). However, Dreyfuss and associates[148,160] found the Patrick test to be reliable with 85% agreement and a κ coefficient of 0.62. The sensitivity was found to be 69%, and a specificity of 16% was demonstrated. Werner and coworkers[178] found the sensitivity to be poor (<35%) but specificity to be good (>90%). In their 2002 review, Cattley and associates[181] concluded that the Patrick test was invalid and unreliable.

Van der Wurff[166,174] determined the sensitivity to be low (57%) in a review of data from Rantanen and Airaksinen.[175] Broadhurst and Bond[186] reported 77% sensitivity and 100% specificity in their study of Patrick's sign when correlated with double-blinded fluoroscopic SIJ joint block.

This test can also be performed with the patient in a sidelying position. The upper leg (test leg) is hyperextended at the hip. The examiner stabilizes the pelvis while extending the hip of the uppermost leg. This results in anterior rotation of the innominate and SIJ on the test side. Pain indicates SIJ pathology, but it may also be caused by an L2 to L4 nerve root lesion.[19,188]

Dreyfuss and coworkers[148,160] determined that this test was 68% sensitive and 35% specific, with a κ coefficient of 0.61 and 82% agreement. Others have challenged the discriminative information provided by the Gaenslen test in the evaluation of a patient with LBP.[177] In a 2005 study, Laslett and associates[26] found that the Gaenslen test did not add any diagnostic value to a prior battery of provocative maneuvers. Werner and colleagues[178] found the sensitivity to be poor (<35%) but specificity to be good (>90%), and a 2002 review by Cattley and others[181] determined it to show agreement on validity.

CRANIAL SHEAR TEST

Mennell[191,192] and Laslett and Williams[171,172] described the cranial shear test, but the original description could not

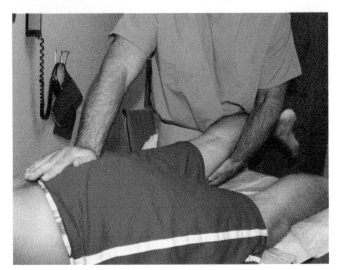

Figure 7.21 Cranial shear test.

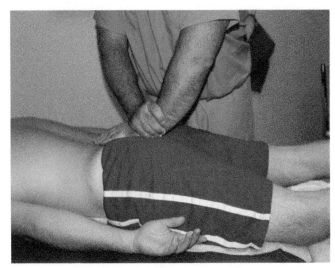

Figure 7.23 Midline sacral thrust.

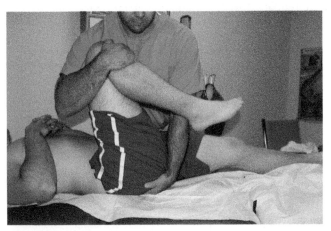

Figure 7.22 Thigh thrust (posterior shear, PPPP, P4, posterior pelvic pain provocation test).

be found. It has been described by Mennell as follows (Fig. 7.21):

> This test consists of the patient lying in the prone position and the examiner applies a pressure to the sacrum near the coccygeal end, directed cranially. The ilium is held immobile through the hip joint as the examiner applies counter pressure against legs in the form of traction force—directed caudad. The test is considered positive if the maneuver aggravates the patient's typical pain.

Laslett and Williams[171,172] found more than 80% intertester agreement for the cranial shear test, with a κ coefficient of 0.61.

THIGH THRUST (POSTERIOR SHEAR, PPPP, P4, POSTERIOR PELVIC PAIN PROVOCATION) TEST

(Video 7-21)

The thigh thrust test, also known as the posterior shear, PPPP, P4, or posterior pelvic pain provocation test, is performed as follows (Fig. 7.22):

The examiner applies a posterior shearing force to the sacroiliac joint through the femur with the patient prone and the hip flexed to 90 degrees with a bent knee. Axial pressure is applied along the length of the femur, using it as a lever to push the ilium posteriorly. One hand is placed beneath the sacrum to stabilize it.

Laslett and Williams[171] describe it as avoiding excessive adduction of the hip because this may normally make the position uncomfortable; Broadhurst and Bond[186] describe the test with the femur adducted to midline. Laslett and Williams[171] found 94% interexaminer agreement with a κ coefficient of 0.88 (highly substantial).

Broadhurst and Bond[186] performed a double-blinded trial to determine the sensitivity and specificity of pain provocative tests for SIJ dysfunction. Forty patients were subsequently randomized in a double-blind study to be injected fluoroscopically with either lidocaine or normal saline. None of the patients who received normal saline had any pain suppression. Positive pain relief was determined by 70% pain reduction, and the thigh thrust/posterior shear test was found to be 100% specific and 80% sensitive.

Dreyfuss and others[160] compared this test followed by diagnostic injection requiring 90% pain reduction and found that this test was 42% sensitive and 45% specific, with a κ coefficient of 0.64 (substantial agreement) between medical doctors and doctors of chiropractic. A 2002 review by Cattley and others[181] believed the thigh thrust was valid and reliable when taking into account multiple studies. Stuber[180] in a 2007 systematic review determined that the thigh thrust/posterior shear was found to have greater than 60% specificity and sensitivity in at least one study and was a candidate for inclusion in a provocative test array.

MIDLINE SACRAL THRUST

Laslett and Williams[171] described the test as follows (Fig. 7.23):

> Pressure is applied directly to the sacrum while the patient lies prone. The force is directed anteriorly against the ilia, which are fixed against the examining couch.

Laslett and Williams[171] found an interrater reliability of 78% with a κ coefficient of 0.52. Dreyfuss and coworkers[160] questioned the utility of this test because there was no correlation among subjects who had a positive shear test with those who had a positive diagnostic fluoroscopically guided injection. They found this test to have a specificity of 40% and a sensitivity of 51%, with an interexaminer (MD and DC) κ coefficient of 0.30. A 2002 review by Cattley and associates[181] felt the midline sacral thrust was invalid and unreliable. Stuber[180] in 2007 reviewed six studies and found that the sacral thrust test was found to have greater than 60% specificity and sensitivity in at least one study.

ACTIVE STRAIGHT-LEG RAISE AND ACTIVE ASSISTED STRAIGHT-LEG RAISE (Video 7-22)

Mens and colleagues[193] described the active straight-leg raise (ASLR) test as follows:

> ASLR was performed in the supine position with straight legs relaxed in lateral rotation, and feet 20 cm apart. The test was performed after the instruction: "Try to raise your legs, one after the other, above the couch for 5 cm without bending the knee." The patient was asked whether she felt weakness, pain or any other unpleasant feelings during the test and whether she noticed any difference between the two sides. The examiner assessed the velocity of raising, the appearance of a tremor of the leg, the amount of rotation of the trunk, and verbal and non-verbal emotional expressions of the patient.

Impairment was scored on a four-point scale:

0 The patient feels no restriction.
1 The patient reports decreased ability to raise the leg, but the examiner assesses no signs of impairment.
2 The patient reports decreased ability to raise the leg, and the examiner assesses signs of impairment.
3 Inability to raise the leg

In a pilot study of 25 patients and 2 assessors, Mens and others[193] found the intertester reliability was high (Kendall's Tb = 0.81).

Mens and coworkers[193] also described assisted ASLR in the same trial, using a sacroiliac belt. The tightening of the belt produced pain improvement in 20 of 21 patients. This study was limited to nonpregnant female patients who had developed pelvic pain during pregnancy or within 3 weeks after delivery. This study also showed a significant association between impaired ASLR and radiographically measured pelvic joint mobility.

Mens and colleagues[23] later compared the reliability of the ASLR to the thigh thrust (P4/posterior pelvic pain provocation) test, again in patients whose pain had begun during pregnancy or in the early postpartum period. Intraobserver test–retest reliability was measured with Pearson's correlation coefficient between two ASLR scores 1 week apart and was 0.87 (high); the ICC was 0.83. ASLR sensitivity was 100%, and specificity was 94%. Sensitivity of the thigh thrust (P4/posterior pelvic pain provocation) was 69%. There was not high agreement between the thigh thrust test and the ASLR (correlation coefficient 0.27), meaning that perhaps the two tests measure different aspects of postpartum posterior pelvic pain.

COMBINED TESTS

Cibulka and others[194] examined the sensitivity, specificity, and positive and negative predictive values of four commonly used SIJ tests: (1) the standing flexion test, (2) sitting PSIS palpation, (3) supine long sitting test, and (4) prone knee flexion tests. SIJ dysfunction was considered positive if at least three of the four test results were positive. A total of 219 patients with and without low back and SIJ-mediated pain were examined. The combination of these tests yielded a sensitivity of 0.82, specificity of 0.88, positive predictive value of 0.86, and negative predictive value of 0.84. However, individual test results were not documented, so no conclusions can be made about their isolated validity.

In 2002, Riddle and Freburger[153] examined the interrater reliability of these same four different assessments of pelvic asymmetry or SIJ motion in 65 subjects with LBP and unilateral buttock pain and found that the reliabilities of the four tests (standing flexion, prone knee flexion, supine long sit, sitting PSIS test) were too low for clinical use, with κ coefficients for individual tests ranging from 0.19 to 0.37, and κ coefficients for composite analysis of the four tests ranging from 0.11 to 0.23.

Laslett and Williams[171,172] examined the intertester reliability of seven pain provocative tests commonly used to diagnose SIJ pathology: (1) distraction, (2) compression, (3) posterior shear, (4) pelvic rotation, (5) pelvic torsion, (6) sacral thrust, and (7) cranial shear test. Fifty-one patients with low pain, with or without radiation into the lower limb, were assessed by two examiners. Intertester reliability was determined for each test; however, combinations of these tests were not reported (Table 7.8).

Slipman and others[195] determined the clinical validity of provocative SIJ maneuvers in making the diagnosis of SIJ dysfunction. Consecutive patients who described LBP, including the region of the sacral sulcus, had a positive Patrick's test result, ipsilateral sacral sulcus tenderness on palpation, and response to anesthetic SIJ block. The positive predictive value of provocative SIJ maneuvers in determining the presence of SIJ dysfunction was determined to be 60%. However, the negative predictive value was not reported. The authors thought that these results do not support the use of provocative SIJ maneuvers to confirm a diagnosis of SIJ dysfunction. Rather, these physical

Table 7.8 Intertester Reliability of Sacroiliac Joint Tests

Sacroiliac Test	Kappa Coefficient	Agreement (%)
Distraction	0.69	88.2
Compression	0.73	88.2
Sacral thrust	0.52	78.0
Thigh thrust	0.88	94.1
Pelvic torsion right	0.75	88.2
Pelvic torsion left	0.72	88.2
Cranial shear	0.61	84.3

Reproduced with permission from Laslett M, Williams M. The reliability of selected pain provocation tests for sacroiliac joint pathology. Spine. 1994;19:1243-1249.

examination techniques can, at best, enter SIJ dysfunction into the differential diagnosis (Table 7.9).

Young and associates[196] performed a prospective validity study with 81 patients referred for diagnostic injection and found a significant odds ratio of 27.9 (*P*<0.001) for patients with three or more positive pain provocation tests; the provocation tests consisted of distraction, compression, sacral thrust, thigh thrust, and the Gaenslen test. In this study, SIJ pain was also associated with pain rising from sitting, unilaterally sided pain, and with the lack of midline pain.

Because SIJ provocation tests have been found to be positive in patients with disc disorders and found to improve when the disc disorder resolves, Laslett and others[182] performed a blinded validity study examining the addition of a McKenzie evaluation with sacroiliac provocation tests in 48 patients referred for diagnostic spinal injection. The presence of centralization or peripheralization phenomenon was incorporated with provocative sacroiliac maneuvers, and the diagnostic accuracy of this clinical examination and reasoning process were found superior to SIJ provocation tests alone, providing a sensitivity of 91%, specificity of 83%, and positive LR of 6.97.

Laslett and coworkers[26] in a blinded validity study evaluated a series of sacroiliac provocation tests singly and in combination (composites), using diagnostic injection of the SIJ as the diagnostic standard. An optimum composite was determined that provided a sensitivity of 94% and specificity of 78% when any two of four selected tests were used (see distraction, Fig. 7.18; thigh thrust, Fig. 7.22; compression, Fig. 7.17; sacral thrust, Fig. 7.23), and a diagnostic algorithm for SIJ pain using these tests was developed (Fig. 7.24).

AUTHORS' PREFERRED APPROACH

When a patient presents with LBP, key historical points we consider are location, duration, and exacerbating and relieving positions or maneuvers. Special attention is placed on whether pain is localized or radiating. Midline or radicular appearing pain exacerbated by sitting, coughing, and sneezing is considered a clue to a discogenic source; off-midline pain provoked with transitional movements such as sit-to-stand raises suspicion for sacroiliac pathology, and pain with flexion/extension changes can be concerning for spondylolisthesis.

Our physical exam begins by observing hip height asymmetries and whether a lateral shift is present. Typically, to detect a lateral shift, a thumb is placed on the L5 to S1 space and another above the thoracolumbar junction to observe whether the higher level is displaced either away or towards the side of their pain. For efficiency, the lumbar segments are palpated sequentially at this point to detect tenderness or step-off deformities. Occasionally, to detect more subtle shifts, the examiner will distance themselves approximately 3 to 5 feet away to obtain a sense of the overall gestalt.

Lumbar ROM is assessed next, with special attention noted as to whether extension involves the lumbar segments appropriately or if "hinging" occurs mainly at the thoracolumbar junction. During flexion, similar attention is paid to the lumbar motion to determine if flexion is pelvis dominant or lumbar dominant, indicating resistance to lumbar segment flexion or to posterior kinetic chain tightness, respectively.

If lumbar flexion or extension produces pain (either axially or with peripheralization), the examiner notes the angle at which pain is first noted, and then the patient is asked to perform a repetitive movement in the opposing direction (ie, pain with flexion, will perform 10 repetitions standing lumbar extensions or prone press-ups). After this, the pain-provoking direction will be repeated to assess for change in point of onset, allowing indication that a mechanical derangement may be present. With the patient still standing at this point, if concern for SIJ pathology exists, a Gillet test will be performed. While not fully indicative of SIJ dysfunction, if positive results are present, it will be supportive, and this also allows rapid assessment of single-legged balance/core stability. Should there be concern, palpatory exam of the PSIS region may find local tenderness; however, in our experience, SIJ pain is also associated with tenderness of gluteal musculature, extending to the greater trochanter at times.

Because of the possibility of hip/spine syndrome, if lateral flexion causes pain, occasionally the examiner will support the patient by the hips and ask the patient to raise the painful side's foot off the floor and repeat the lateral flexion with the hip unloaded. If pain remits, this may indicate hip/SIJ pathology; if pain remains present, it may support stenosis via discogenic or spondylotic etiologies. Finally, oblique extension is performed to load the posterior elements, assessing for reproduction of either axial LBP or radicular symptom onset. As the patient is still standing at this point, he or she will be asked to place the hands against the wall for support and then attempt to achieve 10 of 10 single-legged heel raises to assess symmetry of strength and effort. We find this to be more sensitive for weakness than toe walking because often compensation is present that shows normal appearing toe walk, and weakness is only found with the single-legged heel raises.

Moving the patient to a seated position, manual muscle testing is then performed for the key muscle groups of hip flexors, knee extensors, dorsiflexion, great toe extension, and ankle eversion. Seated slump maneuver is easily incorporated at this point because the patient will have the knee extended already. The result is considered positive if relief of leg pain is noted with neck extension, and equivocal if it does not improve or if only back pain is present and improves.

Moving the patient to a supine position, bilateral hip flexion range is assessed, as are SLR, FAIR, and FABERE. Thigh thrust and active SLR are easily incorporated at this point also. During active SLR, it is noted whether the ASIS of the hip drops during leg lift, which can indicate poor lumbopelvic stability amenable to core strengthening.

If the patient is noted to have a mechanical directional preference that relieves or improves his or her end-range pain, he or she will often be sent for formal mechanical diagnosis and treatment by a McKenzie practitioner because this can find an answer typically within four to six visits. If three or more SIJ provocation tests are present in the setting of transitional pain, the patient will be considered for trial of sacroiliac belt or diagnostic sacroiliac injection.

Table 7.9 Sacroiliac Joint Provocative Maneuvers

Test	First Author	Kappa Coefficient	Agreement	Sensitivity	Specificity	Comments
Compression	Laslett and Williams[171,172]	0.73 (good)	>90%[a]			
	Potter and Rothstein[152]		76%[a]			
	Strender et al.[173]	0.26 (poor)				
	Rantanen and Airaksinen[175]			19%		
	Blower and Griffin[176]					
	Russell et al.[177]			7%	90%	
	Werner et al.[178]			<35%	>90%	With diagnostic block
	Szadek et al.[179]					Systematic review; Positive odds ratio: 3.88
	Stuber[180]					Review: Consider use
	Cattley et al.[181]			>60%	>60%	Review: invalid/ unreliable
Gapping (Distraction)	Potter and Rothstein[152]		94%			
	Laslett[171,172]	0.69 (good)	88%			
	McCombe[170]	0.36 (poor)				
	Laslett[26]			60%	81%	Found to have highest positive predictive value
	Russel et al.[177]		11%	90%		
	Rantanen and Airaksinen[175]			15%		
	Van der Wurff[166,174]		11–21%	90–100%		
Patrick's (FABERE)	Dreyfuss[160]	0.62[a]	85%[a]	69%	16%	
	Deursen[185]	0.38				
	Rantanen and Airaksinen[175]			57%		
	Broadhurst[186]			77%	100%	With diagnostic block
	Strender[173]	0.50[a]	95%[a]			
	Werner et al.[178]			<35%	>90%	
	Cattley[181]					Review: invalid/ unreliable
Gaenslen test	Laslett and Williams[171]	0.72	63%			
	Dreyfuss et al.[160]	0.61[a]	82%[a]	68%	35%	
	Russel et al.[177]			21%	72%	
	Laslett et al.[26]			50–53%	71–77%	
	Werner et al.[178]			<35%	>90%	
	Cattley et al.[181]					Review: valid
Cranial shear	Laslett and Williams[171]	0.61	84.3			
Thigh thrust (posterior shear/P4)	Laslett and Williams[171]	0.88	94%[a]			
	Broadhurst and Bond[186]			80%	100%	With diagnostic block
	Dreyfuss et al.[160]	0.64		42%	45%	With diagnostic block
	Cattley et al.[181]					Review: valid/reliable
	Stuber[180]			>60%	<60%	Review: Consider use
	Mens et al.[193]			69%		Pelvic pain peri- or postpartum
Active SLR	Mens et al.[193]	Kendall's Tb = 0.81 (high)[a]				Pelvic pain peri- or postpartum
	Mens et al.[193]	Pearson's = 0.87 (high)[b]		100%	94%	Pelvic pain per or postpartum
Midline sacral thrust	Laslett and Williams[171]	0.52	78%[a]			
	Dreyfuss et al.[160]	0.30		51%	40%	
	Stuber[180]			>60%	>60	Review: Consider use
	Cattley et al.[181]					Review: invalid/ unreliable

[a]Interexaminer.
[b]Intraexaminer.

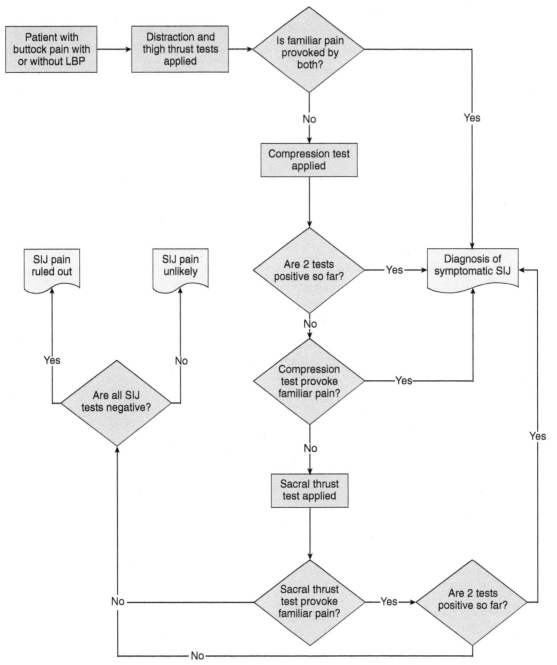

Figure 7.24 Sacroiliac joint (SIJ) diagnostic algorithm. (Used with permission from Laslett el. Man Ther. 2005 Aug;10(3):207-218.) *LBP,* Low back pain.

REFERENCES

1. Prather H. Pelvis and sacral dysfunction in sports and exercise. *Phys Med Rehabil Clin N Am.* 2000;11:805-836, viii.
2. Crenshaw AH, Hamilton JF. Rheumatoid spondylitis. *South Med J.* 1952;45:1055.
3. Forestier J. Quoted in Romanus R, Yden S: *Pelvo-Spondylitis Ossificans.* Munksgaard: Copenhagen; 1955.
4. Knutsson F. Changes in the sacro-iliac joints in morbus bechterew and osteitis condensans. *Acta Radiol.* 1950;33:557.
5. Polley HF, Slocumb CH. Rheumatoid spondylitis: a study of 1035 cases. *Ann Intern Med.* 1947;26:240.
6. Vleeming A, Stochart R, Vokers ACW, et al. The sacro-iliac joint: anatomical, biomechanical and radiological aspects. *J Man Med.* 1990;5:100-102.
7. Vleeming A, Van Wingerden JP, Dijkstra PF, et al. Mobility in the sacroiliac joints in the elderly: a kinematic and radiological study. *Clin Biomech (Bristol, Avon).* 1992;7:170-176.
8. Malanga GA, Nadler SF. Nonoperative treatment of low back pain. *Mayo Clin Proc.* 1999;74:1135-1148.
9. Ebraheim NA, Pananilam TG, Waldrop JT, et al. Anatomic consideration in the anterior approach to the sacroiliac joint. *Spine.* 1994;19:721-725.
10. Greenman PE. Clinical aspects of sacroiliac function in walking. *J Man Med.* 1990;5(3):125-130.
11. Schwarzer AC, Aprill CN, Bogduk N. The sacroiliac joint in chronic low back pain. *Spine.* 1995;20:31-37.
12. Vanelderen P, Szadek K, Cohen SP, et al. Sacroiliac joint pain. *Pain Pract.* 2010;10:470-480.

13. Ebraheim NA, Lu J, Biyani A, et al. The relationship of lumbosacral plexus to the sacrum and the sacroiliac joint. *Am J Orthop.* 1997;26:105-110.

14. Bernard TN, Kirkaldy-Willis WH. Recognizing specific characteristics of nonspecific low back pain. *Clin Orthop.* 1987;217:266-280.

15. Magee DJ. *Orthopedic Physical Assessment.* Philadelphia: W.B. Saunders; 1992.

16. Simons DG, Travell JG. Myofascial origins of low back pain. 1: Principles of diagnosis and treatment. *Postgrad Med.* 1983;73:66, 68-70, 73 passim.

17. Simons DG, Travell JG. Myofascial origins of low back pain. 2: Torso muscles. *Postgrad Med.* 1983;73:81-92.

18. Simons DG, Travell JG. Myofascial origins of low back pain. 3: Pelvic and lower extremity muscles. *Postgrad Med.* 1983;73:99-105, 108.

19. Daum WJ. The sacroiliac joint an under appreciated pain generator. *Am J Orthop.* 1995;24:475-478.

20. Fortin JD, Dwyer AP, West S, et al. Sacroiliac joint: pain referral maps upon applying a new injection arthrography technique. 1: Asymptomatic volunteers. *Spine.* 1994;19:1475-1482.

21. Fortin JD, Falco FJ. The Fortin finger test: an indicator of sacroiliac pain. *Am J Orthop.* 1997;26:477-480.

22. Delpalma MJ, Ketchum JM, Trussell BS, et al. Does the location of low back pain predict its source? *PM R.* 2011;3:33-39.

23. Mens JM, Vleeming A, Snijders CJ, et al. Reliability and validity of the active straight leg raise test in posterior pelvic pain since pregnancy. *Spine.* 2001;26:1167-1171.

24. O'Haire C, Gibbons P. Inter-examiner and intra-examiner agreement for assessing sacroiliac anatomical landmarks using palpation and observation: pilot study. *Man Ther.* 2000;5:3-20.

25. Macrae IF, Wright V. Measurements of back movement. *Ann Rheum Dis.* 1969;28:584-589.

26. Laslett M, Aprill CN, McDonald B, et al. Diagnosis of sacroiliac joint pain: validity of individual provocation tests and composites of tests. *Man Ther.* 2005;10:207-218.

26a. Duniec L, Nowakowski P, Kosson D, et al. Anatomical landmarks based assessment of intravertebral space level for lumbar puncture is misleading in more than 30%. *Anaesthesiol Intensive Ther.* 2013;45:1-6.

27. Locks Gde F, Almeida MC, Pereira AA. Use of the ultrasound to determine the level of lumbar puncture in pregnant women. *Rev Bras Anestesiol.* 2010;60:13-19.

28. Clare HA, Adams R, Maher CG. Reliability of detection of lumbar lateral shift. *J Manipulative Physiol Ther.* 2003;26:476-480.

29. Phillips FM. Lumbar spine. In: Reider B, ed. *The Orthopaedic Physical Examination.* 2nd ed. Philadelphia: Elsevier Saunders; 2005. 335-361.

30. Deyo RA, Rainville J, Kent DL. What can the history and physical examination tell us about low back pain? *JAMA.* 1992;268:760-765.

31. Gonnella C, Paris SV, Kutner M. Reliability in evaluating passive intervertebral motion. *Phys Ther.* 1982;62:436-444.

32. McCombe PF, Fairbank JC, Cockersole BC, et al. 1989 Volvo Award in Clinical Sciences. Reproducibility of physical signs in low-back. *Spine.* 1989;14:908-918.

33. Spangfort EV. Lasègue's sign in patients with lumbar disc herniation. *Acta Orthop Scand.* 1971;42:459-460.

33a. Spangfort EV. The lumbar disc herniation. A computer-aided analysis of 2,504 operations. *Acta Orthop Scand Suppl.* 1972;142:1-95.

34. Troke M, Moore AP, Maillardet FJ, et al. A normative database of lumbar spine ranges of motion. *Man Ther.* 2005;10:198-206.

35. Mellor FE, Thomas PW, Thompson P, et al. Proportional lumbar spine inter-vertebral motion patterns: a comparison of patients with chronic, non-specific low back pain and healthy controls. *Eur Spine J.* 2014;23:2059-2067.

36. Laird RA, Gilbert J, Kent P, et al. Comparing lumbo-pelvic kinematics in people with and without back pain: a systematic review and meta-analysis. *BMC Musculoskeletal Disord.* 2014;15:229.

37. White AA, Panjabi MM. *Clinical Biomechanics of the Spine.* Philadelphia: JB Lippincott; 1978.

38. Pearcy MJ, Portek J, Shepherd J. Three dimensional x-ray analysis of normal measurement in the lumbar spine. *Spine.* 1984;9:294.

39. Pearcy MJ, Tibrewal SB. Axial rotation and lateral bending in the normal lumbar spine measured by three-dimensional radiography. *Spine.* 1984;9:582.

40. Nadler SF, Campagnolo DI, Tomaio AC, et al. High lumbar disc: diagnostic and treatment dilemma. *Am J Phys Med Rehabil.* 1998;77:538-544.

41. Nadler SF, et al. The crossed femoral nerve stretch test to improve diagnostic sensitivity for the high lumbar radiculopathy: two case reports. *Arch Phys Med Rehabil.* 2001;82:522-523.

42. McGill SM. *Low Back Disorders: Evidence-based Prevention and Rehabilitation.* Champaign, IL: Human Kinetics; 2002.

43. Caillet R. *Low Back Pain Syndrome.* 4th ed. Philadelphia: FA Davis; 1988.

44. Littlewood C, May S. Measurement of range of movement in the lumbar spine – what methods are valid? A systematic review. *Physiother.* 2007;93:201-211.

45. Burdett RG, Brown KE, Fall MP. Reliability and validity of our instruments for measuring lumbar spine and pelvic positions. *Phys Ther.* 1986;66:677-684.

46. Portek I, Pearcy MJ, Reader GP, et al. Correlation between radiographic and clinical measurements of lumbar spine movement. *Br J Rheumatol.* 1983;22:197-205.

47. Mayer TG, Tencer AF, et al. Use of noninvasive techniques for quantification of spinal range of motion in normal subjects and chronic low back dysfunction patients. *Spine.* 1984;9:588-595.

48. Saur PMM, Ensink FB, Frese K, et al. Lumbar range of motion: reliability and validity of the inclinometer technique in the clinical measurement of trunk flexibility. *Spine.* 1996;21:1332-1338.

49. Merrit J, McLean T, Erickson R. Measurement of trunk flexibility in normal subjects: reproducibility of three clinical methods. *Mayo Clin Proc.* 1986;61:192-197.

50. Supik LF, Broom MJ. Sciatic tension signs and lumbar disc herniation. *Spine.* 1994;19:1066-1069.

51. Thomas M, Grant N, Marshall J, et al. Surgical treatment of low backache and sciatica. *Lancet.* 1983;2:1437-1439.

52. Robinson HS, Mengshoel AM. Assessments of lumbar flexion range of motion. *Spine.* 2014;39:E270-E275.

52a. Aartun E, Degerfalk A, Kentsdotter L, et al. Screening of the spine in adolescents: inter- and intra-rater reliability and measurement error of commonly used clinical tests. *BMC Musculoskeletal Disord.* 2014;15:37.

53. Thomas E, Silman AJ, Papageorgiou AC, et al. Association between measures of spinal mobility and low back pain: an analysis of new attenders in primary care. *Spine.* 1998;23:343-347.

54. Schober P. The lumbar vertebral column and backaches. *Much Med Wschr.* 1937;84:336.

55. Biering-Sorensen F. Physical measurements as risk indicators for low-back trouble over a one-year period. *Spine.* 1984;9:106-119.

56. Mooney V. Physical measurement of the lumbar spine. *Phys Med Rehabil Clin N Am.* 1998;9:391-410.

57. Rezvani A, Ergin O, Karacan I, et al. Validity and reliability of the metric measurements in the assessment of lumbar spine motion in patients with ankylosing spondylitis. *Spine.* 2012;37:E1189-E1196.

58. Moll JMH, Wright V. Normal range of spinal mobility: an objective clinical study. *Ann Rheum Dis.* 1971;30:381-386.

59. Williams R, Binkley R, Bloch R, et al. Reliability of the modified-modified Schober and double inclinometer methods for measuring lumbar flexion extension. *Phys Ther.* 1993;73:26-37.

60. Reynolds PM. Measurement of spinal mobility: a comparison of three methods. *Rheumatol Rehabil.* 1975;14:180-185.

61. Fitzgerald GK, Wynveen KJ, Rheault W, et al. Objective assessment with establishment of normal values for lumbar spinal range of motion. *Phys Ther.* 1983;63:1776-1781.

62. Gill K, Krag MH, Johnson GB, et al. Repeatability of four clinical methods for assessment of lumbar spinal motion. *Spine.* 1988;13:50-53.

63. Miller SA, Mayer T, Cox R, et al. Reliability problems associated with the modified Schober technique for true lumbar flexion measurement. *Spine.* 1992;17:345-348.

64. Stankovic R, Johnell O, Maly P, et al. Use of lumbar extension, slump test, physical and neurological examination in the evaluation of patients with suspected herniated nucleus pulposus: a prospective clinical study. *Man Ther.* 1999;4:25-32.

65. Viitanen JV, Kokko ML, Heikkila S, et al. Assessment of thoraco-lumbar rotation in ankylosing spondylitis: a simple tape method. *Clin Rheumatol.* 1999;18:152-157.

66. Rahali-Khachlouf H, Poiraudeau S, Fermanian J, et al. Validité et reproductibilité des mesures cliniques rachidiennes dans la spon-dylarthrite ankylosante. *Ann Readapt Med Phys.* 2001;44:205-212.

67. Victor M, Ropper AH, Adams RD. *Adams & Victor's Principles of Neurology.* 7th ed. New York: McGraw-Hill Professional; 2001.

68. Van Adrichem JAM, Van der Korst JK. Assessment of the flexibility of the lumbar spine: a pilot study in children and adolescents. *Scand J Rheumatol.* 1973;2:87-91.

69. Tousignant M, Poulin L, Machand S, et al. The Modified–Modified Schober Test for range of motion assessment of lumbar flexion in patients with low back pain: a study of criterion validity, intra- and inter-rater reliability and minimum metrically detectable change. *Disabil Rehabil.* 2005;27:553-559.

70. Loebl WY. Measurement of spinal posture and range of spinal movement. *Ann Phys Med.* 1967;9:103-110.

70a. Anderson GBJ, Cocchiarella L. *AMA Guides to the Evaluation of Permanent Impairment.* 5th ed. 2000.

71. Nattrass CL, Nitschke JE, Disler PB, et al. Lumbar spine range of motion as a measure of physical and functional impairment: an investigation of validity. *Clin Rehabil.* 1999;13:211-218.

72. Dillard J, Trafimow J, Andersson GB, et al. Motion of the lumbar spine: reliability of two measurement techniques. *Spine.* 1991;16:321-324.

73. Ng JK, Kippers V, Richardson CA, et al. Range of motion and lordosis of the lumbar spine: reliability of measurement and nor-mative values. *Spine.* 2001;26:53-60.

74. Dopf CA, Mandel SS, Geiger DF, et al. Analysis of spine motion variability using a computerized goniometer compared to physical examination: a prospective clinical study. *Spine.* 1994;19:586-595.

75. Keeley J, Mayer TG, Cox R, et al. Quantification of lumbar func-tion. 5: reliability of range-of-motion measures in the sagittal plane and in-vivo torso rotation measurement technique. *Spine.* 1986;11:31-35.

76. Mellin G. Correlations of spinal mobility with degree of chronic low back pain after correction for age and arthometric factors. *Spine.* 1987;12:464-468.

77. Mellin G. Measurement of thoracolumbar posture and mobility with a Myrin inclinometer. *Spine.* 1986;11:759-762.

78. Mellin G. Method and instrument for noninvasive measurements of thoracolumbar rotation. *Spine.* 1987;12:28-31.

79. MacDermid JC, Arumugam V, Vincent JI, et al. The reliability and validity of the computerized double inclinometer in measuring lumbar mobility. *Open Orthop J.* 2014;8:355-360.

80. Bedekar N, Suryawanshi M, Rairikar S, et al. Inter and intra-rater reliability of mobile device goniometer in measuring lumbarflex-ion range of motion. *J Back Musculoskelet Rehabil.* 2014;27:161-166.

81. Kolber M, Pizzini M, Robinson A, et al. The reliability and concur-rent validity of measurements used to quantify lumbar spine mobility: an analysis of an iPhone® application and gravity based inclinometry. *Int J Sports Phys Ther.* 2013;8:129-137.

82. Ohlen G, Spangfort E, Tingvall C. Measurement of spinal con-figuration and mobility with Debrunner's Kyphometer. *Spine.* 1989;14:580-583.

83. Hakelius A, Hindmarsh J. The comparative reliability of preopera-tive diagnostic methods in lumbar disc surgery. *Acta Orthop Scand.* 1972;43:234-238.

84. Hakelius A. Prognosis in sciatica. *Acta Orthop Scand.* 1970;129(suppl):1-70.

85. Kerr RSC, Cadoux-Hudson TA, Adams CB, et al. The value of accurate clinical assessment in the surgical management of the lumbar disc protrusion. *J Neurol Neurosurg Psychiatry.* 1988;51:169-173.

86. Kortelainen P, Puranen J, Koivisto E, et al. Symptoms and signs of sciatica and their relation to the localization of the lumbar disc herniation. *Spine.* 1985;10:8-92.

87. Knutsson B. Comparative value of electromyographic, myelo-graphic, and clinical–neurological examinations in diagnosis of lumbar root compression syndrome. *Acta Orthop Scand.* 1961;49(suppl):1-134.

88. Lauder TD. Physical examination signs, clinical symptoms, and their relationship to electrodiagnostic findings and the presence of radiculopathy. *Phys Med Rehabil Clin N Am.* 2002;13:451-467.

89. Ortiz-Corredor F. Clinical examination and electromyographic abnormalities in patients with lower back pain. *Rev Neurol.* 2003;37:106-111.

90. Suri P, Rainville J, Katz JN, et al. The accuracy of the physical examination for the diagnosis of midlumbar and low lumbar nerve root impingement. *Spine.* 2011;36:63-73.

91. Kosteljanetz M, Esperen JO, Halburt H, et al. Predictive value of clinical and surgical findings in patients with lumbago-sciatica: a prospective study (part 1). *Acta Neurochir (Wien).* 1984;73:67-76.

92. Iizuka Y, Iizuka H, Tsutsumi S, et al. Foot drop due to lumbar degenerative conditions: mechanism and prognostic factors in herniated nucleus pulposus and lumbar spinal stenosis. *J Neuro-surg Spine.* 2009;10:260-264.

93. Al Nezari NH, Anthony G, Schneiders AG, et al. Neurological examination of the peripheral nervous system to diagnose lumbar spinal disc herniation with suspected radiculopathy: a systematic review and meta-analysis. *Spine J.* 2013;13:657-674.

94. O'Keeffe ST, Smith T, Valacio R, et al. A comparison of two tech-niques for ankle jerk assessment in elderly subjects. *Lancet.* 1994;344:1619-1620.

95. Andersson GB, Deyo RA. History and physical examination in patients with herniated lumbar discs. *Spine.* 1996;21(suppl 24):10S-18S.

95a. Iversen T, Solberg TK, Romner B, et al. Accuracy of physical examination for chronic lumbar radiculopathy. *BMC Musculoskelet Disord.* 2013;14:206.

96. Frost JJ. *Contribution a l'étude clinique de la sciatique.* Thèse no. 33, Faculté de Médecine, Paris, 1881.

97. Lindblom K, Hultqvist G. Absorption of protruded disc tissue. *J Bone Joint Surg Am.* 1950;32:557-560.

98. Karbowski K, Radanov BP. Historical perspective: the history of the discovery of the sciatica stretching phenomenon. *Spine.* 1995;20:1315-1317.

99. Inman VT, Saunders JB. The clinico-anatomical aspects of the lumbosacral region. *Radiology.* 1942;38:669-678.

100. Falconer MA, McGeorge M, Begg AC. Observations on the cause and mechanism of symptom production in sciatica and low back pain. *J Neurol Neurosurg Psychiatry.* 1948;11:13-26.

101. Goddard MD, Reid JD. Movements induced by straight leg raising in the lumbosacral roots, nerves and plexus and in the intrapelvic section of the sciatic nerve. *J Neurol Neurosurg Psychiatry.* 1965;28:12-18.

102. Rade M, Könönen M, Vanninen R, et al. 2014 young investigator award winner: in vivo magnetic resonance imaging measurement of spinal cord displacement in the thoracolumbar region of asymptomatic subjects: part 1: straight leg raise test. *Spine.* 2014;39:1288-1293.

103. Fahrni WH. Observation on straight leg raising with special reference to nerve root adhesions. *Can J Surg.* 1966;9:44-48.

104. Shiqing X, Quanzhi Z, Dehao F. Significance of the straight leg raising test in the diagnosis and clinical evaluation of lower lumbar intervertebral disc protrusion. *J Bone Joint Surg.* 1987;69A:517-522.

105. Kosteljanetz M, Bang F, Schmidt-Olsen S. The clinical significance of straight leg raising (Lasègue's sign) in the diagnosis of pro-lapsed lumbar disc: interobserver variation and correlation with surgical findings. *Spine.* 1988;13:393-395.

106. Iglesias-Casarrubios P, Alday-Anzola R, Ruíz-López P, et al. Laseg-ue's test as prognostic factor for patients undergoing lumbar disc surgery. *Neurocirugia (Astur).* 2004;152:138-143.

107. Deville WL, van der Windt DA, Dzaferagic A, et al. The test of Lasègue: systematic review of the accuracy in diagnosing herni-ated discs. *Spine.* 2000;25:1140-1147.

108. Jönsson B, Strömqvist B. The straight leg raising test and the severity of symptoms in lumbar disc herniation. *Spine.* 1995;20:27-30.

109. Jönsson B, Strömqvist B. Symptoms and signs in degeneration of the lumbar spine: a prospective, consecutive study of 300 oper-ated patients. *J Bone Joint Surg.* 1993;75B:381-385.

110. Capra F, Vanti C, Donati R, et al. Validity of the straight-leg raise test for patients with sciatic pain with or without lumbar pain using magnetic resonance imaging results as a reference standard. *J Manipulative Physiol Ther.* 2011;34:231-238.

111. van der Windt DA, Simons E, Riphagen II, et al. Physical examination for lumbar radiculopathy due to disc herniation in patients with low-back pain. *Cochrane Database Syst Rev.* 2010;(2):CD007431.

112. Charnley J. Orthopaedic signs in the diagnosis of disc protrusion, with special reference to the straight leg raising test. *Lancet.* 1951;260:186-192.

113. Magee DJ. *Orthopedic Physical Assessment.* Philadelphia: W.B. Saunders; 1992.

114. Edgar MA, Park WM. Induced pain patterns on passive straight leg raising in lower lumbar disc protrusion. *J Bone Joint Surg.* 1974;56B:658-666.

115. Gurdjian ES, Webster JE, Ostrowski AZ, et al. Herniated lumbar intervertebral discs: an analysis of 1176 operated cases. *J Trauma.* 1961;1:158-176.

116. Aronson HA, Dunsmore RH. Herniated upper lumbar discs. *J Bone Joint Surg Am.* 1963;45:311-317.

117. Albeck MJ. A critical assessment of clinical diagnosis of disc herniation in patients with monoradicular sciatica. *Acta Neurochir (Wien).* 1996;138:40-44.

118. Hirsch C, Nachemson A. The reliability of lumbar disk surgery. *Clin Orthop.* 1963;29:189-195.

119. Hudgins WR. The crossed straight leg raising test: a diagnostic sign of herniated disc. *J Occup Med.* 1979;21:407-408.

120. Poiraudeau S, Foltz V, Drapé JL, et al. Value of the bell test and the hyperextension test for diagnosis in sciatica associated with disc herniation: comparison with Lasègue's sign and the crossed Lasègue's sign. *Rheumatology (Oxford).* 2001;40:460-466.

121. Cyriax J. Perineuritis. *Br Med J.* 1942;1:578-580.

122. Walsh J, Hall T. Agreement and correlation between the straight leg raise and slump tests in subjects with leg pain. *J Manipulative Physiol Ther.* 2009;32:184-192.

123. Abdullah AF, Wolber PG, Warfield JR, et al. Surgical management of extreme lateral lumbar disc herniations. *Neurosurgery.* 1988;22:648-653.

124. Christodoulides AN. Ipsilateral sciatica on the femoral nerve stretch test is pathognomonic of an L4/5 disc protrusion. *J Bone Joint Surg Br.* 1989;71:88-89.

125. Porchet F, Frankhauser H, de Tribolet N. Extreme lateral lumbar disc herniation: a clinical presentation of 178 patients. *Acta Neurochir (Wien).* 1994;127:203-209.

126. Kummel BM. Nonorganic signs of significance in low back pain. *Spine.* 1996;21:1077-1081.

127. Carleton RN, Abrams MP, Kachur SS, et al. Waddell's symptoms as correlates of vulnerabilities associated with fear-anxiety-avoidance models of pain: pain-related anxiety, catastrophic thinking, perceived disability, and treatment outcome. *J Occup Rehabil.* 2009;19:364-374.

128. Waddell G, McCulloch JA, Kummel E, et al. Nonorganic physical signs in low-back pain. *Spine.* 1980;5:117-125.

129. Fajersztajn J. Ueber das gekreutzte ischiaphanomen. *Wien Klin Wochenschr.* 1901;14:41-47.

130. Woodhall B, Hayes G. The well leg raising test of Fajersztajn in the diagnosis of ruptured lumbar intervertebral disc. *J Bone Joint Surg.* 1950;32A:786-792.

131. Khuffash B, Porter RW. Cross leg pain and trunk list. *Spine.* 1989;14:602-603.

132. Vucetic N, Svensson O. Physical signs in lumbar disc hernia. *Clin Orthop.* 1996;333:192-201.

133. Cram RH. A sign of the sciatic nerve root pressure. *J Bone Joint Surg Br.* 1953;35:192195.

134. Wassermann S. Ueber ein neues Schenkelnersymptom nebstr Bemerkungen zur Diagnostik der Schenkelnerverkrankungen. *Dtsch Z Nervenbeilk.* 1918/19;43:140-143.

135. Dyck P. The femoral nerve traction test with lumbar disc protrusions. *Surg Neurol.* 1976;6:163-166.

136. Estridge MN, Rothe SA, Johnson NG. The femoral stretching test: a valuable sign in diagnosing upper lumbar disc herniation. *J Neurosurg.* 1982;57:813-817.

137. Geraci MC, Alleva JT. Physical examination of the spine and its functional kinetic chain. In: Cole AJ, Herrring SA, eds. *The Low Back Pain Handbook.* Philadelphia: Hanley & Belfus; 1996:60.

138. Penning L, Wilmink JT. Biomechanics of lumbosacral dural sac: a study of flexion–extension myelography. *Spine.* 1981;6:398-408.

139. Trainor K, Pinnington MA. Reliability and diagnostic validity of the slump knee bend neurodynamic test for upper/mid lumbar

140. Kreitz BG, Cote P, Yong-Hing K. Crossed femoral stretching test: a case report. *Spine.* 1996;21:1584-1586.

141. Waddell G, et al. Normality and reliability in the clinical assessment of backache. *Br Med J (Clin Res Ed).* 1982;284:1519-1523.

142. Sturesson B, Selvik G, Uden A. Movements of the sacroiliac joints: a roentgen stereophotogrammetric analysis. *Spine.* 1989;14:162-165.

143. Sturesson B, Uden A, Vleeming A. A radiostereometric analysis of movements of the sacroiliac joints during the standing hip flexion test. *Spine.* 2000;25:364-368.

144. Colachis SC, Worden RE, Bechtol CO, et al. Movement of the sacroiliac joint in the adult male: a preliminary report. *Arch Phys Med Rehabil.* 1963;44:490-499.

145. Frigerio NA, Stowe RS, Howe JW. Movement of the sacroiliac joint. *Clin Orthop Relat Res.* 1974;100:370. Communications: 1981;155:293-297.

146. Gemmel HA, Johnson BH. Incidence of sacroiliac joint dysfunction and low back pain in fit college students. *J Manipulative Physiol Ther.* 1990;13(2):63-67.

147. Mierau DR, Cassidy JD, Hamin T. Sacroiliac joint dysfunction and low back pain in school aged children. *J Manipulative Physiol Ther.* 1984;7:81-84.

148. Dreyfuss P, Dreyer S, Griffin J, et al. Positive sacroiliac screening tests in asymptomatic adults. *Spine.* 1994;19:1138-1143.

149. Mitchell FL, Morgan PS, Pruzzo NA. *An Evaluation and Treatment Manual of Osteopathic Muscle Energy Techniques.* Valley Park, MO: Mitchell, Moran & Pruzzo Associates; 1979.

150. Vincent-Smith B, Gibbons P. Inter-examiner and intra-examiner reliability of the standing flexion test. *Man Ther.* 1999;4:87-93.

151. Bourdillon JF. Detailed examination. In: *Spinal Manipulation.* 4th ed. London: William Heinemann Medical Books; 1987:58-72.

152. Potter NA, Rothstein JM. Intertester reliability for selected clinical tests of the sacroiliac joint. *Phys Ther.* 1985;65:1671-1675.

153. Riddle DL, Freburger JK. Evaluation of the presence of sacroiliac joint region dysfunction using a combination of tests: a multi-center intertester reliability study. *Phys Ther.* 2002;82:772-781.

154. Levangie PK. Four clinical tests of sacroiliac joint dysfunction: the association of test results with innominate torsion among patients with and without low back pain. *Phys Ther.* 1999;79:1043-1057.

155. DiGiovanna EL, Schiowitz S. *An Osteopathic Approach to Diagnosis and Treatment.* Philadelphia: JB Lippincott; 1991.

156. Solonen KA, Rokkanen P. Changes in the hip joint caused by asymmetry of the lower limbs: an experimental study on bipedal rats. *Ann Chir Gynaecol Fenn.* 1967;56:189-192.

157. Solonen KA. Perforation of the anterior annulus fibrosus during operation for prolapsed disc. *Ann Chir Gynaecol Fenn.* 1975;64:385-387.

158. Solonen KA. The sacroiliac joint in the light of anatomical, roentgenological, and clinical studies. *Acta Othrop Scand Suppl.* 1957;27(suppl):1-115.

159. Beal MC. The sacroiliac problem: review of anatomy, mechanics, and diagnosis. *J Am Osteopath Assoc.* 1982;81:667-679.

160. Dreyfuss P, Michaelsen M, Pauza K, et al. The value of medical history and physical examination in diagnosing sacroiliac joint pain. *Spine.* 1996;21:2594-2602.

161. Gillet H, Liekens M. *Belgian Chiropractic Research Notes.* 11th ed. Huntington Beach, CA: Motion Palpation Institute; 1981.

162. Meijne W, van Neerbos K, Aufdemkampe G, et al. Intraexaminer and interexaminer reliability of the Gillet test. *J Manipulative Physiol Ther.* 1999;22:4-9.

163. Wiles MR. Reproducibility and inter-examiner correlation of motion palpation findings of the sacroiliac joints. *J Can Chiropr Assoc.* 1980;24:56-69.

164. Herzog W, Read LJ, Conway PJ, et al. Reliability of motion palpation procedures to detect sacroiliac joint fixations. *J Manipulative Physiol Ther.* 1989;12:86-92.

165. Carmichael JP. Inter- and intra-examiner reliability of palpation for sacroiliac joint dysfunction. *J Manipulative Physiol Ther.* 1987;10:164-171.

166. Van der Wurff P, Meyne W, Hagmeijer RH. Clinical tests of the sacroiliac joint. *Man Ther.* 2000;5:89-96.

167. Maigne JY, Aivaliklis A, Pfefer F. Results of sacroiliac joint double block and value of sacroiliac pain provocation tests in 54 patients with low back pain. *Spine.* 1996;21:1889-1892.

168. Murakami E, Aizawa T, Noguchi K, et al. Diagram specific to sacroiliac joint pain site indicated by one-finger test. *J Orthop Sci.* 2008;13:492-497.

169. Newton DRL. Discussion on the clinical and radiological aspect. *Proc R Soc Med.* 1957;50:850-853.

170. McCombe PF, Fairbank JC, Cockersole BC, et al. Volvo Award in Clinical Sciences. Reproducibility of physical signs in low-back. *Spine.* 1989;14:908-918.

171. Laslett M, Williams M. The reliability of selected pain provocation tests for sacroiliac joint pathology. *Spine.* 1994;19:1243-1249.

172. Laslett M. The value of the physical examination in diagnosis of painful sacroiliac joint pathologies. *Spine.* 1998;23:962-964.

173. Strender LE, Sjoblom A, Sundell K, et al. Interexaminer reliability in physical examination of patients with low back pain. *Spine.* 1997;22:814-820.

174. Van der Wurff P, Hagmeijer RH, Meyne W. Clinical tests of the sacroiliac joint—a systemic methodological review. 1: reliability. *Man Ther.* 2000;5:30-36.

175. Rantanen P, Airaksinen O. Poor agreement between so-called sacroiliac joint tests in ankylosing spondylitis patients. *J Manip Med.* 1989;4:62-64.

176. Blower PW, Griffin AJ. Clinical sacroiliac tests in ankylosing spondylitis and other causes of low back pain: two studies. *Ann Rheum Dis.* 1984;43:192-195.

177. Russel AS, Maksymowych W, LeClercq S. Clinical examination of the sacroiliac joints: a prospective study. *Arthritis Rheum.* 1981;24:1575-1577.

178. Werner CM, Hoch A, Gautier L, et al. Distraction test of the posterior superior iliac spine (PSIS) in the diagnosis of sacroiliac joint arthropathy. *BMC Surg.* 2013;13:52.

179. Szadek KM, van der Wurff P, van Tulder MW, et al. Diagnostic validity of criteria for sacroiliac joint pain; a systematic review. *J Pain.* 2009;10:354-368.

180. Stuber KJ. Specificity, sensitivity, and predictive values of clinical tests of the sacroiliac joint: a systematic review of the literature. *J Can Chiropr Assoc.* 2007;51:30-41.

181. Cattley P, Winyard J, Trevaskis J, et al. Validity and reliability of clinical tests for the sacroiliac joint. A review of literature. *Australas Chiropr Osteopathy.* 2002;10(2):73-80.

182. Laslett M, Young SB, Aprill CN. Diagnosing painful sacroiliac joints: A validity study of a McKenzie evaluation and sacroiliac provocation tests. *Aust J Physiother.* 2003;49:89-97.

183. Patrick HT. Brachial neuritis and sciatica. *JAMA.* 1917;LXIX: 2176-2179.

184. Kenna C, Murtagh J. Patrick or FABERE test to test hip and sacroiliac joint disorders. *Aust Fam Physician.* 1989;18:375.

185. Deursen van LLJM, Patijn J, Ockhuysen AL, et al. The value of some clinical tests of the sacroiliac joint. *J Manual Med.* 1990;5:96-99.

186. Broadhurst NA, Bond MJ. Pain provocation tests for the assessment of sacroiliac joint dysfunction. *J Spinal Disord.* 1998;11: 341-345.

187. Gaenslen FJ. Sacro-iliac arthrodesis. *JAMA.* 1927;89:2031-2035.

188. Gross J, Fetto J, Rosen E. *Musculoskeletal Examination.* Cambridge, MA: Blackwell Science; 1996.

189. Hoehler FK, Tobis JS. Low back pain and its treatment by spinal manipulation: measures of flexibility and asymmetry. *Rhematol Rehabil.* 1982;21:21-26.

190. Hseih CY, Walker JM, Gillis K. Straight leg raising test: compression of three instruments. *Phys Ther.* 1983;63:1429-1432.

191. Mennell J. *Joint Pain: Diagnosis and Treatment Using Manipulative Techniques.* Boston: Little, Brown; 1964.

192. Mennell J. The science and art of joint manipulation. In: *The Spinal Column.* Vol. II. Philadelphia: Blakiston Co.; 1952.

193. Mens JM, Vleeming A, Snijders CJ, et al. The active straight leg raising test and mobility of the pelvic joints. *Eur Spine J.* 1999;8:468-473.

194. Cibulka MT, Koldehoff R. Clinical usefulness of a cluster of sacroiliac joint tests in patients with and without low back pain. *J Orthop Sports Phys Ther.* 1999;29:83-89, discussion 90-92.

195. Slipman CW, Sterenfeld EB, Chou LH, et al. The predictive value of provocative sacroiliac joint stress maneuvers in the diagnosis of sacroiliac joint syndrome. *Arch Phys Med Rehabil.* 1998;79: 288-292.

196. Young S, Aprill C, Laslett M. Correlation of clinical examination characteristics with three sources of chronic low back pain. *Spine J.* 2003;3:460-465.

Physical Examination of the Pelvis and Hip

8

Brian Krabak, MD, MBA, FACSM | Walter Sussman, DO |
J. W. Thomas Byrd, MD

INTRODUCTION

The hip joint is one of the more stable joints of the body. The stability stems from the intimacy of the head of the femur within the acetabulum like a ball in a socket. This results in a paradox. Most traumatic injuries require substantial force. However, because of the limited tolerances associated with the constrained anatomy, slight incongruences can lead to early age wear as exemplified both by dysplasia and femoroacetabular impingement. In general, injuries to the hip joint result in difficulty with ambulation. However, pain in the hip region may be referred from other areas such as the sacroiliac joint (SIJ) or lumbar spine. Therefore, careful examination of the hip and the surrounding regions is essential.

INSPECTION, PALPATION, AND RANGE OF MOTION

The initial examination should occur with the individual standing. The examiner should document any soft tissue or bony contour abnormalities, edema, skin discoloration, or scars. In addition, the examiner should note the alignment of the lower extremities. Excessive external rotation at the ankle is potentially indicative of femoral retroversion, while excessive internal rotation ("toeing in") is potentially indicative of femoral anteversion. Patients with intra-articular hip pathology may stand with the involved hip and ipsilateral knee in a slightly flexed position to unload the involved limb. The individual should then be examined for any asymmetry of shoulder height, spinal alignment, iliac crest height, and both femoral and tibial height. Any asymmetry may be indicative of an underlying scoliosis or leg length discrepancy. Compensatory lumbar lordosis may be present in cases of a tight iliopsoas. Similarly, the patient should be examined while supine to further assess for any obvious asymmetries.

A general assessment of the patient's gait in both the sagittal and frontal planes is essential. Abnormal gait patterns, such as hip hiking, circumduction, or excessive trunk extension, may be evidence of muscle weakness, leg length discrepancy, or pain. With intra-articular pathology, the patient may have a shortened stance phase of gait on the affected side, avoidance of hip extension, and shifting of the torso over the involved hip, creating an abductor lurch. Any of these findings should prompt a more focused examination. In addition, the examiner will get a sense of the patient's overall posture and balance while ambulating.

Palpation of the hip area is generally divided into anterior, medial, lateral, and posterior regions. The examiner should be familiar with the deep anatomy and correlating bony landmarks, and any areas of tenderness should be noted. Asking the patient to locate the area of maximal tenderness with one finger can help focus the palpatory examination. While structures should be palpated in a systematic manner, the examiner shoulder reserve the area identified by the patient using the "one-finger test" for last in order to build the patient's trust by not stimulating pain at the beginning.

Often palpation is more useful for extra-articular problems, but deep palpation over the anterior hip capsule may cause pain in cases of intra-articular pathology. In addition, the anterior examination should include palpation of the anterior superior iliac spine and the insertion of the sartorius, anterior hip flexor region, and both the pubic rami and pubic symphysis. The femoral artery and lymph nodes are easily palpated in the femoral triangle, roughly half the distance between the anterior superior iliac spines (ASIS) and pubic symphysis distal to the inguinal ligament.

Laterally, the iliac crest, greater trochanter, insertion site of the gluteus minimus and gluteus medius, muscle belly of the gluteus medius, and origin of the tensor fascia lata should be palpated. Tenderness over the greater trochanter may be indicative of greater trochanter pain syndrome, a common source of lateral hip pain. Posterior palpation should include the posterior superior iliac spine, SIJ, ischial tuberosities and the origin of the hamstrings, and the piriformis and overlying gluteus maximus muscles.

Active and resisted range of motion (ROM) of the hip is generally assessed with the patient either in a sitting or supine position. The exception is hip abduction, which is most easily performed in the lateral position. Stabilization of the pelvis is important when assessing ROM of the hip. Resisted hip flexion with the knee flexed isolates the iliopsoas, while the rectus femoris, which crosses both the hip and knee joint, is recruited when the knee is extended. There can be a wide range of what is considered "normal," so of greater importance is assessing for asymmetry from one side to the other.

MUSCLE TIGHTNESS OR PATHOLOGY OF THE LUMBOPELVIC REGION (TABLE 8.1)

Table 8.1   Tests for Periarticular Hip Pathology

Test	Description	Reliability/Validity Tests	Comments
Thomas Test	The patient lies supine while the examiner checks for excessive lordosis. The examiner flexes one of the patient's hips, bringing the knee to the chest to flatten out the lumbar spine, and the patient holds the flexed hip against the chest. If there is no flexion contracture, the hip being tested (the straight leg) remains on the examining table. If a contracture is present, the patient's leg rises off the table. The angle of contracture can be measured.	Bartlett et al. 1985[4] Interrater reliability: 0.89–0.93, mean difference 1.1–5.1 degrees Intrarater reliability: 0.70–0.90, mean difference 1.9–9.2 degrees Kilgour et al. 2003[5] Intrarater reliability: 0.17–0.66 CP and 0.09–0.91 control McWhirk and Glanzman 2006[6] Interrater reliability: 0.58, mean absolute difference 3.96 Mutlu et al. 2007[7] Interrater reliability: 0.95 Intrarater reliability: 0.99 Glanzman et al. 2008[8] Intrarater reliability: 0.98 Lee et al. 2011[9] Interrater reliability: 0.5 CP and 0.2 control Herrero et al. 2011[10] Intrarater reliability: 0.83–0.95 Interrater reliability: 0.375–0.475	Reliability of 2 experienced therapists examining 15 children with spastic diplegic CP, 15 with meningomyelocele and 15 healthy children Reliability of 1 pediatric therapist examining 25 children with spastic diplegic CP, 25 healthy controls Reliability of 2 therapists with varying experience examining 46 legs of 25 children with spastic CP Reliability of 3 therapists examining 38 children with spastic diplegic CP on 2 different occasions Reliability of 2 therapists with varying experience examining 50 legs of 25 patients with spastic CP Reliability of 3 examiners of 37 children with CP and 36 healthy controls Reliability of 5 therapists examining 7 children (14 limbs) with spastic CP during 2 different sessions
Prone hip extension (Staheli test)	The patient lies prone with the pelvis on the table and the hips at the edge of the table. The examiner supports the uninvolved leg and extends the involved leg until the pelvis rises off the table. The angle of extension can be measured.	Bartlett et al. 1985[4] Interrater reliability: 0.82–0.93, mean difference 1.1–5.8 degrees Intrarater reliability: 0.80–0.92, mean difference 2.1–9.6 degrees Kilgour et al. 2003[5] Intrarater reliability: intrasessional 0.78–0.91 CP and 0.8–0.92 control; intersessional 0.55–0.8 CP and 0.04–0.2 control Glanzman et al. 2008[8] Intrarater reliability: 0.98 Lee et al. 2011[9] Interrater reliability: 0.2 CP and 0.1 control	Reliability of 2 experienced therapists examining 15 children with spastic diplegic CP, 15 with meningomyelocele and 15 healthy children Reliability of 1 pediatric therapist examining 25 children with spastic diplegic CP, 25 healthy controls. Two measurements were taken at the initial visit (intrasessional) and again at 7 days (intersessional) by a pediatric PT Reliability of 2 therapists with varying experience examining 50 legs of 25 patients with spastic CP Reliability of 3 examiners of 37 children with CP and 36 healthy controls
Modified Thomas test	The patient is positioned at the end of the examination table with the uninvolved leg flexed to flatten the lordotic curve, and the involved leg is allowed to extend with gravity. The degree of hip extension is measured.	Ashton et al. 1978[11] Interrater reliability: 0.33–0.52 moderate CP and 0.4–0.516 severe CP Harvey 1998[12] Intrarater reliability: 0.91 Clapis et al. 2008[13] Interrater reliability: 0.89–0.92 Intrarater reliability: 0.86–0.92 Cejudo et al. 2015[14] Intersession reliability: 0.87–0.91 Wakefield et al. 2015[15] Interrater reliability: GON 0.3–0.65; TRIG 0.91–0.94 Intrarater reliability, GON 0.51–0.54; TRIG 0.9–0.95	Reliability of 16 therapists examined 2 children with moderate and 2 children with severe CP Reliability of 3 measurements of the modified Thomas test as a measure of iliopsoas flexibility of 117 elite athletes (tennis, basketball, rowing, running) Reliability of 2 therapists using inclinometer and goniometric measurements of hip extension in 42 healthy subjects Reliability of 2 therapists across 3 sessions examining 90 asymptomatic athletes Reliability of 2 examiners using goniometric (GON) and trigonometric (TRIG) measurements in 22 healthy college students

Table 8.1   Tests for Periarticular Hip Pathology (Continued)

Test	Description	Reliability/Validity Tests	Comments
Pelvifemoral angle	The patient is side-lying with the hip to be measured upward. The examiner passively extends the hip with the knee in 30 degrees of flexion. Mundale method: Stationary arm perpendicular to the ASIS-iliac spine line. Moveable arm along the axis of the femur forming an angle stationary arm. Milch angle: Stationary arm along the ASIS-ischial tuberosity line. Moveable arm along the axis of the femur, forming the pelvifemoral angle.	Bartlett et al. 1985[4] Mundale: Interrater reliability: 0.63–0.91, mean difference 5.8–7.8 degrees Intrarater reliability: 0.79–0.84, mean difference 7.1–10.9 degrees Milch: Interrater reliability: 0.78–0.92, mean difference 3.6–4.3 degrees Intrarater reliability: 0.73–0.77, mean difference 6.7–7.8 degrees	Reliability of 2 experienced therapists examining 15 children with spastic diplegic CP, 15 with meningomyelocele and 15 healthy children
Ely test	The patient lies prone while the examiner passively flexes the patient's knee. Upon flexion of the knee, the patient's hip on the same side spontaneously flexes, indicating that the rectus femoris muscle is tight on that side and that the test is positive. The two sides should be tested and compared.	Peeler and Anderson 2008[16] Intrarater reliability: 0.69	Interrater reliability: 0.66 Reliability of 3 therapists examining 54 healthy subjects in 2 distinct sessions
Rectus femoris contracture test (modified Thomas test)	The patient lies prone while the examiner passively flexes the patient's knee. Upon flexion of the knee, the patient's hip on the same side spontaneously flexes, indicating that the rectus femoris muscle is tight on that side and that the test is positive. The two sides should be tested and compared. The patient lies supine with the knees bent over the end or edge of the examining table. The patient flexes one knee onto the chest. The angle of the test knee should remain at 90 degrees. A contracture may be present if the test knee extends slightly.	Harvey 1998[12] Intrarater reliability: 0.94 Peeler and Anderson 2008[16] Intrarater reliability: 0.67 Atamaz et al. 2011[17] Intrarater reliability: 0.84–0.91 Interrater reliability: 0.75–0.87 Peeler and Leiter 2013[18] Intrarater reliability: 0.98 Interrater reliability: 0.97	Reliability of 3 measurements of quadriceps flexibility of 117 elite athletes Interrater reliability: 0.5 3 therapists assessing 57 healthy subjects during 2 different sessions Reliability of 2 examiners assessing 66 healthy subjects in a test-retest design Ten therapists scoring the degree of rectus femoris flexibility from digital photographs of 28 healthy college students being examined with the modified Thomas test
Ober test	Original Ober test: The patient lies on the side, with the thigh next to the table flexed to obliterate any lumbar lordosis. The upper leg is flexed at a right angle at the knee. The examiner grasps the ankle lightly with one hand and steadies the patient's hip with the other. The upper leg is abducted widely and extended so that the thigh is in line with the body. If there is an abduction contracture, the leg will remain more or less passively abducted. Modified Ober test: Peformed as above, but knee is fully extended before allowing gravity to bring the leg into adduction.	Melchione and Sullivan 1993[19] Intrarater reliability: 0.94 Interrater reliability: 0.73 Gajdosik et al. 2003[20] Intrarater reliability: 0.83–0.87 Intrarater reliability: 0.82–0.92 Reese and Bandy 2003[21] Intrarater reliability: 0.90 Intrarater reliability: 0.91	Two therapists examining 10 subjects with anterior knee pain using the modified Ober test with a test-retest design Reliability of one therapist taking 3 measurements using the Ober and modified Ober tests examining 49 healthy subjects Reliability of the Ober and modified Ober tests in a study of 61 subjects examined by 1 therapist using an inclinometer during 2 distinct sessions

Continued on following page

Table 8.1   Tests for Periarticular Hip Pathology (Continued)

Test	Description	Reliability/Validity Tests	Comments

Piriformis test	SLR or *Lasègue's sign:*
	The patient is supine; examiner passively lifts extended leg.
	Pace test/active piriformis test:
	The patient is seated. The examiner places his or her hands on the lateral aspect of the knee and asks the patient to push the hands apart. Pain with resisted abduction–external rotatation is a positive test.
	Passive pirifomris stretch:
	The patient is side-lying with the nontest leg against the table, and the patient flexes the test hip to 60 degrees with the knee flexed. The examiner applies a downward pressure to the knee, which the patient resists. Pain is elicited in the muscle if the piriformis is tight. The traditional variation described by Pace was with the patient seated. This test can also be performed with the patient in a seated position as described by Martin.[22]
		Martin 2011[22]
		  Straight-leg raise
		
		  Active piriformis test
		
		Seated piriformis stretch
		  Sensitivity: 52%
		  Specificity: 90%
		  +LR: 5.22
		  –LR: 0.53
		  OR: 9.82
			Validity of 3 different tests for piriformis syndrome in retrospective study. Examination performed on 35 patients with unexplained posterior hip pain evaluated by single examiner and diagnosis confirmed with endoscopic evaluation

Popliteal angle	The popliteal angle is measured with the patient supine and the hip flexed 90 degrees. The examiner attempts to extend the knee until firm resistance is met while the hip is maintained at 90 degrees (passive knee extension [PKE] method). This can also be performed with the patient actively extending the knee (AKE method). The popliteal angle is the angle from the tibia to the femur.	Gajdosik and Lusin 1983[23]
		  Intrarater reliability: 0.99
		
		Sullivan et al. 1992[24]
		  Intrarater reliability: 0.99
		  Interrater reliability: 0.93
		Davis et al. 2008[25]
		  Intrarater reliability: 0.94
		
		Atamaz et al. 2011[17]
		  Intrarater reliability: 0.68–0.73
		  Interrater reliability: 0.61–0.79
		Hamid et al. 2013[26]
		  Intrarater reliability: 0.75–0.97
		  Interrater reliability: 0.81–0.87
		
		Reurink et al. 2013[27]
		  AKE method
		  Interrater reliability: 0.89 injured;
		    0.76 uninjured knee
		  PKE method
		  Interrater reliability: 0.77 injured;
		    0.69 uninjured knee
			Reliability of single examiner using AKE method in 15 healthy subjects during 2 sessions
			Reliability of 2 examiners using the AKE method before and after stretching while examining 12 subjects
			Reliability and correlation of PKE, sacral angle, SLR, and sit and reach in test-retest design assessing 81 college-age subjects
			Reliability of 2 examiners using PKE method to assess 66 healthy subjects in a test-retest design
			Reliability of a sports physician and therapists examining 16 healthy subjects using the AKE method in a test-retest design
			Reliability of 2 examiners using the AKE and PKE methods and an inclinometer in assessing 50 athletes with an acute hamstring injury confirmed by MRI

Table 8.1   Tests for Periarticular Hip Pathology (Continued)

Test	Description	Reliability/Validity Tests	Comments
Trendelenburg test	The patient is observed standing on one limb. The test result is felt to be positive if the pelvis on the opposite side drops. A positive Trendelenburg test result is suggestive of a weak gluteus muscle or an unstable hip on the affected side.	Bird 2001[28] Sensitivity: 72.7% Specificity: 76.9% Intrarater reliability: 0.676 (95% CI; 0.270–1.08)	Twenty-four women with GTPS examined in both standing and ambulation, compared to MRI finding of gluteus medius tear
		Altman 2001[29] Sensitivity: 37% Specificity: 81%	Two hundred twenty-seven consecutive patients with clinical plus radiographic diagnosis of hip OA, compared with control group without hip OA. Intraobserver κ: 0.676 (95% CI; 0.270–1.08); 24 women underwent MRI for gluteus medius tear
		Burnett et al. 2006[30] Sensitivity: 38%	Retrospective review of clinical findings in 66 consecutive patients with arthroscopically confirmed labral tear
		Woodley 2008[31] Sensitivity: 23% Specificity: 94% +LR: 3.64 −LR: 0.82	Cross-sectional study of 40 patients with with GTPS, clinical findings compared with MRI
		Lequesne 2008[32] Sensitivity: 100% Specificity: 97%	Prospecitve study of 17 patients with GTPS, compared with MRI using sustained or fatigue Trendelenburg test
		Clohisy et al. 2009[33] Sensitivity: 33%	Prospective evaluation of 51 patients with symptomatic FAI
		Youdas et al. 2010[34] Sensitivity: 55% Specificity: 70% +LR: 1.83 Intrarater reliability: 0.63–0.69	20 patients with hip OA, and 20 healthy adults examined by 2 therapists using a goniometer over the ASIS and the axis of the femur

ASIS, Anterior superior iliac spines; *CI,* confidence interval; *CP,* cerebral palsy; *FAI,* femoroacetabular impingement; *GTPS,* greater trochanteric pain syndrome; *LR,* likelihood ratio; *MRI,* magnetic resonance imaging; *OA,* osteoarthritis; *OR,* odds ratio; *PT,* physical therapist; *SLR,* straight-leg raise.

THOMAS TEST (Video 8-1)

In 1876, Hugh Owens Thomas described a novel method to help differentiate "morbus coxae," or inflammatory disease of the hip, from "abscesses, sciatica, or hysterical simulation" of hip joint pain. He described the test as follows[1]:

> Having undressed the patient and laid him on his back upon a table or other hard plane surface, the surgeon takes the sound limb and flexes it, so that the sound knee joint is in contact with the chest. Thus he makes certain that the spine and back of the pelvis are lying flat on the table; an assistant maintains the sound limb in this fixed position; the patient is then urged to extend, as far as he is able, the diseased limb, and this he will be able to do in a degree varying with the previous duration of the infection. … By noticing the amount of flexion, the surgeon will, with practice, soon be able to guess the previous duration of the disease.

Since Thomas's original description, this test has become a common method of assessing fixed flexion deformities of the hip. Several modified versions of this test have been described in an attempt to isolate the hip joint and account for the impact of lumbar lordosis and/or pelvic tilt on motion at the hip. In 1936, Cave and Roberts[2] described a variant of the original Thomas test that is similar to the current description. In this method, the patient is positioned supine with the involved leg flat against the table and the uninvolved leg maximally flexed bringing the knee to the chest to flatten out any lumbar lordosis. If a contracture is present, the involved leg will rise off the table, and the angle of contracture can be measured (Fig. 8.1).

The lack of a "gold standard" for measuring hip flexion makes validating the Thomas test challenging, but a number of subjects have assessed the reliability of the Thomas test. In children with spastic cerebral palsy (CP), most studies have shown an excellent intrarater reliability with an intraclass coefficient (ICC) value of more than 0.80,[4,7,8,10] although not all studies have shown such a high intrarater reliability.[5] The interrater reliability has been fair in most, but not all, studies.[4,6,7,9,10]

MODIFIED THOMAS TEST

In 1978, Ashton and colleagues[11] described a variation of the Thomas test in which the patient is positioned at the end of the examination table, the uninvolved leg is flexed to flatten the lordotic curve, and the involved leg is extended

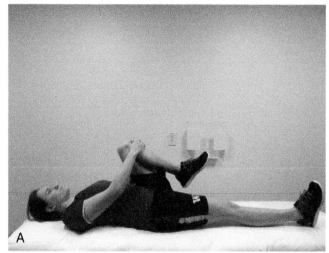

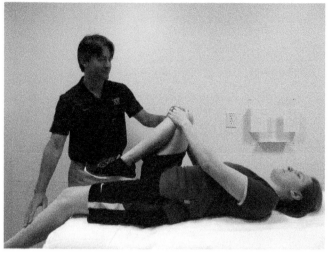

Figure 8.2 Normal Modified Thomas test.

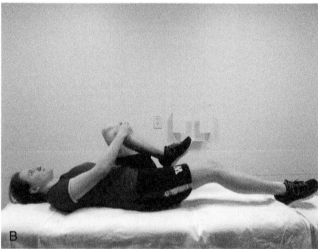

Figure 8.1 A, Normal Thomas test result. **B,** Iliopsoas tightness demonstrated by Thomas test.

(Fig. 8.2). In this study, therapists examined 4 children with spastic CP and found this method to lack interrater and intrarater reliability.

Harvey[12] used this "modified Thomas test" to assess the flexibility of the iliopsoas, as well as the quadriceps and tensor fascia lata (TFL)/iliotibial (IT) band, in 117 elite athletes. Harvey performed the modified Thomas test in the following manner:

> [T]he subject sat on the end of the plinth, rolled back onto the plinth, and held both knees to the chest. This ensured that the lumbar spine was flat on the plinth and the pelvis was in posterior rotation. The subject held the contralateral hip in maximal flexion with the arms, while the tested limb was lowered towards the floor.

The mean angle of hip extension, reflecting the flexibility of the iliopsoas, was −11.9 degrees, and the intrarater reliability was excellent (ICC = 0.91). Eland and associates[35] advocated stabilizing the pelvis and eliminating any regional motion by applying "enough pressure to maintain the position of the [anterior superior iliac spine] during extension." This counterbalances the weight and leverage of the

lower extremity and prevents anterior rotation of the innominate bone during the test.

A number of studies have examined the reliability of the modified Thomas test in healthy subjects. Clapis and colleagues[13] examined 42 asymptomatic subjects and found a high interrater and intrarater reliability using both an inclinometer and goniometer (r = 0.86 to 0.93; ICC = 0.86 to 0.92; r = 0.089 to 0.92; ICC = 0.91 to 0.93). Cejudo and coworkers[14] also found the modified Thomas test to be highly reliable when examining 60 futsal and 30 handball players (intersession reliability of 0.87 to 0.91). Wakefield and coworkers[15] examined 22 asymptomatic college students using a protocol similar to Clapis and associates[13] and compared measurements using a tape measure and trigonometric principles. In Wakefield's study,[15] the reliability of the goniometric measurements was low (intrarater ICC = 0.51 to 0.54; interrater ICC = 0.30 to 0.65; confidence interval [CI], 95%), but the reliability of the trigonometric technique was excellent (intrarater ICC = 0.90 to 0.95; interrater ICC = 0.91 to 0.94; CI, 95%).

PRONE HIP EXTENSION (STAHELI TEST)

In 1945, West[36] advocated measuring hip extension with the patient in a prone position on the examination table to "stabilize the torso." In the original description, the axis of the goniometer was centered over the greater trochanter, with the reference arm placed along the midaxillary line and the movable arm along the lateral midline of the femur. Moore[37] reported a similar method with the patient either in a prone or side-lying position.

Staheli[38] presented the "prone hip extension test," with the patient in a prone position with both hips comfortably flexed over the end of the examining table. The examiner stabilizes the noninvolved leg, places one hand on the pelvis, and gradually extends the involved thigh with the other hand (Fig. 8.3). The precise point at which the pelvis begins to rise marks the end of the hip motion and the beginning of spine motion. At this point, the examiner measures the degree of hip extension. The reliability of the prone hip extension test has been fair in most studies. In

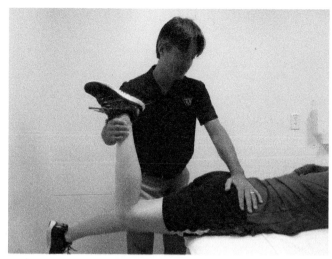

Figure 8.3   Prone hip extension.

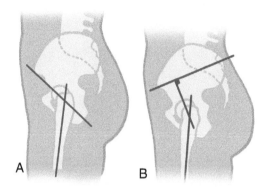

Figure 8.4   Measurements of the pelvifemoral angle. **A,** Milch angle. **B,** Mundale angle. (Reproduced with permission from Bartlett MD, Wolf LS, Shurtleff DB, et al. Hip flexion contractures: a comparison of measurement methods. *Arch Phys Med Rehabil.* 1985;66:620-625.)

Kilgour and coworkers'[5] study, the prone hip extension test was performed during the initial visit (intrasessional) and again in 7 days (intersessional). The intrasessional reliability was higher (spastic CP ICC = 0.78 to 0.91; control ICC = 0.80 to 0.92) than that of the intersessional reliability (spastic CP ICC = 0.55 to 0.80; control ICC = 0.04 to 0.20). Lee and associates[9] found the prone hip extension test to have an interrater reliability ICC value of 0.198 (CI, 95%; 0.012 to 0.437) in the spastic CP group and 0.107 (CI, 95%; 0.033 to 0.294) in the control.

Thurston[39] proposed a similar prone method but differed in the initial positioning of the patient. In Thurston's method, instead of positioning the legs over the end of the examination table, the affected leg is positioned off the side of the table. Similar to Staheli's description, the examiner steadies the pelvis, extends the affected leg until the pelvis begins to move, and then measures the angle of fixed flexion deformity. Thurston compared this new method with the Thomas test, and the degree of flexion contracture and variability in measurements was consistently larger using the Thomas tests compared with Thurston's method, 5 to 20 degrees and 0.5 to 4.5 degrees, respectively.

MEASUREMENTS OF THE PELVIFEMORAL ANGLE

In 1942, Milch[40] argued that lumbar and pelvic rotation compromised the validity of the Thomas test and "merely determines the amount of hip extension possible at any given degree of pelvic flexion. Since [pelvic rotation] cannot be fixed as a standard of reference, the whole procedure loses its validity." As an alternative, Milch proposed using the pelvifemoral angle to measure hip extension. In this test, the patient is placed in a side-lying position, and the examiner passively extends the involved upper hip. Milch's pelvifemoral angle is formed by the Nelaton line, a line between the ASIS and ischial tuberosity, and the axis of the extended femur (Fig. 8.4A).

Mundale and others[41] described another method for measuring the pelvifemoral angle. In the original article, the authors argued that this method better took into account the position of the innominate bone. To establish the position of the innominate bone, the ASIS and posterior superior iliac spines are used as fixed landmarks. A perpendicular line is drawn from the line connecting the iliac spines, through the greater trochanter. The Mundale pelvifemoral angle is measured between the perpendicular line and a line along the axis of the extended femur (Fig. 8.4B).

The reliability of the aforementioned methods to assess hip flexor flexibility (Thomas test, Staheli's prone hip extension test, and both Mundale's and Milch's pelvifemoral angle measurements) were evaluated by Bartlett and associates.[4] In this study, two therapists examined 45 children aged 4 to 19 years (15 with CP and spastic diplegia, 15 with meningomyelocele, and 15 healthy children). In the cohort of patients with meningomyelocele, the Thomas test had the smallest mean intrarater difference (6.4 degrees, r = 0.90), and the Mundale had the largest (10.9 degrees, r = 0.79). For the cohort of CP patients, the prone hip extension test had the largest variability of intrarater difference (9.6 degrees, r − 80) and the Mundale method the lowest (7.1 degrees, r = 0.84). When all four tests were compared in the CP group, there was no significant difference in the reliability of the techniques. In the healthy group, the prone hip extension and Thomas test had the smallest intrarater difference (2.1 degrees and 1.9 degrees, respectively) compared with the Mundale and Milch methods (7.1 degrees and 7.8 degrees, respectively), which required identifying multiple bony landmarks. The authors concluded that no single measurement technique was superior in all cases.

ELY TESTS AND RECTUS FEMORIS CONTRACTURE TEST (Videos 8-2, 8-3)

Although the original description of the Ely test could not be found, several sources have described the Ely test as a method to assess flexibility of the rectus femoris muscle. In the Ely test, the patient lies prone. The examiner passively flexes the patient's knee, and if the ipsilateral hip spontaneously flexes, the test result is considered positive, indicating that the rectus femoris muscle is tight (Fig. 8.5). Both sides should be tested and compared.

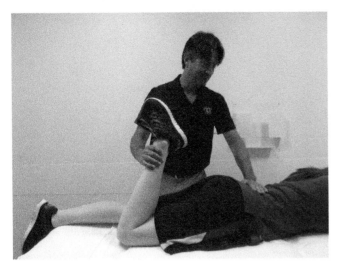

Figure 8.5 Normal Ely test result.

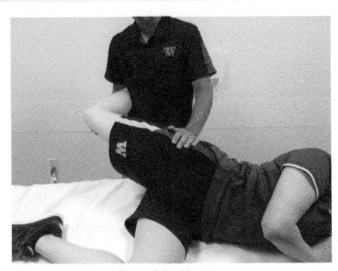

Figure 8.6 Ober test.

The reliability of Ely's test was examined by Peeler and Anderson.[16] In this study, 54 healthy subjects were examined by three therapists during two distinct sessions, and the Ely test demonstrated only moderate levels of intrarater and interrater reliability (ICC = 0.69 and 0.66, respectively). In Atamaz and associates' study,[17] two examiners examined 66 healthy subjects in a test-retest design, and the interrater and intrarater reliability ranged from an ICC = 0.75 to 0.87 and 0.84 to 0.91, respectively.

A different test used to identify tightness of the rectus femoris muscle is the rectus femoris contracture test. This test is also referred to as the modified Thomas test in the literature because the positioning is the same as that used to measure iliopsoas flexibility (see Fig. 8.2). Magee describes the test in the following manner[3]:

> The patient lies supine with the knees bent over the end or edge of the examining table. The patient flexes one knee onto the chest and holds it. The angle of the test knee should remain at 90 degrees when the opposite knee is flexed to the chest. If it does not (i.e., the test knee extends slightly), a contracture is probably present. The examiner may attempt to passively flex the knee to see whether it will remain at 90 degrees of its own volition. The examiner should always palpate for muscle tightness when doing any contracture test. If there is no palpable tightness, the probable cause of restriction is tight joint structures (e.g., the capsule). The two sides should be tested and compared.

Ferber and colleagues[42] presented normative values for rectus femoris flexibility using the rectus femoris contracture test. The average inclinometer angle was −10.6 degrees ±9.6 degrees (−9.5 to 11.7 degrees, 95% CI). When declared a negative test result by the examiner, the average angle was −15.5 degrees ±5.8 degrees, and when declared a positive test result, the average angle was −0.3 degrees ±7.0 degrees.

In Harvey's[12] study, the flexibility of three muscles (iliopsoas, TFL/IT band, and quadriceps) were assessed. A total of 117 elite athletes were examined while in the modified Thomas test position, and the intrarater reliability of two measurements of passive quadriceps length was

excellent (ICC = 0.94). Peeler and Anderson[16] evaluated the reliability of the rectus femoris contracture test in a test-retest design. Fifty-seven healthy subjects were examined by three therapists during two sessions 7 to 10 days apart. The interrater and intrarater reliability was modest (ICC = 0.5 and 0.67, respectively). In 2013, Peeler and Leiter[18] presented another study assessing the flexibility of the rectus femoris in 28 active university students. The subjects were photographed while being evaluated by a therapist, and 10 examiners then used the digital photographs to score the degree of rectus femoris flexibility. The interrater and intrarater reliability of the measurements from the digital photographs was excellent (0.97 and 0.98, respectively).

OBER TEST (Video 8-4)

In 1936, Frank R. Ober,[43] an American orthopedic surgeon, described the role of the IT band and TFL as a source of sciatica after observing that certain patients experienced relief of their pain after surgical release of the fascia. Ober surmised "that the relief of symptoms in these cases might be due to releasing the fascial pull exerted through the fascia lata and its attachments to the gluteus maximus muscle." Ober described a method of identifying tightness of the TFL and IT band, as follows[43]:

> The patient lies on his side, with the thigh next to the table and flexed enough to obliterate any lumbar lordosis. The upper leg is flexed at a right angle at the knee. The examiner grasps the ankle lightly with one hand and steadies the patient's hip with the other. The upper leg is abducted widely and extended so that the thigh is in line with the body. If there is any abduction contracture, the leg will remain more or less passively abducted, depending upon the shortening of the iliotibial band. This band can be easily felt with the examining fingers between the crest of the ilium and the anterior aspect of the trochanter. (Fig. 8.6, Video 8-4)

In the original article, Ober described flexing the involved knee 90 degrees, abducting and extending the hip, and then allowing the force of gravity to bring the leg into adduction. Ferber and associates[42] presented normative values for IT band flexibility using the Ober test. The average inclinometer angle was −24.6 degrees ±7.3 degrees (−23.8 to 25.4 degrees, 95% CI), and when the examiner declared the test result as negative, the average angle was −27.1 degrees ±5.5°, and when the test result was positive, the average angle was −16.3 degrees ±6.9 degrees.

Kendall[44] described a similar test but with the knee fully extended to 0 degrees as opposed to flexed as originally described. This variation has come to be known as the modified Ober test. In a study by Melchione and Sullivan,[19] two therapists examined 10 subjects with anterior knee pain using the modified Ober test in a test-retest study design and reported an intrarater and interrater reliability ICC of 0.94 and 0.73, respectively.

Reese and Bandy[21] and Gajdosik and coworkers[20] examined the reliability of both the Ober test and the modified Ober test and did not find a significant difference between the reliability of the two tests. In a study by Reese and Bandy,[21] 61 subjects were examined by one therapist using an inclinometer in a test-retest design, and the ICC values for intrarater reliability were 0.90 for the Ober test and 0.91 for the modified Ober test. In a study by Gajdosik and associates,[20] three measurements were taken while examining 49 subjects without lower extremity symptoms during a single session. The ICC values for intrarater reliability ranged from 0.83 to 0.87 for the Ober test and 0.82 to 0.92 for the modified Ober test.

PIRIFORMIS TESTS (Video 8-5)

In 1928, Yeoman published the first reference to the piriformis muscle as a source of sciatic pain.[45] Usually the sciatic nerve emerges from the pelvis through the greater sciatic foramen and passes beneath the piriformis muscle. In a subset of patients, the piriformis muscle or sciatic nerve splits, altering the "normal" relationship. The various relationships between the piriformis muscle and sciatic nerve were first described in 1896 in the English literature by Parsons and Keith[46] and include[47] (1) the sciatic nerve passing above or below the piriformis muscle, (2) the sciatic nerve splitting and passing around the muscle, or (3) the piriformis muscle splitting to surround the nerve.

Provocative tests for piriformis syndrome elicit symptoms by compressing the sciatic nerve beneath the piriformis muscle, and over the years, a number of tests have been described to assess for piriformis syndrome. While the piriformis muscle is an external rotator, in flexion, the piriformis tendon becomes an abductor. Therefore, tests for intra-articular hip pathology that place the hip in flexion–adduction–internal rotation may also stretch the piriformis and provoke symptoms in cases of piriformis syndrome.[48,49]

The historic lack of a "gold standard" to compare the diagnostic accuracy of these clinical tests has led to a lack of literature on the sensitivity and specificity of piriformis provocative tests. Martin and associates[50] conducted the only currently available study that has studied the validity of provocative maneuvers for piriformis syndrome. In this retrospective study, the accuracy of the straight-leg raise (SLR), active piriformis test, and seated piriformis stretch were assessed in 33 patients and compared with endoscopic findings of sciatic nerve entrapment. The specific results for

each test are described subsequently. Combing the active piriformis test and seated piriformis stretch test resulted in a sensitivity of 0.91, specificity of 0.80, positive likelihood ratio (+LR) of 4.57, −LR of 0.11, and diagnostic odds ratio of 42.00.

ACTIVE PIRIFORMIS TEST (PACE TEST)

Albert H. Freiberg is often credited with publishing the first description of piriformis syndrome provocative maneuvers. Freiberg found that sciatic pain could be attributed to piriformis syndrome if (1) the SLR test result was positive, (2) if there was marked tenderness at the sciatic notch, or (3) if internal rotation of an extended hip reproduced symptoms. The Freiberg test was initially described in 1934 as follows[51]:

> Clinical evidence of [piriformis] spasm has been found in the presence of limitation of motion in inward rotation of the thigh, if looked for with the patient's hip joints fully extended but not hyperextended.

A variation of the Freiberg test has been described that places the hip into flexion, adduction, and internal rotation, putting tension on the deep rotators and compressing the sciatic nerve.[48,52]

The Pace test is a variation of the Freiberg test and involves flexion, adduction, and internal rotation of the hip. This test was first described by Pace and Nagle in 1976 as follows[53]:

> A more consistent finding in piriformis syndrome is that of pain and weakness on resisted abduction-external rotation of the thigh … With the patient seated, the examiner places his hands on the lateral aspects of the knees and asks the patient to push the hands apart.

Pain and weakness with resisted abduction and external rotation of the hip is a positive test result. In one study, the active piriformis test has a sensitivity of 0.78, specificity of 0.80, +LR 3.90, −LR 0.27, and odds ratio of 14.4 for sciatic nerve entrapment.[22]

A variant of the Pace test has been described with the patient in a side-lying position. In this test, the patient lies on the nonaffected side, and the involved knee is flexed with the foot on the table behind the nonaffected knee. The patient is instructed to push the involved heel down into the table, thus actively abducting and externally rotating the involved leg while the examiner provides resistance.[54]

PASSIVE PIRIFORMIS STRETCH TEST

A passive piriformis stretch test has also been described and can be performed with the patient in a side-lying or seated position. Magee described the side-lying test (Fig. 8.7) as follows[3]:

> [The patient is placed] in the side-lying position with the non-test leg against the table. The patient flexes the test hip to 60 degrees with the knee flexed, while the examiner applies a downward pressure to the knee. Pain is elicited in the muscle if the piriformis muscle is tight. Radiation of pain down the leg will occur if the substance of the piriformis muscle compromises the sciatic nerve.

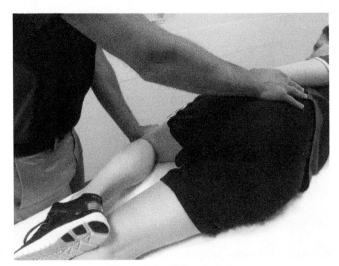

Figure 8.7   Piriformis test.

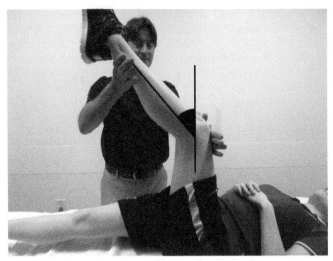

Figure 8.9   Popliteal angle measurement.

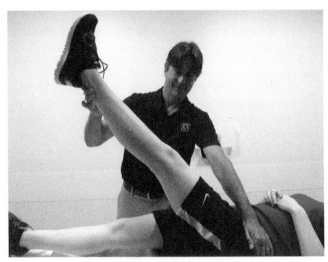

Figure 8.8   Straight-leg raise.

In the seated version, also known as the seated piriformis stretch test, the patient is sitting with the hip in 90 degrees of flexion. While palpating the sciatic notch, the examiner extends the knee and passively adducts and internally rotates the hip, stretching the piriformis muscle.[55] In a positive test result, the patient reports reproduction of the posterior gluteal and leg pain. Martin and colleagues[22] used the seated version in studying the validity of passive stretch for identifying patients with sciatic nerve entrapment. In this study, the seated piriformis stretch test had a sensitivity of 0.52, specificity of 0.90, +LR 5.22, −LR 0.53, and odds ratio of 9.82.[22]

STRAIGHT-LEG RAISE (LASÈGUE'S SIGN)

Freiberg hypothesized that pain during an SLR (Fig. 8.8), or Lasègue's sign, was due to the close relationship between the neurovascular bundle and piriformis muscle. While many authors attributed the positive SLR to stretching of the sciatic nerve, cadaveric studies have shown the sciatic nerve experiences a proximal excursion of 28 mm when the hip is flexed.[56] Abnormal contraction of the piriformis muscle or adhesions between the piriformis and nerve may

limit the ability of the sciatic nerve to glide or stretch and provoke sciatic pain. Martin and coworkers[50] reported that the SLR had a sensitivity of 0.15, specificity of 0.95, +LR 3.20, −LR 0.90, and odds ratio of 3.59 for an endoscopic finding of sciatic nerve entrapment. While not always positive in cases of piriformis syndrome, Martin and colleagues[50] still recommended using this test clinically to alert the examiner to the presence of radicular pain.

POPLITEAL ANGLE OR KNEE EXTENSION ANGLE
(Video 8-6)

The popliteal angle has been used in the pediatric literature as an indirect measurement of hamstring flexibility. In 1966, Koenigsberger[57] was the first to use the terminology "popliteal angle" when measuring knee extension in premature infants. Since muscle tone increases longitudinally as the neurologic system develops, the popliteal angle can be used to help estimate cerebral maturation and thus gestational age when unknown.[57,58] In addition to gestational age, hamstring hypertonicity in an infant can alert the clinician to potential neuromuscular pathology, such as CP. In one study of 1843 infants, a popliteal angle of less than 100 degrees had a sensitivity of 51% and a specificity of 92% in identifying children who will go on to be diagnosed with CP.[59]

A variety of methods have been proposed to measure the popliteal angle, but many descriptions are vague and fail to describe the exact position of the hip or contralateral limb.[60] In 1979, Bleck[61] described a method of measuring the popliteal angle which is commonly used today (Fig. 8.9). According to Bleck[61]:

> … the popliteal angle is measured with the patient supine and the hip flexed 90 degrees. The examiner attempts to extend the knee until firm resistance is met while the hip is maintained at 00 degrees. The popliteal angle is the acute angle between the lower leg and an imaginary line extending up from the flexed femur.

The angle measured by Bleck has also been named the *knee extension angle* and differed from earlier descriptions of the popliteal angle, which measured the angle at the popliteal fossa.[60] The popliteal and knee extension angles are complementary, and their sum is 180 degrees. Variations of Bleck's method involve placing the hip in full flexion instead of 90 degrees. Authors also differ in whether the noninvolved hip should be in full extension or flexed until lumbar lordosis is relieved.[60] In addition to differences in positioning, articles differ in whether the knee extension should be active (AKE) or passive (PKE).

A number of other clinical tests with comparable intrarater reliability have been used to measure hamstring muscle flexibility (sacral angle [SA], SLR, sit and reach test [SR]), but these methods have potentially confounding variables.[25] These variables include inconsistencies in pelvic positioning, limitations due to neural stretch, and tightness of the hip joint capsule or contralateral hip flexors and have made some suggest the popliteal angle as the gold standard measurement for assessing hamstring length.[25]

In Davis and coworkers[25] study, four investigators took three measurements of hamstring length in 81 college-age subjects using the PKE and three other hamstring examination techniques (SA, SLR, SR) in a test-retest design with 1 week between the two tests. There was excellent intrarater reliability for the PKE (ICC = 0.94) and the other three tests, but among the 4 tests, there was poor to fair correlation (Pearson's correlation coefficient, r = 0.45 to 0.65). Atamaz and coworkers[17] presented 66 healthy subjects evaluated by two examiners using the PKE test in a test-retest design. There was good to very good interrater and intrarater reliability with and ICC ranging from 0.68 to 0.73 and 0.61 to 0.79, respectively.

In 1982, Gajdosik and Lusin[23] investigated the intrarater reliability of the AKE test in 15 healthy subjects during two testing sessions and found excellent reliability with a Pearson correlation coefficient of r = 0.99. Sullivan and coworkers[24] used the AKE method when assessing the results of two different hamstring stretching techniques. Two examiners examined 12 subjects before and after the stretching session, and the ICC values for interrater and intrarater reliability were 0.93 and 0.99, respectively. Hamid and colleagues[26] examined the reliability of the AKE method. In this study, a sports physician and therapists evaluated 16 healthy subjects; each angle was measured twice, and all subjects were measured at two different sessions. The interrater and intrarater reliability ICC values ranged from 0.81 to 0.87 and 0.75 to 0.97. Reurink and associates[27] evaluated the reliability of the AKE and PKE tests in examining 50 consecutive athletes with an acute hamstring injury confirmed by magnetic resonance imaging (MRI). Two testers (out of a pool of eight clinicians) used an inclinometer to examine each subject during a single session, and the intertester reliability ICCs for the AKE test were 0.89 and 0.76 for the injured and uninjured leg, respectively. For the PKE test, the intertester reliability ICCs were 0.77 and 0.69, respectively.

TRENDELENBURG SIGN OR TEST

Friedrich Trendelenburg originally described the Trendelenburg test in 1895 to explain the waddling gait pattern of children with developmental dysplasia of the hip and progressive muscular atrophy[62]:

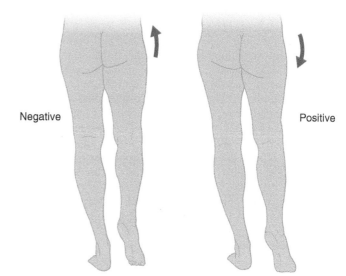

Figure 8.10 Trendelenburg sign. (Adapted with permission from Goldstein B, Chavez F. Applied anatomy of the lower extremities. *Phys Med Rehabil State Art Rev.* 1996;10:601-630.)

The pelvis hangs down on the swinging side, and the upper part of the body leans far over to the standing side to restore balance. From what has been said, the cause of the pelvis hanging down can only be that the abductors of the standing leg cannot keep the pelvis horizontal.

While initially described as an assessment of abductor function during gait, the Trendelenburg test now is often performed by instructing the patient to stand on the affected leg, while the examiner assesses pelvic movement. Contraction of the hip abductors during single-leg stance should prevent a downward tilting of the contralateral pelvis, but in a positive Trendelenburg test, the pelvis drops suggesting gluteus medius or minimus weakness (Fig. 8.10).

There is some evidence that the nonstance leg should be flexed to 30 degrees while maintaining single-leg posture. In one study, when hip flexion was to 90 degrees, the authors found a higher rate of false-negative test results compared with 30 degrees of flexion. The authors hypothesized that at 90 degrees, there is increased pelvic rotation that elevates the iliac crest or results in contraction of the latissimus dorsi, psoas major, or quadratus lumborum to stabilize the pelvis.[63]

While various methods for performing the Trendelenburg test have been described in textbooks,[63] only a few studies have looked at the validity of the Trendelenburg test. The Trendelenburg test has been studied as a clinical test to identify patients with intra-articular hip pathology, but it lacks sensitivity. In two studies of patients with early hip osteoarthritis (OA), the Trendelenburg test had a sensitivity of 0.37 to 0.55, specificity of 0.70 to 0.81, and +LR of 1.83.[29,34] As a tool to identify patients with femoroacetabular impingement or labral pathology, the Trendelenburg test also lacked sensitivity (0.33 to 0.38 in two uncontrolled studies.)[30,33]

The reliability and validity of the Trendelenburg test is better for greater trochanteric pain syndrome (GTPS). The gluteus medius is the primary pelvic stabilizer and is commonly implicated as a source of pain or weakness in GTPS.

In 2001, Bird and colleagues[28] examined 24 women with clinical evidence of GTPS using the Trendelenburg test with the patient standing and while walking. For this study, the pelvic tilt was only regarded as abnormal if the tilt was seen in both standing and with ambulation, and clinical findings were compared with MRI findings (partial or complete gluteus medius tear). The Trendelenburg test had a sensitivity of 0.73, specificity of 0.77, and intraobserver kappa score (κ) of 0.676 (95% CI; 0.270 to 1.08). Woodley and associates[31] assessed the validity of the Trendelenburg test in a prospective cross-sectional study of 40 patients with lateral hip pain. Unlike Bird and others' study,[28] this study only looked at the results of a standing Trendelenburg test. Clinical findings were compared with MRI findings, and the Trendelenburg test had a sensitivity of 0.23, specificity of 0.94, +LR of 3.64, and −LR of 0.82 (95% CI) in predicting gluteal tendon pathology.

In 2008, Lequesne and associates[32] tested the validity of the sustained single-leg stance test, or "fatigue" Trendelenburg test in which the patient holds the single-leg stance for 30 seconds. The sustained single-leg stance test was first described by Hardcastle and Nade in 1985.[63] Although performed the same way, the Trendelenburg test result is positive if the pelvis drops, and the "fatigue" Trendelenburg test result is positive if it reproduces lateral hip pain. Lequesne and colleagues found a sensitivity and specificity of 1.0 and 0.97, respectively.[32]

RESISTED INTERNAL ROTATION OF THE THIGH (RESISTED EXTERNAL DEROTATION)

In GTPS, reproduction of pain can also be provoked at the extremes of rotation by stretching the gluteus medius and minimus tendons[28,31,64,65] or with resisted hip abduction.[31,64,66-69] External rotation has long been recognized to elicit pain in cases of GTPS. In 1961, Gordon[66] presented a series of 61 cases of clinical trochanteric bursitis and tendinopathy. Gordon found that external rotation and abduction, as achieved with the FABER maneuver, elicited pain in 35 of the patients. In 2001, Bird and coworkers[28] reported that resisted internal rotation (active external rotation) had a sensitivity and specificity of 0.55 and 0.69 for GTPS, respectively. In this study, the leg was in neutral rotation, not in a position of extreme rotation.

In 2008, Lequesne and coworkers[32] described a similar maneuver that placed the hip in extreme external rotation (Fig. 8.11) to maximize the stretching of the gluteus medius and minimus tendons:

> Patients were asked to lie supine on a table with the hip and knee flexed at 90° and the hip in external rotation (a position that is usually painful in patients with [trochanteric tendinobursitis]). After slightly diminishing the external rotation just enough to relieve the pain (if any), patients were asked to return actively to neutral rotation, that is, to place the leg along the axis of the bed, against resistance. The test result was considered positive when the test reproduced spontaneous pain.

In this study, 17 patients with suspected GTPS were examined prospectively with the sustained Trendelenburg test and resisted external derotation and compared with MRI

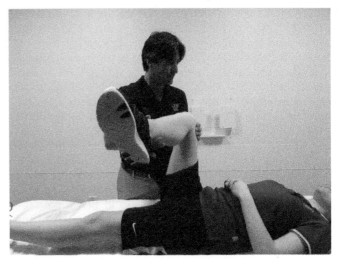

Figure 8.11 Resisted external derotation.

findings. The resisted external derotation test had a very good sensitivity and specificity of 0.88 and 0.97 for the diagnosis of gluteus medius tendinopathy and/or greater trochanteric bursitis.

TESTS FOR INTRA-ARTICULAR OR PERIARTICULAR HIP JOINT PATHOLOGY (TABLE 8.2)

Often the examination for intra-articular pathology begins with passive ROM testing. Loss of internal rotation is one of the earliest signs of intra-articular pathology,[70] and the ligamentous forces limiting internal rotation varies with the degree of hip flexion or extension.[71] In one study, passive internal rotation of less than or equal to 25 degrees had a sensitivity of 0.76, specificity of 0.61, +LR of 1.9, and −LR of 0.39 in predicting hip OA.[72] Another study used less than 15 degrees of internal rotation as the cutoff and had a sensitivity of 0.66 and specificity of 0.72 in predicting hip OA.[29] Loss of flexion may also be useful for detecting hip OA, with one study showing hip flexion of less than or equal to 115 degrees having a sensitivity of 0.96 and specificity 0.18.[29] Limited internal rotation has also been correlated with radiographic findings for femoroacetabular impingement (FAI). Kapron and coworkers[73] reported limited internal rotation was correlated with an alpha angle greater than 50 degrees and head-neck offset of less than 8 mm in asymptomatic collegiate football players (sensitivity, 0.80 to 0.85; specificity, 0.34 to 0.51).

As with passive ROM testing, many of the provocative maneuvers lack the sensitivity to be used in isolation. Multiple provocative maneuvers should be used in combination as part of the examination for intra-articular pathology.

FABERE TEST

FABERE is the acronym for flexion, abduction, external rotation, and extension, which describes the positioning of the hip used when first described in 1917. The FABER test is also known as the Patrick test or Patrick-FABER test, after Hugh Talbot Patrick, an American neurologist credited with

Table 8.2   Tests for Intra-articular Hip Joint Pathology

Test	Description	Reliability/Validity Tests	Comments
FABER test (Patrick test)	The patient is placed in the supine position, and the examiner flexes, abducts, and externally rotates the hip ankle resting on the contralateral knee. The examiner then stabilizes the pelvis by applying pressure to the contralateral ilium. Pressure is then applied dorsally to the knee to further external rotation at the hip. The test result is considered positive if this positioning recreates the patient's groin pain.	Sutlive et al. 2008[72] Sensitivity: 57% Specificity: 71% +LR: 1.9 −LR: 0.61 Interrater reliability: 0.90	Reliability and validity of 2 PT students examining 72 symptomatic subjects with a radiographic diagnosis of OA
		Theiler et al. 1996[75] Interrater reliability: 0.66	Reliability of 3 rheumatologists examining 49 patients with radiographic diagnosis of hip OA
		Cliborne et al. 2004[76] Intrarater reliability: 0.87	Reliability of 2 PT students examining 22 patients with radiographic diagnosis of hip OA and 17 asymptomatic controls
		Cibere et al. 2008[77] Interrater reliability: 0.6–0.8	Reliability of 6 examiners (4 rheumatologists and 2 orthopedic surgeons) examining 6 patients with clinical and radiographic diagnosis of hip OA
		Mitchell et al. 2003[78] Sensitivity: 88%	Retrospective case series, 25 consecutive patients examined with FABER and scour testing who underwent arthroscopy
		Martin et al. 2008[79] Sensitivity: 60% Specificity: 18% +LR: 0.73 −LR: 2.2 PPV: 0.45 NPV: 0.29	Validity of FABER and in predicting >50% improvement in hip pain after intra-articular injection in 49 patients with intra-articular pathology
		Troelsen et al. 2009[80] Sensitivity: 41% Specificity: 100% PPV: 1.0 NPV: 0.9	Validity of FABER, Stinchfield and FADDIR for labral tears diagnosed by MRI arthrogram in 18 patients with a history of acetabular dysplasia treated with osteotomy
		Clohisy et al. 2009[33] Sensitivity: 69%	Validity of single examiner performing 5 provocative maneuvers on 51 patients with symptomatic FAI/labral pathology diagnosed clinically and radiographically
		Maslowski et al. 2010[81] Sensitivity: 82% Specificity: 25% PPV: 0.46 NPV: 0.64	Validity of FABER and 3 other maneuvers in predicting 80% improvement in the VAS after fluoroscopically guided anesthetic hip injection in 50 patients with various intra-articular pathologies
Resisted straight-leg raise (Stinchfield test)	The patient is positioned supine with the knee extended and hip actively flexed to 20 to 30 degrees. The examiner then provides a downward force resisting the hip flexion. The test result is considered positive if it reproduces the patient's groin pain.	Maslowski et al. 2010[81] Sensitivity: 59% Specificity: 32% PPV: 0.41 NPV: 0.50	See FABER section
		Clohisy et al. 2009[33] Sensitivity: 56.1%	See FABER section

Continued on following page

Table 8.2   Tests for Intra-articular Hip Joint Pathology (Continued)

Test	Description	Reliability/Validity Tests	Comments
Impingement testing Anterior impingement test (FADDIR/FAIR)	The patient is supine or in a lateral recumbent position, and the leg is passively moved into 90 degrees of flexion, adduction, and internal rotation. In a positive test result, the patient has reproduction of pain or apprehension.	Ito et al. 2004[82] Sensitivity: 96%	Validity of single orthopedic surgeon examining 25 patients with symptomatic FAI confirmed on MRI and surgically
		Burnett et al. 2006[30] Sensitivity: 95%	Retrospective review of 66 consecutive patients with arthroscopically confirmed labral tear
		Martin et al. 2008[79] Sensitivity: 60% Specificity: 18% +LR: 0.73 −LR: 2.2 PPV: 0.45 NPV: 0.29	See FABER section
		Sink et al. 2008[83] Sensitivity: 100%	Retrospective review of 35 adolescent athletes with chronic hip pain and a radiographic diagnosis of FAI/labral pathology
		Troelsen et al. 2009[80] Sensitivity: 59% Specificity: 100% PPV: 1.0 NPV: 0.13	See FABER section
		Clohisy et al. 2009[33] Sensitivity: 88%	See FABER section
Flexion-internal rotation	Variation of anterior impingement test where the hip and knee are flexed to 90 degrees and internally rotated without adduction.	Nogier et al. 2010[84] Sensitivity: 0.2–0.7 Specificity: 0.44–0.86 PPV: 0.63–0.67 NPV: 0.44–0.53	Prospective multicenter study of 292 patients with FAI
Flexion-internal rotation-axial compression or internal rotation over pressure (IROP)	Variation with flexion-internal rotation test in which the examiner performs the internal rotation over pressure.	Maslowski et al. 2010[81] Sensitivity: 91% Specificity: 18% PPV: 0.47 NPV: 0.71	See FABER section
		Narvani et al. 2003[85] Sensitivity: 75% Specificity: 43% PPV: 0.27 NPV: 0.86	Case series of 18 patients with hip pain examined with IROP test; 4 were diagnosed with labral tear on MRI arthrogram
Passive supine rotation test (log roll)	The patient is positioned supine, the hip is in neutral, and the leg is passively rotated internally. The examiner notes any side-to-side difference.	Clohisy et al. 2009[33] Sensitivity: 30%	See FABER section
Flexion-extension maneuvers	These maneuvers have several different names and variations, but all involve moving the knee from flexion to extension. Variations include: Fitzgerald's test Quadrant/Scour Test DIRI/DEXRIT tests	Cliborne et al. 2004[76] Interrater reliability: 0.87	Hip quadrant/Scour test See FABER section
		Sutlive et al. 2008[72] Sensitive: 62% Specificity: 75% +LR: 2.4 −LR: 0.51	Hip quadrant/Scour test See FABER section
		Maslowski et al. 2010[81] Sensitivity: 50% Specificity: 29% PPV: 0.38 NPV: 0.42	Hip quadrant/Scour test See FABER section

Table 8.2   Tests for Intra-articular Hip Joint Pathology (Continued)

Test	Description	Reliability/Validity Tests	Comments
Posterior impingement test	The patient is positioned at the edge of the table with the nonaffected leg held in flexion and the affected leg in full extension off the end of the table. The affected hip is then passively abducted and externally rotated to approximate the femoral neck and the posterior acetabular wall.	Clohisy et al. 2009[33] Sensitivity: 22%	See FABER section
Axial hip distraction	With the patient supine, the examiner abducts the hip 30 degrees and applies long-axis traction by holding the leg just above the ankle. Reproduction on pain symptoms may indicate an intra-articular process.	There are no studies to be found that investigated the specificity, sensitivity, or reliability of this test.	

DEXRIT, Dynamic external rotatory impingement test; *DIRI,* dynamic internal rotatory impingement test; *FABERE,* flexion, abduction, external rotation and extension; *FAI,* femoroacetabular impingement; *FADDIR* or *FAIR,* flexion-adduction-internal rotation; *LR,* likelihood ratio; *MRI,* magnetic resonance imaging; NPV, negative predictive value; PPV, positive predictive value; *PT,* physical therapy; VAS, visual analog scale.

first describing the test.[74] In modern literature, the final "E" is often left off, and the test is described as the FABER maneuver.

With this test, the patient is placed in the supine position, and the affected hip joint is passively flexed, abducted, and externally rotated with the knee flexed. The ankle is placed just above the contralateral patella forming a figure "4." The examiner then stabilizes the pelvis by applying pressure to the contralateral ilium and applies a downward pressure on the ipsilateral knee causing further external rotation of the affected hip (Fig. 8.12). This position also stresses the surrounding soft tissue, inguinal ligament, pubic symphysis, SIJ, and lumbar spine. The FABER test can reproduce pain in any of these structures. While the location of pain can help the examiner differentiate between a lumbar, sacroiliac, or intra-articular pain progenitor, the FABER maneuver is considered positive for intra-articular hip joint pathology when the test recreates groin pain.

The diagnostic accuracy of the FABER test has been studied for hip OA and various other intra-articular disorders. In Sutlive and associates prospective study, 72 subjects with symptomatic hip OA were examined by two physical therapy doctoral students. The FABER test had a sensitivity of 0.57 (95% CI; 0.34 to 0.77), specificity of 0.71 (95% CI; 0.56 to 0.82), +LR of 1.9 (95% CI; 1.3 to 3.0), −LR of 0.61 (95% CI; 0.36 to 1.0), and interrater reliability ICC value of 0.90 (95% CI; 0.78 to 0.93) for predicting hip OA.[72] Three other studies also reported the reliability of the FABER test in patients with hip OA but not the validity. Theiler and associates presented a series of 49 patients, and the authors found an interrater reliability of 0.66.[75] In Cliborne and coworkers' study, 22 patients and 17 asymptomatic subjects were examined before and after mobilizing the joint, and the intrarater reliability was excellent with an ICC value of 0.87 (0.78 to 0.94, 95% CI).[76] Cibere and

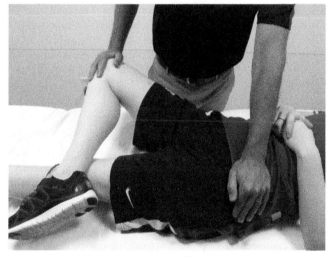

Figure 8.12   Patrick (FABERE) test.

coworkers presented the interrater reliability while examining 6 patients and found the test to be reliable (κ score = 0.6 and 0.8).[77]

For FAI or labral pathology, three uncontrolled studies have assessed the validity of the FABER test. Mitchell and coworkers[78] presented a retrospective case series of 25 consecutive patients who underwent hip arthroscopy for suspected hip pathology. Of the 25 patients, 17 had a recorded FABER test, and the sensitivity for labral pathology was 0.88. In Clohisy and colleagues,[33] one examiner prospectively evaluated 51 patients with symptomatic FAI and labral pathology with five provocative maneuvers (FABER, resisted SLR, log role, posterior impingement test and anterior and posterior impingement signs), and the FABER test had a sensitivity of 0.69. Troelsen and others[80] examined 18 patients with a history of acetabular dysplasia and osteotomy before a hip MRI arthrogram using three provocative maneuvers, including the FABER test. Of these patients, 17 had evidence of a labral tear, and the FABER test had a sensitivity of 0.41, specificity of 1.0, PPV of 1.0, and NPV of 0.9. Finally, Philippon and others[86] presented 122 patients who underwent arthroscopic surgery for suspected FAI and chondrolabral dysfunction. All patients in this series had either a positive anterior impingement test or FABER test result, but the sensitivity and specificity of the FABER test alone were not reported.

In two studies, various intra-articular pathologies were grouped together. Martin and colleagues[79] prospectively examined 49 patients with radiographic evidence of labral pathology, arthritic changes, FAI, or acetabular dysplasia before a diagnostic intra-articular anesthetic injection. Neither the FABER nor flexion–internal rotation–adduction tests predicted an intra-articular pain generator, as defined by a greater than 50% improvement in hip pain after the injection. The FABER tests had a sensitivity of 0.6 (95% CI; 0.41 to 0.77), specificity of 0.18 (95% CI; 0.07 to 0.39), +LR of 0.73 (95% CI; 0.5 to 1.1), –LR of 2.2 (95% CI; 0.8 to 6), PPV of 0.45, and NPV of 0.29. Maslowski and colleagues[81] examined 50 patients with a variety of hip pathologies (osteoarthritis, FAI, labral tears, and avascular necrosis [AVN]), who underwent four provocative maneuvers (FABER, internal rotation over pressure [IROP], Stinchfield, and scour) before and after a fluoroscopically guided intra-articular hip injection. Using an 80% improvement in the visual analog scale (VAS) after the injection, the authors found the FABER maneuver had a sensitivity of 0.82, specificity of 0.25, PPV of 0.46, and NPV of 0.64.

RESISTED STRAIGHT LEG RAISE (STINCHFIELD TEST) (Video 8-7)

The resisted SLR has also been referred to as the resisted hip flexion test or Stinchfield test. The origin of this maneuver is unknown, but it is named after Frank Stinchfield, an orthopedic surgeon whose academic career focused on hip joint arthroplasty.[87]

The test is performed with the patient supine and the knee extended. The patient actively flexes the hip to 20 to 30 degrees, and the examiner then provides a downward force resisting the hip flexion (Fig. 8.13). The test is thought to increase pressure on the labrum as the iliopsoas contracts and is considered a positive test result if it reproduces the patient's groin pain. This test also assesses the strength of the iliopsoas and rectus femoris muscles, and caution should be used in interpreting a positive test result.

In three studies, the validity of the resisted straight leg has been fair. In 2009, Troelsen and colleagues[80] examined 18 patients before an MRI arthrogram using three provocative maneuvers, including the resisted straight-leg maneuver. While 17 of the patients had confirmed labral tears on MRI arthrogram, only 1 patient had a positive resisted straight-leg maneuver. In 2010, Maslowski and coworkers[81] examined 50 patients with various intra-articular hip pathologies (osteoarthritis, FAI, labral tears, AVN) before and after a fluoroscopically guided intra-articular anesthetic hip injection. The resisted straight-leg maneuver and three other

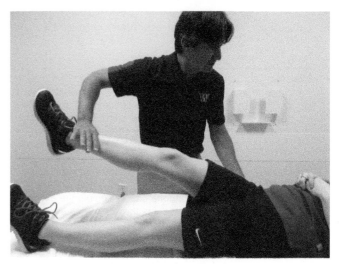

Figure 8.13 Stinchfield test.

provocative maneuvers were used in this study, and the resisted straight leg maneuver had a sensitivity of 0.59, specificity of 0.32, PPV of 0.41, and NPV of 0.50 for identifying an intra-articular hip pain generator (defined as an 80% decrease in pain). Clohisy and coworkers[33] prospectively evaluated 51 patients with symptomatic FAI and labral pathology with five provocative maneuvers, and the resisted straight-leg test had a sensitivity of 0.56. Both the Maslowski[81] and Clohisy[33] studies lacked a control group.

IMPINGEMENT TESTING

Abnormal contact between the femoral head and acetabular rim in terminal hip motion can result in femoroacetabular impingement or FAI. Because the acetabular labrum provides joint stability at the extremes of motion, the labrum and adjacent cartilage can be impinged between the bony structures. Aberrant bony morphology of the proximal femur and/or acetabulum can lead to continued abutment of the bony structures of the hip and early chondral and/or labral lesions. Most provocative maneuvers involve trying to reproduce this impingement by approximating the bony structures in flexion, internal rotation, and adduction, and many different variations of this basic maneuver have been described.

ANTERIOR IMPINGEMENT TEST

The anterior impingement test, also known as the flexion–adduction–internal rotation (FADDIR or FAIR) test (Fig. 8.14), is the most commonly described clinical test for FAI or labral pathology.[88] The anterior impingement test was first described in 1991 by Klaue and coworkers[89] as a test for labral tears in dysplastic hips:

[I]n most cases pain can be elicited by passive movement of the thigh into full flexion, adduction and internal rotation. This combination brings the proximal and anterior part of the femoral neck into contact with the rim of the acetabulum, at exactly the point where the labrum is likely to be damaged. The test exerts a shear force on the limbus at its attachment to the acetabular bony margin and if a tear is present, the dislocation of the limbus may be palpable. Sometimes the

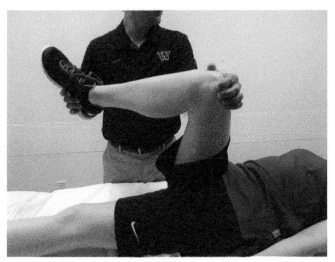

Figure 8.14 Flexion-adduction-internal rotation (FADDIR) test.

opposite movements, passive hyperextension with external rotation, may also produce pain and a sensation of apprehension.

Klaue and coworkers[89] performed the test with the patient supine, but the test has also been described with the patient in a lateral position.[90,91] In Klaue and associates,[89] the validity of this test was not reported.

The anterior impingement test was one of a number of provocative tests performed by Martin and others,[79] Troelsen and colleagues,[80] and Clohisy and associates.[33] Martin and colleagues[79] looked at the diagnostic accuracy of the anterior impingement test in 49 patients with various intra-articular hip pathologies, including labral pathology, arthritic changes, FAI, and acetabular dysplasia. The authors reported a sensitivity of 0.78 (95% CI; 0.59 to 0.89), specificity of 0.10 (95% CI; 0.03 to 0.29), +LR 0.86 (95% CI; 0.67 to 1.1), and −LR 2.3 (95% CI; 0.52 to 10.4) in predicting a response to an intra-articular anesthetic hip injection. Troelsen and associates[80] examined 18 patients before an MRI arthrogram using three provocative maneuvers. Seventeen of the patients had a labral tear on imaging, and the anterior impingement had a sensitivity of 0.59, specificity of 1.0, PPV of 1.0, and NPV of 0.13.[80] Clohisy and coworkers[33] prospectively evaluated 51 patients with symptomatic FAI and labral pathology with five provocative maneuvers, and the anterior impingement test reproduced hip pain in 88% of subjects compared with FABER (98%), resisted SLR (56%), log roll (30%) and positive impingement test result (21%).

A number of other studies have reported just the sensitivity of the anterior impingement test. Ito and associates[82] presented a series of 25 patients with symptomatic FAI, confirmed radiographically and surgically. The anterior impingement test result was positive in 24 of the patients (sensitivity, 0.96). Burnett and coworkers[30] retrospectively reviewed 66 consecutive patients with a labral tear confirmed by arthroscopy and reported a sensitivity of 0.95. Sink and colleagues[83] retrospectively reviewed 35 adolescent athletes with FAI and/or labral pathology, and all of the patients had a positive impingement test result (sensitivity, 1.0). Finally, Philippon and associates[86] prospectively examined 122 patients with FAI using both the anterior impingement and FABER test before hip arthroscopy. All of the patients had either a positive impingement or FABER test result, but the sensitivity and specificity of the anterior impingement test alone were not reported.

FLEXION–INTERNAL ROTATION TEST

A variation of the anterior impingement test has been reported where the hip is flexed to 90 degrees and internally rotated without adduction.[84,92-95] Hase and Ueo[93] presented a series of 10 patients with an acetabular labral tear diagnosed by arthroscopy, and 7 of these patients had pain with the flexion–internal rotation test. Chan and colleagues[92] imaged 30 patients with intra-articular hip pain that was provoked with the flexion–internal rotation test. Of the 30 patients with suspected labral tears, 25 had evidence of a tear on MRI arthrogram, and 17 ultimately underwent arthroscopic hip surgery. While this test was not designed to assess the sensitivity and specificity of the flexion–internal rotation test, when compared with MRI arthrogram, the accuracy of the clinical examination was 0.83. Nogier and others[84] presented a prospective multicenter study of 292 patients with mechanical hip pain from FAI. The impingement test result was positive in 18% to 65% of the cases depending on the variation used, but pain was predominantly found in flexion–internal rotation. In 65% of cases, pain was predominantly associated with flexion–internal rotation (sensitivity = 0.70; specificity = 0.44), and exclusively so, in 18% of cases (sensitivity = 0.20; specificity = 0.86).

FLEXION–INTERNAL ROTATION–AXIAL COMPRESSION OR INTERNAL ROTATION OVER PRESSURE

Maslowski and associates[81] tested the internal rotation over pressure (IROP) test with three other provocative maneuvers in 50 patients with various hip pathologies and described the IROP tests as follows:

> IROP testing was also performed with the subject supine. The affected hip was flexed to 90 degrees and the knee flexed to 90 degrees. The examiner internally rotated the hip by rotating the leg laterally while stabilizing the knee at the same time. Internal rotation over pressure was administered with further gentle rotation of the ipsilateral leg. The pelvis was stabilized, when necessary, by the examiner's other hand at the contralateral anterior superior iliac spine to reduce contralateral ilial rotation. The test was positive if it recreated the patient's hip pain.

In this study, the IROP have a relatively high sensitivity but low specificity for detecting intra-articular hip pathology (sensitivity = 0.91, specificity = 0.18, PPV = 0.47, NPV = 0.71).

Narvani and associates[85] presented a case series of 18 patients with hip pain. Four of these patients had a labral tear on MRI arthrogram, and 3 of them had reproduction of pain with IROP. Of the 14 patients without a tear on MRI arthrogram, 8 also had a positive test result. IROP had a sensitivity of 0.75 (95% confidence; 19.4% to 99.4%), specificity of 0.43 (17.7% to 71.7%), PPV of 0.27, and NPV of 0.86. Because the rate of a positive test result was not significantly different in patients with a tear on MRI arthrogram and those without, the authors did not find this maneuver useful in the diagnosis of labral tears.

FLEXION–ADDUCTION–AXIAL COMPRESSION TEST

Hase and Ueo[93] described eliciting pain when applying an axial compression to the hip joint when the hip was flexed to 90 degrees and slightly adducted but not internally rotated. All 10 patients included in this case series had pain with this maneuver, but no other studies have looked at the validity of this test.

PASSIVE SUPINE ROTATION TEST (LOG ROLL)

(Video 8-8)

This test assesses hip rotation with the patient supine and the hip in neutral. Since this test is passive, the femoral head can be moved within the acetabulum and capsule without significantly stressing the surrounding structures.[96] The examiner passively rotates the hip internally and externally and notes any pain or restricted motion in the involved hip compared with the other side. Clohisy and associates[33] prospectively evaluated 51 patients with symptomatic FAI and labral pathology with five provocative maneuvers, and the log roll test had a sensitivity of 0.30.

FLEXION-EXTENSION MANEUVERS

The flexion-extension maneuvers are dynamic and have been compared to the McMurray test of the knee. These maneuvers have several different names, but all involve moving the hip from flexion to extension. These tests have subtle variations in whether there is a rotational and/or abduction/adduction component to the examination.[88]

FITZGERALD'S TEST

In 1995, Fitzgerald[97] described 55 patients diagnosed with labral tears. In 54 of these patients, Fitzgerald was able to elicit a sharp, catching pain with the following maneuver[97]:

> The hip was initially brought into acute flexion, external rotation, and full abduction and was then extended with internal rotation and adduction. This maneuver precipitated pain with or without an associated click in patients with an anterior labral tear. Extension with abduction and external rotation from the fully flexed, adducted, and internally rotated position reproduced sharp pain with or without an associated click in those patients with a posterior labral tear. No further studies have assessed this test for validity.

QUADRANT TEST (HIP SCOUR TEST) (Video 8-9)

The hip quadrant test, or scour test, attempts to load as much of the acetabular surface as possible. Maitland's description of the quadrant test emphasized the importance of determining whether joint loading reproduced symptoms or if any irregularity of motion could be detected by the examiner.[98]

The test is performed with the patient lying in a supine position. The examiner flexes and adducts the hip to end range where resistance is felt. The examiner then moves the hip into abduction while maintaining the flexed position in a circular arc and applying a posterior compressive force in the direction of the femoral shaft The four quadrants tested can be divided into the following arc of motion:

1. Flexion/abduction/external rotation to extension/abduction/external rotation

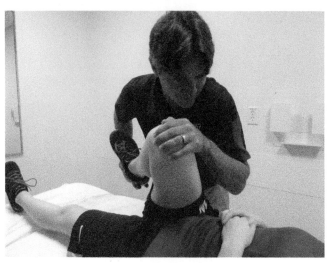

Figure 8.15   Scour test.

2. Flexion/adduction/external rotation to extension/adduction/external rotation
3. Flexion/abduction/internal rotation to extension/abduction/internal rotation
4. Flexion/adduction/internal rotation to extension/adduction/internal rotation

Any irregularity in motion, reproduction of pain, locking, crepitus, clicking, or apprehension is considered a positive test result and may indicate intra-articular pathology. Painful quadrant testing may also be secondary to psoas bursitis or tendinopathy, and restricted motion can be due to a tight hip capsule or gluteal muscles.

Maslowski and coworkers[81] prospectively examined 50 patients with various intra-articular hip pathologies using four provocative maneuvers before and after a fluoroscopically guided anesthetic intra-articular hip injection. The scour test (Fig. 8.15, Video 8-9) was performed as follows: The hip is maximally flexed and adducted. Then, with a compressive force applied to the joint in the direction of the shaft of the femur, the examiner moves the femur through a circular arc of motion. The maneuver is considered positive if it recreates pain. In this study,[81] the scour test was not useful in predicting a positive response to the diagnostic intra-articular injection (sensitivity = 0.50, specificity = 0.29, PPV = 0.36, NPV = 0.42).

Mitchell and associates[78] examined 25 consecutive patients who underwent hip arthroscopies after either a positive diagnostic anesthetic hip injection or hip MRI arthrogram and found that "the only consistently positive clinical test result was a restricted and painful hip quadrant compared with the contralateral hip." In Sutlive and associates' prospective study[72] of 72 patients with hip OA, the scour test had a sensitivity of 0.62 (95% CI, 0.39 to 0.81), specificity of 0.75 (95% CI, 0.6 to 0.85), +LR of 2.4 (95% CI, 1.4 to 4.3), and LR of 0.51 (95% CI, 0.29 to 0.89). Cliborne and others[76] included the scour test as one of four provocative maneuvers while examining 22 patients with hip OA and 17 asymptomatic subjects. The interrater reliability ICC value was 0.87 (95% CI, 0.76 to 0.93), but the sensitivity and specificity were not reported.

Variations of the hip quadrant test are the dynamic internal rotatory impingement test (DIRI) and the dynamic external rotatory impingement test (DEXRIT). These tests are distinguished from the traditional hip quadrant testing by (1) having the patient hold the nonaffected leg in more than 90 degrees of flexion to eliminate lumbar lordosis and (2) not applying a compressive force when passively ranging the hip joint.[88] In the DIRI test, the affected hip is brought into full flexion and then extended in a wide arc maintaining adduction and internal rotation. The DEXRIT brings the hip into abduction and external rotation when extending the hip from full flexion to extension. When performed together, the DIRI and DEXRIT tests have been referred to as the McCarthy test in the literature.[90,91,99] No validation studies have been found for the DIRI and DEXRIT test.

POSTERIOR AND LATERAL RIM IMPINGEMENT TEST

While the majority of acetabular labral tears are located in the anterior or anterosuperior regions of the acetabulum,[100] posterior labral tears can occur, and they present with pain in positions of extension and external rotation. The posterior impingement test is performed with the patient positioned at the edge of the examination table with the nonaffected leg held in flexion and the affected leg off the table in full extension. The affected hip is then passively abducted and externally rotated to approximate the femoral neck and the posterior acetabular wall.[101] A variation of this includes the lateral rim impingement test in which the patient is positioned in a lateral position and the hip is brought from flexion into extension in continuous abduction.[101] The FABER test places similar stress on the acetabular rim.

In Clohisy and associates,[33] one examiner prospectively evaluated 51 patients with symptomatic FAI and/or labral pathology with five provocative maneuvers, including the posterior impingement test. Clohisy and colleagues[33] did not explain how they performed the posterior impingement test, but when compared with radiographs, this maneuver had a sensitivity of 0.22.

AXIAL HIP DISTRACTION (Video 8-10)

Axial hip distraction (Fig. 8.16) has also been called the caudal glide, foveal distraction, or axial distraction test. The patient is in a supine position, and the examiner abducts the hip 30 degrees and applies long-axis traction by holding the leg just above the ankle. If knee pathology is suspected or evident, the examiner should place his or her hands around the thigh just proximal to the knee.[3,90,91] The examiner should feel for giving way or telescoping as the traction is applied.[3] Relief of the patient's symptoms is reported to be a sign of an underlying intra-articular process. The test result may also be positive in cases of hip instability from capsular laxity.[102] No sensitivity, specificity, or reliability studies have been performed on this test.

ATHLETIC PUBALGIA TESTS (TABLE 8.3)

Historically known as sports hernia or sportsman's groin, athletic pubalgia is due to an injury of the lower abdominal and/or adductor muscles. Chronic repetitive abduction movements of the thigh and/or hyperextension of the

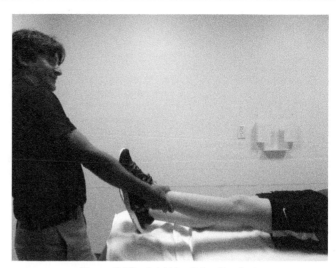

Figure 8.16   Axial hip distraction test.

trunk place torque on the common aponeurosis of the rectus abdominis and adductor tendons at the pubic symphysis.[99] Commonly presenting as chronic inguinal pain in athletes, clinical examination should include ruling out a fascial hernia.

RESISTED SIT-UP (Video 8-11)

Contraction of the abdominal muscles, as occurs with coughing, sneezing, or abdominal contraction can aggravate symptoms.[103-105] The resisted sit-up (Fig. 8.17) is performed with the patient supine and the examiner placing a hand on the patient's chest to provide resistance.[91] The test result is positive if it reproduces pain at the insertion of the rectus abdominis or in the groin.

In one series of 157 athletes with inguinal pain, 72 patients (46%) had pain with resisted abdominal contraction.[106] No studies were found that investigated the specificity, sensitivity, or reliability of this test.

RESISTED HIP ADDUCTION (Video 8-12)

Resisted contraction[106,107] or stretching[108,109] of the hip adductors has been associated with athletic pubalgia. Verrall and coworkers[110] studied the reliability and validity of resisted hip adduction for diagnosing athletic pubalgia in a cross-sectional prospective study. Three provocative tests were used to assess 89 Australian rules football players, 61 with and 28 without groin symptoms, and the clinical findings were compared with MRI of the groin.

All three provocative tests were performed with the patient in a supine position. The single adductor test (Fig. 8.18A) was performed with one hip raised in 30 degrees of flexion and the contralateral hip in 0 degrees of flexion. Contracting the adductor muscles of the raised hip, the patient is asked to resist the examiner's abduction force. The single adductor test is performed one leg at a time but performed bilaterally. The bilateral adductor test (Fig. 8.18B) is performed with both legs raised off the table with the hips in 30 degrees of flexion. The patient resists the examiner's bilateral abduction force, contracting both adductor muscles simultaneously. In both tests, pubic pain constitutes a

Table 8.3   Athletic Pubalgia Tests

Test	Description	Reliability/Validity Tests	Comments
Resisted sit-up	Patient is supine. The examiner places a hand on the patient's chest providing resistance as the patient tries to sit up. The test result is positive if it reproduces pain at the insertion of the rectus abdominis or in the groin.	There are no studies found that investigated the specificity, sensitivity, or reliability of this test.	
Resisted hip adduction			
Single adductor test	Patient is supine with one hip raised off the table to 30 degrees, and the adductor muscles are contracted against the examiner. The test result is positive if it reproduces groin pain.	Verrall et al. 2005[110] Sensitivity: 30% Specificity: 93% PPV: 0.78 NPV: 0.45	Compared resisted adduction tests with MRI
Bilateral adductor test	Patient is supine. Both hips raise off the table to 30 degrees and bilateral adductor muscles are contracted simultaneously. Reproduction of pubic pain constitutes a positive test result.	Sensitivity: 54% Specificity: 93% PPV: 0.89 NPV: 0.34	
Squeeze test	Patient is supine, with both hips and knees flexed with the feet flat on the table. The examiner places a clenched fist between the athlete's knees, and the athlete is asked to squeeze the examiner's fist. A positive test result recreates pain in the groin region.	Sensitivity: 43% Specificity: 91% PPV: 0.83 NPV: 0.40	

MRI, magnetic resonance imaging; *NPV*, negative predictive value; *PPV*, positive predictive value.

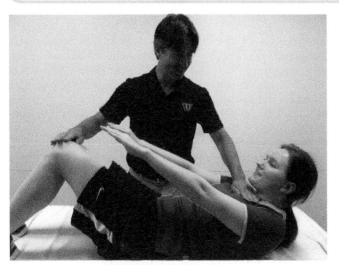

Figure 8.17   Resisted sit-up.

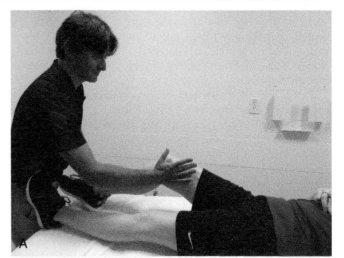

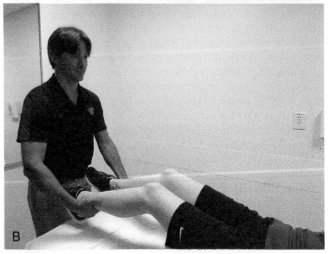

positive test. The squeeze test is performed with both hips flexed to 45 degrees, knees flexed to 90 degrees, and feet flat on the table. The examiner places a clenched fist between the athlete's knees, and the athlete is asked to "squeeze the fist," contracting both adductor muscles simultaneously. A positive test result recreates pain in the groin region.

In Verrall and associates' study,[110] the bilateral adductor test had the highest sensitivity and PPV compared with the other tests, with a sensitivity of 0.54, specificity of 0.93, PPV of 0.89, and NPV 0.34. The single adductor test had a sensitivity of 0.30, specificity of 0.91, PPV of 0.78, and NPV of 0.45. The squeeze test had a sensitivity of 0.43, specificity of 0.91, PPV of 0.83, and NPV of 0.40. When there was

Figure 8.18   A, Single adductor test. **B,** Bilateral adductor test.

associated evidence of pubic bone stress injury, the sensitivity and specificity were similar. The bilateral adductor test had a sensitivity of 0.65 and specificity of 0.92, the single adductor test had a sensitivity of 0.32 and specificity of 0.88, and the squeeze test had a sensitivity of 0.49 and specificity of 0.88.

TESTS FOR LEG-LENGTH DISCREPANCY (TABLE 8.4)

Leg-length discrepancy (LLD) can be classified into two etiologic groups: structural or functional. Structural LLDs are those in which bony asymmetry results in an actual or true difference in leg length. Functional LLDs are due to altered biomechanics in the lower extremity or spine giving the appearance of a leg-length asymmetry when one does not actually exist.[111]

While radiography remains the gold standard for measuring LLD, two clinical methods have been described over the years.[111] The direct method, or the tape measurement method (TMM), directly measures the length of each lower extremity using bony anatomic landmarks. The indirect method uses lift blocks under the short leg until the pelvis appears level on visual examination and then measures the size of the lift necessary to correct the pelvic obliquity.

DIRECT LEG-LENGTH DISCREPANCY METHOD

(Video 8-13)

The commonly used direct technique to determine LLD is measuring between either (1) the ASIS to the medial malleolus (MM) of the tibia (Fig. 8.19A) or (2) the ASIS to the lateral malleolus (LM) (Fig. 8.19B). In many studies of the validity and reliability of these direct techniques, the clinical measurements are compared with a radiographic standard. However, there are inherent methodologic problems with this study design. With the clinical examination, the tape measure rarely takes a straight trajectory because it bows out over the anterior thigh, while the x-ray measurement simply calculates the distance between two anatomic landmarks in space.

In 1955, Nichols and Bailey[126] reported the accuracy, or "observer error," of the ASIS-MM measurement in 50 patients. When a $\frac{1}{2}$-inch difference in LLD was used as an acceptable variation in measurements, there was complete agreement between the examiners in 86% of cases. When a $\frac{1}{4}$-inch difference was used, complete agreement occurred in only 40% of cases. The authors concluded that the "overall degree of accuracy of the measurement of leg lengths is such that differences of $\frac{1}{2}$ inch (12.5 mm) or more may be accepted as diagnostically significant, but differences of less than $\frac{1}{2}$ inch are not reliable unless based on the average of at least four measurements."

A number of studies have looked at the reliability of the direct ASIS-MM method, compared with a radiographic standard. Gogia and Braatz[112] compared the ASIS-MM TMM with radiographic measurement in a series of 30 patients. The authors found the ASIS-MM TM to have a strong interrater and intrarater reliability between examiners and between examiners and x-ray measurements, r = 0.98.

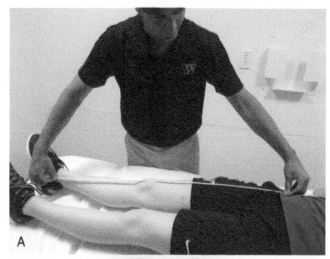

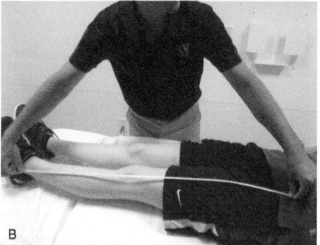

Figure 8.19 A, Leg length measurement from anterior superior iliac spine to the medial malleolus. **B,** Leg length measurement from anterior superior iliac spine to the lateral malleolus.

Beattie and coworkers[113] enrolled 10 subjects with a clinical diagnosis of LLD and 9 controls subjects and compared the direct ASIS-MM TMM with radiographic measurements. In this study, the ASIS-MM TMM had an intrarater reliability of ICC = 0.77 for subjects with suspected LLD and ICC = 0.68 for all enrolled subjects. When two measurements were taken and averaged, the ICC improved to 0.85 and 0.79, respectively. Hoyle and colleagues[114] reported an interexaminer reliability of r = 0.97 to 0.99 and intraexaminer reliability of r = 0.89 to 0.95 for the ASIS to MM method between two physical therapists evaluating 25 subjects compared to an electrogoniometer.

Jamaluddin and associates[115] assessed the reliability and accuracy of the ASIS-MM TMM compared with computed tomography (CT) measurement of LLD. In a cross-sectional study of 35 patients with LLD and 13 patients without, the authors found an interrater reliability between two observes of 0.805 (0.59 to 0.91; 95% CI) when TMM was compared with CT. Neelly and colleagues[116] also compared the ASIS-MM TMM to CT-derived leg length measurements. Unlike the above studies, the authors only measured the unilateral leg length and did not attempt to assess LLD by

Table 8.4 Tests for Leg-Length Discrepancy

Test	Description	Reliability/Validity Tests	Comments

Leg-length discrepancy	Direct (ASIS-MM)	Gogia and Braatz 1986[112]
		  Interrater reliability: 0.98
		  Intrarater reliability: 0.98
			TMM compared with radiographs

		Beattie et al. 1990[113] Intraclass coefficient reliability: 0.77	TMM compared with radiographs

		Hoyle et al. 1991[114]
		  Interrater reliability: 0.97–0.99
		  Intrarater reliability: 0.89–0.95
			TMM compared with electrogoniometer

		Jamaluddin et al. 2011[115] Interrater reliability: 0.92	TMM compared with CT measurement of LLD

		Neelly et al. 2013[116]
		  Interrater reliability: 0.99
		  Intrarater reliability: 0.99
			TMM compared with CT measurement of ipsilateral leg

	Indirect method:
	With lift blocks
		Jonson and Gross 1997[117]
		  Interrater reliability: 0.87
		  Intrarater reliability: 0.70
			Iliac crest palpation with lift blocks and pelvic leveling device

		Gross et al. 1998[118]
		  Interrater reliability: 0.77
		  Intrarater reliability: 0.84
		  Difference of ±5.5–5.8 mm compared with radiographs
			Iliac crest palpation with lift blocks and pelvic leveling device compared to radiographs

	With book correction	Hanada et al. 2001[119]
		  Interrater reliability: 0.91
		  Intrarater reliability: 0.98
			Iliac crest palpation with book correction compared with radiographs

	Direct and indirect methods	Clarke 1972[120] Direct and indirect methods were both inaccurate	Comparison of direct ASIS-MM and indirect block method with radiographs

		Woerman et al. 1984[121]
		  Indirect: difference of ±4 mm compared with radiographs.
		  Direct ASIS-LM method was the most accurate and precise of the direct methods; difference of ±5.2 mm compared to radiographs
			Comparison of direct ASIS-MM, ASIS-LM, U-MM, X-MM, and indirect method of iliac crest palpation with lift blocks with radiographs

		Friberg et al. 1988[122]
		  Direct: difference of ±8.6 mm compared with radiographs
		  Indirect: difference of ±7.5 mm compared with radiographs
			Comparison of ASIS-MM and indirect method with lift blocks with radiographs

		Lampe et al. 1996[123]
		  Direct: difference of ±9.7 mm compared with radiographs
		  Indirect: difference of ±7.8 mm compared with radiographs
			Comparison of ASIS-MM and indirect method with lift blocks with radiographs

		Terry et al. 2005[124]
		  Direct ASIS-LM/MM
		    Interrater reliability: 0.83/0.8
		    Intrarater reliability: 0.88/0.78
		  Indirect
		    Interrater reliability: 0.83
		    Intrarater reliability: 0.86
			Comparison of ASIS-MM, ASIS-LM and indirect method with lift blocks with radiographs

		Badii et al. 2014[125]
		  Direct ASIS-LM
		    Interrater reliability: 48
		    Sensitivity: 45%
		    Specificity: 56%
		  Indirect
		    Interrater reliability: 0.74
		    Sensitivity: 55%
		    Specificity: 89%
			Comparison of ASIS-LM and indirect method with lift blocks with radiographs

ASIS-LM, anterior superior iliac spine to the lateral malleolus; *ASIS-MM,* anterior superior iliac spine to the medial malleolus; *CT,* computed tomography; *LLD,* leg-length discrepancy; *TMM,* tape measurement method; *U-MM,* umbilicus to the medial malleolus; *X-MM,* xiphisternum to the medial malleolus.

measuring the contralateral leg. Two examiners assessed 30 volunteers, and the interrater and intrarater reliabilities for a single measurement were 0.99 and 0.99, respectively.

INDIRECT LEG-LENGTH DISCREPANCY METHOD

Gofton[127] initially described a three-step process of estimating LLD. In the initial step the examiner observes the patient for any findings of LLD:

> The patient stands with his feet parallel and about seven inches apart. The examiner sits behind him. The patient should stand erect and look forward, not downwards. His knees must be straight and the pelvis centered over the feet. If significant leg-length disparity exists, three observations will be made: (1) The upper lateral thigh on the long side will protrude. (2) Scoliosis will be apparent. (3) The examiner's hands placed on top of the iliac crests will rest at different heights. All three of these findings should be present if the estimation of disparity is to be trusted.

If there is evidence of (1) prominence of the upper lateral thigh on the long side, (2) scoliosis, or (3) asymmetry of the iliac crests, then the examiner places a lift or block under the presumed short side to correct the imbalance. The size of the block necessary to correct the pelvis asymmetry indicates the amount of LLD. Finally, Gofton[127] recommended placing the same block under the presumed longer leg as a method of confirmation, and the three original findings should now be exaggerated.

Bourdillon[128] in 1973 described an alternative final step to confirm the presence of a LLD:

> With the patient in the sitting position, the effect of any leg-length discrepancy is eliminated. If, therefore, the right posterior inferior spine appears to be lower than the left in the standing position, but the two appear to be level with the patient sitting, this is additional evidence that the right leg is shorter than the left. If, with the patient sitting, the posterior inferior spine on the right side still appears lower than that on the left, the probable cause is a fixed torsion of the pelvis.

Therefore, in a true structural LLD, the pelvic tilt would correct with the patient sitting. However, if the asymmetry in iliac crest heights was due to a functional LLD, then the pelvic obliquity would be present in both a standing and seated position.

A number of studies have looked at the reliability of assessing iliac crest height, which is a requisite for the indirect method. Mann and coworkers[129] examined the intrarater and interrater agreement for 11 examiners assessing the iliac crest height of 10 subjects in the standing position and found this test to be unreliable, with examiners sometimes not even agreeing on the laterality of which iliac crest was elevated.

Jonson and Gross[117] used 63 healthy naval shipmen to study the reliability of the indirect lift block method and a pelvic leveling device at the iliac crests. The intrarater reliability ICC was 0.87, while the interrater reliability was 0.70 (N = 18). Gross and others[118] using a similar method with lifts and a pelvic leveling device, compared indirect and radiographic measurements of LLD. The authors found an good intrarater reliability (ICC = 0.84), fair interrater reliability (ICC = 0.77), and validity between clinical and radiographic measurements ranging from 0.64 to 0.76 with an absolute difference of 0.55 to 0.58 cm (±0.37 to 0.58). Hanada and others[119] described a similar approach but corrected the LLD with a book opened to the required number of pages and then measured the thickness of the book. The indirect measurement was then compared with the radiographic measurement. The interexaminer ICC was 0.91, intraexaminer ICC was 0.98, and validity when compared with radiographs was 0.76. Fisk and Baigent[130] presented a series of 117 patients with a clinical finding of LLD using the indirect method as described by Bourdillon,[128] and of the 107 who had subsequent radiographs, there was a difference of more than 5 mm in approximately 30% of the cases.

A number of studies have compared the indirect and direct methods. Clarke[120] presented 50 patients thought with have a LLD of at least ½ inch based on clinical findings. While radiography confirmed the diagnosis in all 50 patients, both the direct ASIS-MM TMM and indirect methods were inaccurate. Examiners were within 5 mm of the radiographic measurement in only 20 of the cases using the direct method and 16 cases using the indirect method.

Woerman and Binder-Macleod[121] presented a series of five patients using both direct and indirect methods for LLD compared with radiography. In addition to the ASIS-MM and ASIS-LM method, measurements from the umbilicus (U) and xiphisternum (X) to MM were obtained. Overall, the indirect method was more precise and accurate (difference = 0.4 cm) than any of the direct methods. The ASIS-LM method was the most accurate and precise direct method (difference = 0.52 cm), and the U and X to MM the most inaccurate and imprecise direct method.

Friberg and coworkers[122] found both the direct ASIS-MM TMM and indirect method to be inaccurate and imprecise, with a mean difference of ±8.6 and 7.5 mm compared with radiographs, respectively. In 12% of the direct and 13.4% of the indirect measurements, the examiners in this series incorrectly identified which leg was the short one. Lampe and colleagues[123] studied both direct and indirect methods in 190 children and compared clinical measurements with radiography. The ASIS-MM method was less accurate (difference = 0.97 cm; −1.8–2.1; CI, 95%) than the indirect measurement using lift blocks and iliac crest height (difference = 0.78 cm; −1.4–1.6; CI, 95%). Terry and associates[124] assessed the interobserver and intraobserver reliability in 16 patients among four examiners using the ASIS-LM, ASIS-MM, and indirect methods compared with a radiographic measurement. All had high reliability with an intrarater ICC of 0.88, 0.78, and 0.86 respectively, and an interrater ICC of 0.83, 0.80, and 0.83, respectively. Badii and associates[125] studied the ASIS-LM TMM and indirect method on 20 subjects compared to radiographic measurements of LLD. Measurement errors of more than 5 mm were greatest with the direct method (14/20) compared with the indirect method (2/20). In the direct tape measurement group, 7 of the 20 patients had the wrong leg identified as being shorter compared with radiograph, versus 1 of the 20 in the lift group. The direct ASIS-LM

Table 8.5 Tests for Femoral Stress Fractures

Test	Description	Reliability/Validity Tests	Comments
Fulcrum test	Patient is seated with lower legs dangling. The examiner's arm is used as a gentle pressure is applied to the dorsum of the knee with the opposite hand. The test result is positive if gentle pressure on the knee produces increased discomfort in the thigh.	There are no studies found that investigated the specificity, sensitivity or reliability of this test.	
Hop test	A positive test result occurs when the patient experiences pain in the area of a suspected stress fracture with the performance of a one-legged hop.	There are no studies found that investigated the specificity, sensitivity, or reliability of this test.	

measurement had an interrater reliability of 0.48 (CI, 95%; 0.25 to 0.71), sensitivity of 0.45, and specificity of 0.56, while the lifts had an ICC of 0.74 (CI, 95%; 0.57 to 0.87), sensitivity of 0.55, and specificity of 0.89.

TESTS FOR FEMORAL STRESS FRACTURES (TABLE 8.5)

Femoral shaft stress fractures can present as a vague thigh pain, and often few physical findings are present to assist the clinician. While uncommon, stress fractures of the femoral shaft are usually located in the proximal one-third of the femur.

FULCRUM TEST (Video 4-13)

In 1994, Johnson and colleagues[131] described the fulcrum test to diagnose stress fractures of the femoral shaft. The foundation for this test was four athletes with femoral shaft stress fractures who reported aggravation of anterior thigh pain when they sat on the edge of a desk with the leg dangling in the air or when the affected leg was crossed over the opposite thigh (Fig. 8.20). The fulcrum test was described in the following manner[131]:

> [T]he athlete is seated on the examination table with the lower legs dangling. The examiner's arm is used as a fulcrum under the thigh and is moved from distal to proximal thigh as gentle pressure is applied to the dorsum of the knee with the opposite hand. At the point of the fulcrum under the stress fracture, gentle pressure on the knee produced increased discomfort that was often described as a sharp pain and was accompanied with apprehension.

In the original study, 914 collegiate athletes were followed prospectively over 2 years. Thirty-four stress fractures were diagnosed, and 7 of them (20.6%) were femoral shaft stress fractures. Only one false-positive was found in a patient with a quadriceps strain and one false-negative in a patient with a femoral neck stress fracture. The reliability, sensitivity, and specificity were not assessed.

The test was also useful for management and for assessing healing. Johnson and colleagues found that pain elicited by the test diminished with time and suggested that when the

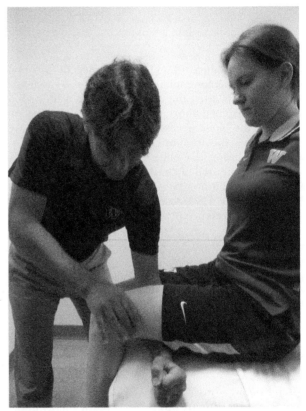

Figure 8.20 Fulcrum test.

patient feels no discomfort "gradual return to a sport appears safe."

HOP TEST

The hop test was originally described by Matheson and colleagues[132] to assess for stress fractures involving the lower extremity. In this original series of 320 athletes, "pain at the site of stress fracture reproduced by one-legged hopping" was considered a positive test result. While the authors found a positive test result to carry a high likelihood of predicting a stress fracture, the authors did not report the validity or reliability of this test.

Clement and associates[133] studied 71 athletes with 74 stress injuries to the femur using a case-controlled design.

During the clinical examination, 70.3% of the patients had pain reproduced in the hip, groin, or anterior thigh when asked to hop on the affected limb. The authors concluded that the hop test was clinically useful in cases of suspected stress injury of the femur. These results should be used cautiously in that the true sensitivity, specificity, and reliability of this test have not been evaluated.

AUTHOR'S PREFERRED APPROACH

Evaluation of the hip requires a comprehensive understanding of the anatomy and biomechanics of the hip and related structures. The scientific evidence of the sensitivity, specificity, and reliability of physical examination maneuvers of the hip is limited, and many of the studies referenced are flawed because of the small sample size, study design, and variable "gold standards" used to confirm the diagnosis.

While many of these tests are imperfect, the authors believe that developing a systematic and thorough approach increases the likelihood of an accurate diagnosis. Many potential pitfalls exist when assessing hip pain, because numerous neurologic, visceral, and vascular etiologies can mimic hip joint pathology. Therefore, the clinician should thoughtfully use these provocative maneuvers in concert with the patient history and all-encompassing examination to come to a treatment plan.

Here we propose one approach to the examination of the hip. The patient should be examined in standing, sitting, supine, lateral, and prone positions. Additional tests can be added to this basic approach depending on the patient's presenting history.

STANDING

The standing examination should include an inspection of gait, posture, and spinal alignment. Both walking and running should be assessed. An assessment of balance with single-leg stance and the Trendelenburg test may be indicative of gluteus medius and minimus weakness or a compensated variant in which the patient shifts over to the involved leg to decrease the force required from the abductors. The Trendelenburg test should be assessed bilaterally. The hop test may be performed if there is concern for a stress fracture. If suspicion exists regarding a LLD, the examiner should perform an indirect measurement of LLD or a direct measurement should be performed with the patient supine.

SITTING

The sitting examination should include a neurologic and vascular examination of both extremities. The seated position allows for stabilization of the pelvis, and hip rotation can easily be assessed. Internal and external rotation should be assessed and compared with the contralateral side. Loss of internal rotation may be a sign of intra-articular pathology. Femoral anteversion may present with increased internal rotation and decreased external rotation.

The active piriformis test (Pace test) and passive piriformis stretch test can also be performed with the patient in a seated position. If clinical suspicion for a femoral shaft stress fracture exists, the fulcrum test would be added to the seated examination.

SUPINE

The supine examination is often key to help distinguish between intra- and extra-articular sources of dysfunction. The examiner should begin by inspecting for any asymmetry in thigh circumference, which may be present with femoral neuropathy or diabetic amyotrophy. Any asymmetry of medial malleolus height should prompt a direct measurement of LLD, either measurement of the ASIS-MM or ASIS-LM. An abdominal examination should also be part of the supine examination, including palpation of pubic rami and pubic symphysis, to screen for athletic pubalgia and referred visceral mimics.

Range of motion testing should include flexion, abduction, adduction, and rotation and be compared with the contralateral side. Stabilizing pelvic motion is necessary to isolate motion at the hip joint. Extension should be tested when the patient is in a prone position. The Thomas test and popliteal angle can be used to test for hip flexor and hamstring tightness, respectively.

While many provocative maneuvers have been described to assess for intra-articular pathology, combining a number of these tests has been shown to increase the validity of the clinical examination. Maslowski and others[81] demonstrated that when combining the FABER, Stinchfield, scour, and IROP tests, the reliability of the examination in predicting a response to an intra-articular hip injection improved. Additionally, the passive supine rotation test (log roll) may be considered as a screening test for assessing intra-articular pathology. Extra-articular causes of hip pain can be assessed with such tests as the FABERE (SIJ), piriformis test (piriformis), SLR (lumbar radiculopathy), and athletic pubalgia tests (resisted hip adduction and resisted sit-up) based on the examiner's differential diagnosis.

LATERAL

The lateral examination should begin with palpation of the lateral structures and resisted hip abduction testing. Pain with this test that localizes to the greater trochanter may indicate involvement of the gluteus medius and minimus tendons. The Ober test or the modified Ober test can also be performed to further assess tightness of the iliotibial band.

PRONE

The prone examination should begin with palpation of the posterior hip structures. Passive ROM may be performed to assess for asymmetries in motion. The Ely test can be performed to test for rectus femoris tightness

REFERENCES

1. Thomas HO. *Diseases of the Hip, Knee, and Ankle Joints and Their Deformities Treated by a New and Efficient Method.* 3rd ed. Liverpool: T. Dobb & Co.; 1876:17-19.
2. Cave EF, Roberts SM. A method for measuring and recording joint function. *J Bone Joint Surg.* 1936;18:455-465.
3. Magee DM. *Orthopedic Physical Assessment.* 4th ed. Philadelphia: W.B. Saunders; 2002:606-640.

4. Bartlett MD, Wolf LS, Shurtleff DB, et al. Hip flexion contractures: a comparison of measurement methods. *Arch Phys Med Rehabil.* 1985;66:620-625.

5. Kilgour G, McNair P, Stott NS. Intrarater reliability of lower limb sagittal range-of-motion measures in children with spastic diplegia. *Dev Med Child Neurol.* 2003;45:391-399.

6. McWhirk LB, Glanzman AM. Within-session inter-rater reliability of goniometric measures in patients with spastic cerebral palsy. *Pediatr Phys Ther.* 2006;18:262-265.

7. Mutlu A, Livanelioglu A, Gunel MK. Reliability of goniometric measurements in children with spastic cerebral palsy. *Med Sci Monit.* 2007;13:CR323-CR329.

8. Glanzman AM, Swenson AE, Kim H. Intrarater range of motion reliability in cerebral palsy: a comparison of assessment methods. *Pediatr Phys Ther.* 2008;20:369-372.

9. Lee KM, Chung CY, Kwon DG, et al. Reliability of physical examination in the measurement of hip flexion contracture and correlation with gait parameters in cerebral palsy. *J Bone Joint Surg Am.* 2011;93:150-158.

10. Herrero P, Carrera P, Garcia E, et al. Reliability of goniometric measurements in children with cerebral palsy: a comparative analysis of universal goniometer and electronic inclinometer. A pilot study. *BMC Musculoskelet Disord.* 2011;12:155-162.

11. Ashton BB, Pickles B, Roll JW. Reliability of goniometric measurements of hip motion in spastic cerebral palsy. *Dev Med Child Neurol.* 1978;20:87-94.

12. Harvey D. Assessment of the flexibility of elite athletes using the modified Thomas test. *Br J Sports Med.* 1998;32:68-70.

13. Clapis PA, Davis SM, Davis RO. Reliability of inclinometer and goniometric measurements of hip extension flexibility using the modified Thomas test. *Physiother Theory Pract.* 2008;24:135-141.

14. Cejudo A, Sainz de Baranda P, Ayala F, et al. Test-retest reliability of seven common clinical tests for assessing lower extremity muscle flexibility in futsal and handball players. *Phys Ther Sport.* 2015;16:107-113.

15. Wakefield CB, Halls A, Difilippo N, et al. Reliability of goniometric and trigonometric techniques for measuring hip-extension range of motion using the modified Thomas test. *J Athl Train.* 2015;50:460-466.

16. Peeler J, Anderson JE. Reliability of the Ely's test for assessing rectus femoris muscle flexibility and joint range of motion. *J Orthop Res.* 2008;26:793-799.

17. Atamaz F, Ozcaldiran B, Ozdedeli S, et al. Interobserver and intraobserver reliability in lower-limb flexibility measurements. *J Sports Med Phys Fitness.* 2011;51:689-694.

18. Peeler J, Leiter J. Using digital photography to document rectus femoris flexibility: a reliability study of the modified Thomas test. *Physiother Theory Pract.* 2013;29:319-327.

19. Melchione WE, Sullivan MS. Reliability of measurements obtained by use of an instrument designed to indirectly measure iliotibial band length. *J Orthop Sports Phy Ther.* 1993;18:511-515.

20. Gajdosik RL, Sandler MM, Marr HL. Influence of knee positions and gender on the Ober test for length of the iliotibial band. *Clin Biomech (Bristol, Avon).* 2003;18:77-79.

21. Reese NB, Bandy WD. Use of an inclinometer to measure flexibility of the iliotibial band using the Ober test and the modified Ober test: differences in magnitude and reliability of measurements. *J Orthop Sports Phy Ther.* 2003;33:326-330.

22. Martin HD, Shears SA, Johnson C, et al. The endoscopic treatment of sciatic nerve entrapment/deep gluteal syndrome. *Arthroscopy.* 2011;27(2):172-181.

23. Gajdosik RL, Lusin GF. Hamstring muscle tightness: reliability of an active knee-extension test. *Phys Ther.* 1983;63:1085-1088.

24. Sullivan MK, Dejulia JJ, Worrell TW. Effect of pelvic position and stretching method on hamstring muscle flexibility. *Med Sci Sports Exerc.* 1992;24:1383-1389.

25. Davis D, Quinn R, Whiteman C, et al. Concurrent validity of four clinical tests used to measure hamstring flexibility. *J Strength Cond Res.* 2008;22:583-588.

26. Hamid MS, Ali MR, Yusof A. Interrater and intrarater reliability of the active knee extension (AKE) test among healthy adults. *J Phys Ther Sci.* 2013;25:957-961.

27. Reurink G1, Goudswaard GJ, Oomen HG, et al. Reliability of the active and passive knee extension test in acute hamstring injuries. *Am J Sports Med.* 2013;41:1757-1761.

28. Bird PA, Oakley SP, Shnier R, et al. Prospective evaluation of magnetic resonance imaging and physical examination findings in patients with greater trochanteric pain syndrome. *Arthritis Rheum.* 2001;44:2138-2145.

29. Altman R, Alarcón G, Appelrouth D, et al. The American College of Rheumatology criteria for the classification and reporting of osteoarthritis of the hip. *Arthritis Rheum.* 1991;34:505-514.

30. Burnett RS, Della Rocca GJ, Prather H, et al. Clinical presentation of patients with tears of the acetabular labrum. *J Bone Joint Surg Am.* 2006;88:1448-1457.

31. Woodley SJ, Nicholson HD, Livingstone V, et al. Lateral hip pain: findings from magnetic resonance imaging and clinical examination. *J Orthop Sports Phy Ther.* 2008;38:313-328.

32. Lequesne M, Mathieu P, Vuillemin-Bodaghi V, et al. Gluteal tendinopathy in refractory greater trochanter pain syndrome: diagnostic value of two clinical tests. *Arthritis Rheum.* 2008;59:241-246.

33. Clohisy JC, Knaus ER, Hunt DM, et al. Clinical presentation of patients with symptomatic anterior hip impingement. *Clin Orthop Relat Res.* 2009;467:638-644.

34. Youdas JW, Madson TJ, Hollman JH. Usefulness of the Trendelenburg test for identification of patients with hip joint osteoarthritis. *Physiother Theory Pract.* 2010;26:184-194.

35. Eland DC, Singleton TN, Conaster RR, et al. The "iliacus test": new information for the evaluation of hip extension dysfunction. *J Am Osteopath Assoc.* 2002;102:130-142.

36. West CC. Measurement of joint motion. *Arch Phys Med.* 1945;26:414-425.

37. Moore ML. The measurement of joint motion. II: The technique of goniometry. *Phys Ther Rev.* 1949;29:256-264.

38. Staheli LT. The prone hip extension test: a method of measuring hip flexion deformity. *Clin Orthop.* 1977;123:12-15.

39. Thurston A. Assessment of fixed flexion deformity of the hip. *Clin Orthop.* 1982;169:186-189.

40. Milch H. Pelvifemoral angle: determination of hip-flexion deformity. *J Bone Joint Surg.* 1942;24:148-153.

41. Mundale MO, Hislop HJ, Rabideau RJ, et al. Evaluation of extension of hip. *Arch Phys Med Rehabil.* 1956;37:75-80.

42. Ferber R, Kendall KD, McElroy L. Normative and critical criteria for iliotibial band and iliopsoas muscle flexibility. *J Athl Train.* 2010;45:344-348.

43. Ober FB. The role of the iliotibial band and fascia lata as a factor in the causation of low back disabilities and sciatica. *J Bone Joint Surg.* 1936;18:105-110.

44. Kendall HO, Kendall FP, Boynton DA. *Posture and Pain.* Baltimore: Williams & Wilkins; 1952.

45. Yeoman W. Relation of arthritis of sacro-iliac joint to sciatica. *Lancet.* 1928;ii:1119.

46. Parsons FG, Keith A. Sixth Annual Report of the Committee of Collective Investigation of the Anatomical Society of Great Britain and Ireland, 1895-96. *J Anat Physiol.* 1896;31:31-44.

47. Beaton LE, Anson BJ. The relation of the sciatic nerve and its subdivisions to the piriformis muscle. *Anat Rec.* 1937;70:1-5.

48. Benson ER, Schutzer SF. Posttraumatic piriformis syndrome: diagnosis and results of operative treatment. *J Bone Joint Surg Am.* 1999;81:941-949.

49. Solheim LF, Siewers P, Paus B. The piriformis muscle syndrome: sciatic nerve entrapment treated with section of the piriformis muscle. *Acta Orthop Scand.* 1981;52:73-75.

50. Martin HD, Kivlan BR, Palmer IJ, et al. Diagnostic accuracy of clinical tests for sciatic nerve entrapment in the gluteal region. *Knee Surg Sports Traumatol Arthrosc.* 2014;22:882-888.

51. Freiberg AH, Vinke TH. Sciatica and the sacro-iliac joint. *J Bone Joint Surg.* 1934;16:126-136.

52. Papadopoulos EC, Khan SN. Piriformis syndrome and low back pain: a new classification and review of the literature. *Orthop Clin North Am.* 2004;35:65-71.

53. Pace JB, Nagle D. Piriformis syndrome. *West J Med.* 1976;124:435-439.

54. Martin HD. Patient history and exam. In: *The Adult Hip: Hip Preservation Surgery.* Philadelphia: Lippincott Williams & Wilkins; 2014:97-120.

55. Byrd JW, Guanche CA. Clinical examination and imaging of the hip. In: *AANA Advanced Arthroscopy: The Hip.* Philadelphia: W.B. Saunders; 2010:3-30.

56. Coppieters MW, Alshami AM, Babri AS, et al. Strain and excursion of the sciatic, tibial, and plantar nerves during a modified straight leg raising test. *J Orthop Res.* 2006;24:1883-1889.

57. Koenigsberger MR. Judgement of fetal age. 1: Neurologic evaluation. *Pediatr Clin North Am.* 1966;13:823-833.

58. Amiel-Tison C. Neurologic evaluation of the maturity of newborn infants. *Arch Dis Child.* 1968;43:89-93.

59. Johnson A, Ashurst H. Is popliteal angle measurement useful in early identification of cerebral palsy? *Dev Med Child Neurol.* 1989; 31:457-465.

60. Reade E, Hom L, Hallum A, et al. Changes in popliteal angle measurement in infants up to one year of age. *Dev Med Child Neurol.* 1984;26:774-780.

61. Bleck EE. *Orthopedic Management of Cerebral Palsy.* Vol 2. Philadelphia: W.B. Saunders; 1979:29-33.

62. Trendelenburg F. Trendelenburg's test 1895. *Clin Orthop.* 1998; 355:3-7.

63. Hardcastle P, Nade S. The significance of the Trendelenburg test. *J Bone Joint Surg Br.* 1985;67:741-746.

64. Ege Rasmussen KJ, Fanø N. Trochanteric bursitis. Treatment by corticosteroid injection. *Scand J Rheumatol.* 1985;14:417-420.

65. Gordon EJ. Trochanteric bursitis and tendinitis. *Clin Orthop.* 1961;20:193-202.

66. Anderson TP. Trochanteric bursitis: diagnostic criteria and clinical significance. *Arch Phys Med Rehabil.* 1958;39:617-622.

67. Arromdee E, Matteson EL. Bursitis: common condition, uncommon challenge. *J Musculoskel Med.* 2001;18:213-224.

68. Kandemir U, Bharam S, Philippon MJ, et al. Endoscopic treatment of calcific tendinitis of gluteus medius and minimus. *Arthroscopy.* 2003;19:E4.

69. Karpinski MRK, Piggott H. Greater trochanteric pain syndrome. *J Bone Joint Surg.* 1985;67B:762-763.

70. Pearson JR, Riddell DM. Idiopathic osteoarthritis of the hip. *Ann Rheum Dis.* 1962;21:31-39.

71. Martin HD, Savage A, Braly BA, et al. The function of the hip capsular ligaments: a quantitative report. *Arthroscopy.* 2008;24: 188-195.

72. Sutlive TG, Lopez HP, Schniker DE, et al. Development of a clinical prediction rule for diagnosing hip osteoarthritis in individuals with unilateral hip pain. *J Orthop Sports Phy Ther.* 2008;38:542-550.

73. Kapron AL, Anderson AE, Peters CL, et al. Hip internal rotation is correlated to radiographic findings of cam femoroacetabular impingement in collegiate football players. *Arthroscopy.* 2012;28: 1661-1670.

74. Patrick HT. Brachial neuritis and sciatica. *JAMA.* 1917;LXIX: 2176-2179.

75. Theiler R, Stucki G, Schütz R, et al. Parametric and non-parametric measures in the assessment of knee and hip osteoarthritis: interobserver reliability and correlation with radiology. *Osteoarthritis Cartilage.* 1996;4:35-42.

76. Cliborne AV, Wainner RS, Rhon DI, et al. Clinical hip tests and a functional squat test in patients with knee osteoarthritis: reliability, prevalence of positive test findings, and short-term response to hip mobilization. *J Orthop Sports Phy Ther.* 2004;34:676-685.

77. Cibere J, Thorne A, Bellamy N, et al. Reliability of the hip examination in osteoarthritis: effect of standardization. *Arthritis Rheum.* 2008;59:373-381.

78. Mitchell B, McCrory P, Brukner P, et al. Hip joint pathology: clinical presentation and correlation between magnetic resonance arthrography, ultrasound, and arthroscopic findings in 25 consecutive cases. *Clin J Sport Med.* 2003;13:152-156.

79. Martin RL, Irrgang JJ, Sekiya JK. The diagnostic accuracy of a clinical examination in determining intra-articular hip pain for potential hip arthroscopy candidates. *Arthroscopy.* 2008;24: 1013-1018.

80. Troelsen A, Mechlenburg I, Gelineck J, et al. What is the role of clinical tests and ultrasound in acetabular labral tear diagnostics? *Acta Orthop.* 2009;80:314-318.

81. Maslowski E, Sullivan W, Forster Harwood J, et al. The diagnostic validity of hip provocation maneuvers to detect intra-articular hip pathology. *PM R.* 2010;2:174-181.

82. Ito K, Leunig M, Ganz R. Histopathologic features of the acetabular labrum in femoroacetabular impingement. *Clin Orthop Relat Res.* 2004;429:262-271.

83. Sink EL, Gralla J, Ryba A, et al. Clinical presentation of femoroacetabular impingement in adolescents. *J Pediatr Orthop.* 2008;28: 806-811.

84. Nogier A, Bonin N, May O, et al. Descriptive epidemiology of mechanical hip pathology in adults under 50 years of age. Prospective series of 292 cases: clinical and radiological aspects and physiopathological review. *Orthop Traumatol Surg Res.* 2010;96: S253-S258.

85. Narvani AA, Tsiridis E, Kendall S, et al. A preliminary report on prevalence of acetabular labrum tears in sports patients with groin pain. *Knee Surg Sports Traumatol Arthrosc.* 2003;11:403-408.

86. Philippon MJ, Briggs KK, Yen YM, et al. Outcomes following hip arthroscopy for femoroacetabular impingement with associated chondrolabral dysfunction: minimum two-year follow-up. *J Bone Joint Surg Br.* 2009;91:16-23.

87. McGrory BJ. Stinchfield resisted hip flexion test. *Hosp Physician.* 1999;35:41-42.

88. Tijssen M, van Cingel R, Willemsen L, et al. Diagnostics of femoroacetabular impingement and labral pathology of the hip: a systematic review of the accuracy and validity of physical tests. *Arthroscopy.* 2012;28:860-871.

89. Klaue K, Durnin CW, Ganz R. The acetabular rim syndrome: a clinical presentation of dysplasia of the hip. *J Bone Joint Surg Br.* 1991;73B:423-429.

90. Martin HD, Shears SA, Palmer IJ. Evaluation of the hip. *Sports Med Arthrosc.* 2010;18:63-75.

91. Plante M, Wallace R, Busconi BD. Clinical diagnosis of hip pain. *Clin Sports Med.* 2011;30:225-238.

92. Chan YS, Lien LC, Hsu HL, et al. Evaluating hip labral tears using magnetic resonance arthrography: a prospective study comparing hip arthroscopy and magnetic resonance arthrography diagnosis. *Arthroscopy.* 2005;21:1250.e1-1250.e8.

93. Hase T, Ueo T. Acetabular labral tear: arthroscopic diagnosis and treatment. *Arthroscopy.* 1999;15:138-141.

94. Petersilge CA, Haque MA, Petersilge WJ, et al. Acetabular labral tears: evaluation with MR arthrography. *Radiology.* 1996;200: 231-235.

95. Santori N, Villar RN. Acetabular labral tears: result of arthroscopic partial limbectomy. *Arthroscopy.* 2000;16:11-15.

96. Martin RL, Enseki KR, Draovitch P, et al. Acetabular labral tears of the hip: examination and diagnostic challenges. *J Orthop Phy Ther.* 2006;36:503-515.

97. Fitzgerald RH. Acetabular labrum tears: diagnosis and treatment. *Clin Orthop.* 1995;311:60-68.

98. Maitland GD. *The Peripheral Joints: Examination and Recording Guide.* Adelaide: Virgo Press; 1979.

99. Domb BG, Brooks AG, Byrd JW. Clinical examination of the hip joint in athletes. *J Sport Rehabil.* 2009;18:3-23.

100. McCarthy J, Noble P, Aluisio FV, et al. Anatomy, pathologic features, and treatment of acetabular labral tears. *Clin Orthop Relat Res.* 2003;406:38-47.

101. Martin HD, Kelly BT, Leunig M, et al. The pattern and technique in the clinical evaluation of the adult hip: the common physical examination tests of hip specialists. *Arthroscopy.* 2010;26:161-172.

102. Philippon MJ. The role of arthroscopic thermal capsulorrhaph in the hip. *Clin Sports Med.* 2001;20:817-829.

103. Hölmich P, Hölmich LR, Bjerg AM. Clinical examination of athletes with groin pain: an intraobserver reliability study. *Br J Sports Med.* 2004;38:446-451.

104. Kachingwe AF, Grech S. Proposed algorithm for the management of athletes with athletic pubalgia (sports hernia): a case series. *J Orthop Sports Phy Ther.* 2008;38:768-781.

105. Woodward JS, Parker A, Macdonald RM. Non-surgical treatment of a professional hockey player with the signs and symptoms of sports hernia: a case report. *Int J Sports Phys Ther.* 2012;7:85-100.

106. Meyers WC, Foley DP, Garrett WE, et al. Management of severe lower abdominal or inguinal pain in high-performance athletes. *Am J Sports Med.* 2000;28:2-8.

107. Hölmich P. Adductor related groin pain in athletes. *Sports Med Arth Rev.* 1998;5:285-291.

108. Fricker PA, Taunton JE, Amman W. Osteitis pubis in athletes. *Sports Med.* 1991;12:266-279.

109. Harris NH, Murray RO. Lesions of the symphysis in athletes. *BMJ.* 1974;4:211-214.

110. Verrall GM, Slavotinek JP, Barnes PG, et al. Description of pain provocation tests used for the diagnosis of sports related chronic

groin pain: relationship of tests to defined clinical (pain and tenderness) and MRI (pubic bone marrow oedema) criteria. *Scand J Med Sci Sports.* 2005;15:36-42.

111. Gurney B. Leg length discrepancy. *Gait Posture.* 2002;15: 195-206.

112. Gogia PP, Braatz JH. Validity and reliability of leg length measurements. *J Orthop Sports Phy Ther.* 1986;8:185-188.

113. Beattie P, Isaacson K, Riddle DL, et al. Validity of derived measurements of leg-length differences obtained by use of a tape measure. *Phys Ther.* 1990;70:150-157.

114. Hoyle DA, Latour M, Bohannon RW. Intraexaminer, interexaminer, and interdevice comparability of leg length measurements obtained with measuring tape and metrecom. *J Orthop Sports Phy Ther.* 1991;14:263-268.

115. Jamaluddin S, Sulaiman AR, Imran MK, et al. Reliability and accuracy of the tape measurement method with a nearest reading of 5 mm in the assessment of leg length discrepancy. *Singapore Med J.* 2011;52(9):681-684.

116. Neely K, Wallmann HW, Backus CJ. Validity of measuring leg length with a tape measure compared to a computed tomography scan. *Physiother Theory Pract.* 2013;29:487-492.

117. Jonson SR, Gross MT. Intraexaminer reliability, interexaminer reliability, and mean values for nine lower extremity skeletal measures in healthy naval midshipmen. *J Orthop Sports Phy Ther.* 1997;25:253-263.

118. Gross MT, Burns CB, Chapman SW, et al. Reliability and validity of rigid lift and pelvic leveling device method in assessing functional leg length inequality. *J Orthop Sports Phy Ther.* 1998;27: 285-294.

119. Hanada E, Kirby RL, Mitchell M, et al. Measuring leg-length discrepancy by the "iliac crest palpation and book correction" method: reliability and validity. *Arch Phys Med Rehabil.* 2001;82: 938-942.

120. Clarke GR. Unequal leg length: an accurate method of detection and some clinical results. *Rheumatol Phys Med.* 1972;11:385-390.

121. Woerman AL, Binder-Macleod SA. Leg length discrepancy assessment: accuracy and precision in five clinical methods of evaluation. *J Orthop Sports Phy Ther.* 1984;5:230-239.

122. Friberg O, Nurminen M, Kouhonen K, et al. Accuracy and precision of clinical estimation of leg length inequality and lumbar scoliosis: comparison of clinical and radiological measurements. *Int Disabil Stud.* 1988;10:49-53.

123. Lampe HIH, Swierstra BA, Diepstraten FM. Measurement of limb length inequality: comparison of clinical methods with orthoradiography in 190 children. *Acta Orthop Scand.* 1996;67:242-244.

124. Terry MA, Winell JJ, Green DW, et al. Measurement variance in limb length discrepancy: clinical and radiographic assessment of interobserver and intraobserver variability. *J Pediatr Orthop.* 2005;25:197-201.

125. Badii M, Wade AN, Collins DR, et al. Comparison of lifts versus tape measure in determining leg length discrepancy. *J Rheumatol.* 2014;41:1689-1694.

126. Nichols PJR, Bailey NTJ. The accuracy of measuring leg-length differences. *Br Med J.* 1955;2:1247.

127. Gofton JP. Studies in osteoarthritis of the hip. IV: biomechanics and clinical considerations. *Can Med Assoc J.* 1971;104:1007-1011.

128. Bourdillon JF. *Spinal Manipulation.* 2nd ed. London: Heinemann; 1973.

129. Mann M, Glasheen-Wray M, Nyberg R. Therapist agreement for palpation and observation of iliac crest heights. *Phys Ther.* 1984;64:334-338.

130. Fisk JW, Baigent ML. Clinical and radiological assessment of leg length. *N Z Med J.* 1975;81:477-480.

131. Johnson AW, Weiss CB, Wheeler DL. Stress fractures of the femoral shaft in athletes: more common than expected. A new clinical test. *Am J Sports Med.* 1994;22:248-256.

132. Matheson GO, Clement DB, McKenzie DC, et al. Stress fractures in athletes: a study of 320 cases. *Am J Sports Med.* 1987;15:46-58.

133. Clement DB, Ammann W, Taunton JE, et al. Exercise-induced stress injuries to the femur. *Int J Sports Med.* 1993;14:347-352.

Physical Examination of the Knee

Anthony Beutler, MD | Francis G. O'Connor, COL, MC, USA, MD, PhD

INTRODUCTION

The knee is particularly susceptible to traumatic injury because of its vulnerable location midway between the hip and the ankle, where it is exposed to the considerable forces transmitted from the ground through the knee to the hip. Thorough examination of all of the knee structures, including the ligaments and menisci, should be included in every knee evaluation. The examiner must rely on numerous physical exam maneuvers to evaluate these structures. It is crucial not only that these maneuvers are performed correctly but also that the examiner is aware of the sensitivity and specificity of the various tests, as well as the limitations of the tests, to make the most accurate diagnosis possible.[1-83] In this chapter, we provide a review of the physical examination of the knee followed by a literature-based review of the diagnostic accuracy of the major provocative tests used to diagnose knee injuries.

INSPECTION

Assessment of the knee should begin with an overall evaluation of lower extremity alignment. Varus–valgus alignment of the lower extremity while weight bearing with the knee in full extension should be noted. Normally, the tibia has a slight valgus angulation compared with the femur, and this angle is usually more pronounced in females. From the side, the knee should be fully extended when the patient is standing. Slight hyperextension of the knee is a normal finding, provided that it is present in both lower extremities. The position of the patella should be noted. When viewing the patella, the examiner should note whether the patella points straight ahead, tilts inward or outward, or is rotated in any way. Rotation and tilt may be caused by tight structures in the lower extremities that alter the position of the patella.

The skin around the knee joint should be inspected for any bruising, abrasions, lacerations, or surgical scars. External signs of injury can give a clue as to the mechanism of injury and internal structures damaged. Signs of swelling in the knee should be observed and may be suggested by the loss of the peripatellar groove on either side of the patella. Generalized swelling may be due to an effusion in the joint, whereas localized swelling may be due to a distended bursa or cyst.

The quadriceps muscle atrophies quickly when there is any type of knee joint pathology. Signs of muscular atrophy should therefore be observed and quantified with circumferential measurements that compare the affected and unaffected sides for differences in muscle girth.

Assessment of gait is an integral component of the comprehensive knee examination. In the traditional, heel-striker gait cycle, the knee comes to full extension only at heel strike. During stance phase, slight flexion occurs, and it is the contraction of the quadriceps at this point that prevents giving way. At toe-off, the knee flexes to about 40 degrees and continues to flex through midswing to approximately 65 degrees. At this point, the quadriceps contract to begin acceleration of the leg, with the knee returning to full extension again at heel strike. At heel strike, the hamstrings must contract in order to decelerate the leg. Abnormalities in gait pattern can occur from various causes. Weak hamstrings may not decelerate the knee properly and result in hyperextension at heel strike. Weakness in the quadriceps can cause a hard heel strike to occur, with excessive hip extension to force the knee into a hyperextended position to prevent buckling. Ligament injuries may result in a varus or valgus thrust or even a buckling of the joint, depending on the extent of the ligament compromise. Finally, pain within the knee joint may cause the patient to walk with an antalgic gait.

RANGE OF MOTION

Active and passive range of motions (ROMs) of the knee should be measured. The neutral position (0 degrees) for the knee joint occurs when the femur and tibia are in a straight, fully extended position. Positive degrees of motion are measured for flexion, and negative degrees of motion are used to describe hyperextension of the knee. Normal ROMs are typically 135 degrees of flexion and as much as 5 to 10 degrees of hyperextension. Given the significant amount of normal individual variation, it is very important to compare the involved and uninvolved sides when determining normal motion for an injured individual.

As the examiner moves the knee through flexion and extension, the movements of the patella as it tracks along the femoral trochlea should be observed. The patella does not follow a straight path as the knee moves but instead follows a curved pattern. The examiner should note whether the patella tilts laterally, tilts anteroposteriorly, or rotates during dynamic knee extension. The examiner should also observe for signs of quadriceps lag, which results from weakness of the quadriceps muscle and causes the patient to have difficulty in completing the last 10 to 15 degrees of knee extension. Although the majority of motion occurs with extension and flexion, the knee does possess the ability to rotate both internally and externally and does so normally as part of the "screw-home" mechanism of full extension. Approximately 10 degrees of rotation in either direction is thought to represent a normal range; significant increases in internal or external rotation may indicate ligament compromise.

Passive ROM testing is particularly useful when the patient is not able to perform the full range of active movements. Flexion is tested with the patient lying prone. The leg is held just proximal to the ankle, and the knee is flexed. There are a number of causes for a decrease in ROM at the knee. The most common cause is an effusion within the knee joint. A large meniscus tear or other intra-articular loose body can act as a mechanical block, preventing full motion of the knee. Osteoarthritic changes can also reduce knee motion, typically with flexion being less affected than extension. On the other hand, significant ligamentous injuries can undermine the normal knee restraints and allow an abnormally increased range of knee motion.

PALPATION

The entire knee should be palpated in a sequential manner and compared with the uninjured side. The presence of an increase in temperature of the skin overlying the joint should be determined before other tests are performed. The skin over the noninflamed knee is typically cooler than the skin overlying surrounding musculature because of the relatively avascular nature of the knee joint. Palpation is the best way to determine the presence of swelling in and around the knee joint. A large joint effusion will be obvious to the examiner, whereas a small effusion can be identified by placing gentle thumb pressure over the lateral aspect of the patellofemoral joint and detecting a fluid wave with the index finger. In the ballottement test, one hand milks fluid from the suprapatellar pouch while the other hand presses down on the patella. The patella's springing back indicates the presence of a larger effusion.

Localized tenderness is helpful in pinpointing the site of injury or pathology in the knee joint. A detailed knowledge of the bony and soft tissue surface anatomy is therefore of critical importance when trying to make a specific diagnosis in the knee. Palpation of the bony and soft tissue structures of the knee can be divided into four quadrants: medial, lateral, anterior, and posterior.

MEDIAL KNEE

BONY STRUCTURES

The bony structures of interest in the medial aspect of the knee include the medial tibial plateau, tibial tubercle, medial femoral condyle, medial femoral epicondyle, and the adductor tubercle. The examiner's thumbs are placed on the anterior portion of the knee and pressed into the

soft tissue depressions on each side of the infrapatellar tendon. Pushing a thumb slightly inferiorly into the soft tissue depression, the examiner palpates the distinct upper edge of the medial tibial plateau. The medial tibial plateau represents one site of attachment for the medial meniscus. Next, the infrapatellar tendon may be followed distally to its insertion into the tibial tubercle. Moving the thumb superior from the starting position in the depressions on each side of the infrapatellar tendon, the medial femoral condyle will become palpable. The femoral condyle is more easily palpated if the knee is flexed to greater than 90 degrees. The adductor tubercle is located on the posterior medial aspect of the medial femoral condyle. It can be located by moving the thumbs posteriorly from the medial surface of the medial femoral condyle.[1]

SOFT TISSUE STRUCTURES

Palpation of the medial meniscus is performed along the medial joint line. The medial edge of the medial meniscus becomes more prominent when the tibia is internally rotated. Tears of the posteromedial portion of the medial meniscus are the most common and are diagnosed clinically in part by the finding of tenderness at the posteromedial corner of the knee. The medial collateral ligament (MCL) is a broad ligament that spans from the medial femoral epicondyle to the tibia. Historically believed to be a relatively straightforward stabilizer against valgus stress, recent anatomic dissections show that the MCL has a deep and superficial layer that performs distinct functions. The superficial MCL attaches to the medial femoral epicondyle proximally and the medial aspect of the tibia distally, approximately 4 cm below the level of the joint line. The superficial MCL is the primary restraint against valgus forces at all angles of knee flexion.[2] The deep fibers of the MCL represent a thickening of the middle third of the joint capsule. The deep MCL is a primary stabilizer of the medial meniscus and functions as a rotational constraint for the tibiofemoral joint. It consists of two subligaments, the meniscofemoral ligament (attaching the medial meniscus to the femur) and the meniscotibial ligament (attaching the medial meniscus to the tibia).[3] Given the complex substructure of the MCL complex, the entire region of the MCL ligament should be palpated from origin to insertion for tenderness.

On the posteromedial side of the knee, the tendons of the sartorius, gracilis, and semitendinosus muscles cross the knee joint and insert into the lower portion of the medial tibial plateau. The pes anserine bursa lies at the common insertion of these muscles and may become a source of pain when the bursa is inflamed (Fig. 9.1).

LATERAL KNEE

BONY STRUCTURES

The bony structures of interest in the lateral aspect of the knee include the lateral tibial plateau, lateral tubercle (Gerdy tubercle), lateral femoral condyle, lateral femoral epicondyle, and head of the fibula. Starting with your thumb in the soft tissue depression just lateral to the infrapatellar tendon, the edge of the lateral tibial plateau can be palpated inferiorly. The lateral tubercle is the large prominence of bone palpable just below the lateral tibial plateau. Moving

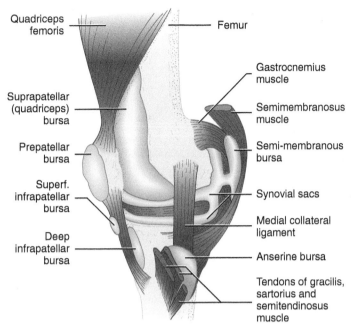

Figure 9.1 The pes anserine bursa and medial knee structures. (Adapted with permission from O'Donoghue DH. *Treatment of Injuries to Athletes.* 4th ed. Philadelphia: W.B. Saunders; 1984:466.)

upward and laterally from the starting point of the depression, the lateral femoral condyle becomes palpable. More of the lateral femoral condyle is palpable when the knee is flexed to greater than 90 degrees. Finally, the fibular head is easily palpable along the lateral aspect of the knee, inferior to the joint line, at about the level of the tibial tubercle.[1]

SOFT TISSUE STRUCTURES

Palpation of the lateral meniscus is performed along the lateral joint line, with the knee in a slightly flexed position (Fig. 9.2). The lateral meniscus is attached to the popliteus muscle and not the lateral collateral ligament (LCL). The LCL is a palpable cord that runs between the lateral femoral condyle and the fibular head (Fig. 9.3). Also inserting on the fibular head is the biceps femoris tendon. The major portion of the biceps femoris inserts deep to the LCL on the lateral fibular head, while a smaller slip of the biceps femoris inserts superficial to the LCL. Thus, at the fibula, the LCL can be palpated as it is "sandwiched" between fibers of the biceps femoris tendon.[4] Additionally, the iliotibial band can be assessed for tenderness at its insertion point on the Gerdy tubercle of the tibia and as it crosses the lateral condyle of the femur. Complaints of "snapping" over the lateral femoral condyle are often associated with a tight iliotibial band. The common peroneal nerve can be palpated as it wraps around the fibula, and the nerve may be assessed for a positive Tinel's sign, indicative of nerve irritation or damage.[5]

ANTERIOR KNEE

BONY STRUCTURES

The bony structures of interest in the anterior knee are the patella and the trochlear groove of the femur. The trochlear groove can be palpated by placing your thumbs over the medial and lateral joint lines and moving upward along the two femoral condyles. The depression of the trochlear groove is palpated in the midline, above the level of the patella. In flexion, the patella is fixed in the trochlear groove and therefore the undersurface of the patella is not easily palpated. In extension, the patella is more mobile, and palpation of the medial and lateral undersurfaces (facets) of the patella is possible in this position.[1]

SOFT TISSUE STRUCTURES

In the anterior aspect of the knee, an assessment of the tone and bulk of the quadriceps muscle should be made because this is the main stabilizing muscle for the knee. Quadriceps strength along with gluteal and core muscular function are important areas along the kinetic chain that are important to evaluate as part of the assessment of the patellofemoral joint. The prepatellar bursa overlies the anterior aspect of the patella (Fig. 9.4). Thickening or swelling of the prepatellar bursa is commonly seen in people who frequently kneel. The patellar tendon is the continuation of the quadriceps tendon from the lower pole of the patella to the tibial tubercle. The superficial infrapatellar bursa lies between the skin and the patellar tendon and is easily palpable on exam. The deep infrapatellar bursa lies beneath the patellar tendon.

POSTERIOR KNEE

The posterior fossa is bounded by the hamstring tendons proximally and the two heads of the gastrocnemius muscle distally. Passing through the posterior fossa are the tibial nerve, the popliteal artery, and the popliteal vein. Examination of the popliteal pulse is best performed with the knee in 90 degrees of flexion, so that the hamstring and calf

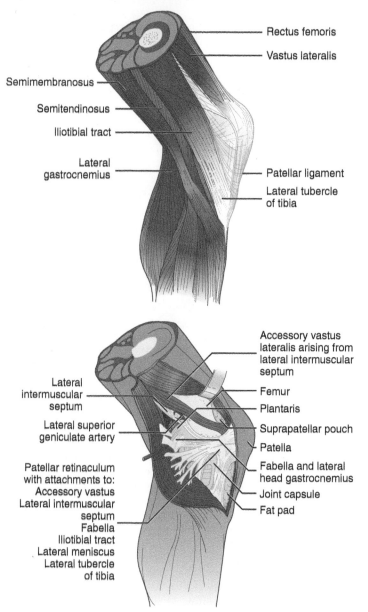

Rectus femoris

Vastus lateralis

Semimembranosus

Semitendinosus

Iliotibial tract

Lateral gastrocnemius

Patellar ligament

Lateral tubercle of tibia

Accessory vastus lateralis arising from lateral intermuscular septum

Lateral intermuscular septum

Lateral superior geniculate artery

Patellar retinaculum with attachments to:
Accessory vastus
Lateral intermuscular septum
Fabella
Iliotibial tract
Lateral meniscus
Lateral tubercle of tibia

Femur

Plantaris

Suprapatellar pouch

Patella

Fabella and lateral head gastrocnemius

Joint capsule

Fat pad

Figure 9.2 The lateral structures of the knee. (Adapted with permission from Pagnani MJ, Warren RF, Arnoczky SP, et al. Anatomy of the knee. In: Nicholas J, Hershman E, eds. *The Lower Extremity and Spine in Sports Medicine.* 2nd ed. St. Louis: Mosby: 1995:607.)

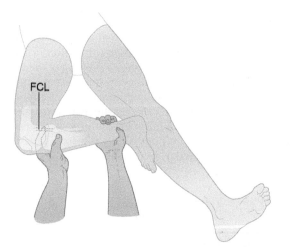

FCL

Figure 9.3 Palpation of the lateral (fibular) collateral ligament (FCL). (Adapted with permission from Zarins B, Fish DN. Knee ligament injury. In: Nicholas J, Hershman E, eds. *The Lower Extremity and Spine in Sports Medicine.* 2nd ed. St. Louis: Mosby; 1995:54.)

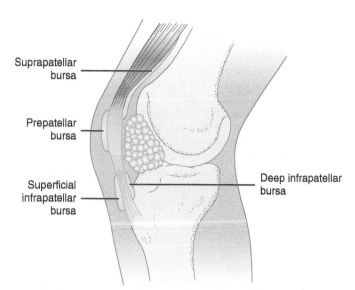

Suprapatellar bursa

Prepatellar bursa

Superficial infrapatellar bursa

Deep infrapatellar bursa

Figure 9.4 The bursa of the knee. (Adapted with permission from Boland AL, Hulstyn MJ. Soft tissue injuries of the knee. In: Nicholas J, Hershman E, eds. *The Lower Extremity and Spine in Sports Medicine.* 2nd ed. St. Louis: Mosby; 1995:909.)

muscles are relaxed. The popliteal artery is the deepest structure in the posterior fossa and travels against the joint capsule. The posterior tibial nerve is the most superficial structure in the popliteal area, with the popliteal vein running directly beneath it. A cystic swelling within the fossa, called a Baker cyst, can present as a usually painless, mobile swelling on the medial side of the fossa. Many Baker cysts directly communicate with the joint. The cyst is an enlargement of the normal gastrocnemius–semimembranosus bursa.

The quadriceps muscle is the primary extensor of the knee and is innervated by the femoral nerve, with primarily L3 and L4 nerve root innervation. Manual testing of the quadriceps muscle can be performed with the patient in the sitting position. The patient should be asked to extend the knee actively. The examiner can use one hand to resist the extension of the leg, while using the other hand to palpate the tone and bulk of the muscle as it is contracting. The primary flexors of the knee are the hamstring muscles, which include the semimembranosus, semitendinosus, and biceps femoris. All of the hamstring muscles are innervated by the tibial portion of the sciatic nerve. The semimembranosus and semitendinosus receive the majority of their innervation from the L5 nerve root, while the biceps femoris receives most of its innervation from the S1 nerve root.

Manual testing of the hamstrings as a group can be performed by having the patient lie prone on the examination table. The patient is instructed to flex his or her knee while you resist this motion by holding the leg just proximal to the ankle joint. The patellar tendon reflex is a deep tendon reflex involving the L2, L3, and L4 neurologic levels, but for clinical application, it is primarily considered an L4 reflex. Sensation should also be assessed in the area of the knee and surrounding areas. Peripheral pulses should be tested in the femoral, popliteal, dorsalis pedis, and posterior tibial arteries. Historically, the incidence of popliteal artery injury following knee dislocation was reported as high as 25%.[6] More recent and more carefully controlled studies place the rate of arterial injury following knee dislocation between 1.3 and 18%[6,7]; however, unrecognized vascular injury may result in catastrophic outcomes. Hence, assessment of vascular system integrity is crucial with all acute knee injuries.[6,7]

The ligaments of the knee joint are the primary structures responsible for maintaining stability of the joint (Fig. 9.5). The knee should be checked for stability in the anteroposterior, medial–lateral, and rotatory directions. It is important to compare tests for stability with the normal contralateral knee, since there can be individual variation in the laxity of the ligaments tested. It can be helpful to evaluate the uninjured knee first, so that the patient has an understanding of what manipulations are going to be performed. In the acute situation, when the mechanism of injury is observed and the patient can be evaluated immediately before pain, guarding, and secondary muscle spasm occur, the assessment of the ligaments can be much easier. Specific tests to assess the anterior cruciate ligament (ACL), posterior cruciate ligament (PCL), LCL, and MCL are described in the following sections, along with a literature review of the sensitivity and specificity of the individual tests.

TESTS FOR THE ANTERIOR CRUCIATE LIGAMENT

The ACL is one of the main stabilizers of the knee with injury often resulting in significant disability. Three of the most commonly applied tests are the anterior drawer test the Lachman test, and the pivot shift test (Table 9.1). The lever sign test or Lelli test is a new test proposed to evaluate ACL injury.

ANTERIOR DRAWER TEST (Video 9-1)

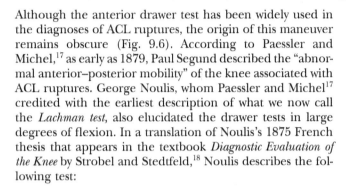

Although the anterior drawer test has been widely used in the diagnoses of ACL ruptures, the origin of this maneuver remains obscure (Fig. 9.6). According to Paessler and Michel,[17] as early as 1879, Paul Segund described the "abnormal anterior–posterior mobility" of the knee associated with ACL ruptures. George Noulis, whom Paessler and Michel[17] credited with the earliest description of what we now call the *Lachman test*, also elucidated the drawer tests in large degrees of flexion. In a translation of Noulis's 1875 French thesis that appears in the textbook *Diagnostic Evaluation of the Knee* by Strobel and Stedtfeld,[18] Noulis describes the following test:

> [With] the patient's leg flexed, the thigh can be grasped with one hand at the lower leg with the other hand keeping the thumbs to the front and fingers to the back. If the lower leg is held in this grip and then moved backwards and forwards, it will be seen that the tibia can be moved directly backwards and forwards.

Noulis observed a great deal of tibia displacement when both cruciate ligaments were severed. The assumption that a positive anterior drawer test indicates a tear of the ACL was not commonly accepted until much later.[19] Increased anterior tibial displacement compared with the uninvolved side is now supported as indicative of a tear of the ACL.

There remain some limitations of this test with sensitivities reported between 18% to 92% and specificities between 78% to 98%.[20] A recent meta-analysis illustrates the difference in test characteristics when performed on patients under anesthesia. In an analysis of 20 available studies, the mean sensitivity and specificity of the anterior drawer test were 38% to 81% in awake patients and 63% to 91% in anesthetized patients, respectively.[21] Differences in accuracy of the test are also noted in those with acute versus chronic injury, with the anterior drawer test being more accurate in chronic injury.[22] Anterior drawer results may also be affected by the presence of concomitant injury.[11] Injuries to other secondary stabilizers that typically limit anterior tibial translation (ie, MCL, anterolateral ligament, and medial meniscus) are known to increase the degree of anterior knee displacement caused by the anterior drawer maneuver.[23] These combined observations suggest that the anterior drawer test may become increasingly sensitive as the secondary restraints of anterior stability are lost. As with other tests of anterior stability, the real-world accuracy of the anterior drawer test depends on the expertise of the examiner. The anterior drawer test exhibited only moderate interrater reliability among providers (x = 0.57).[24]

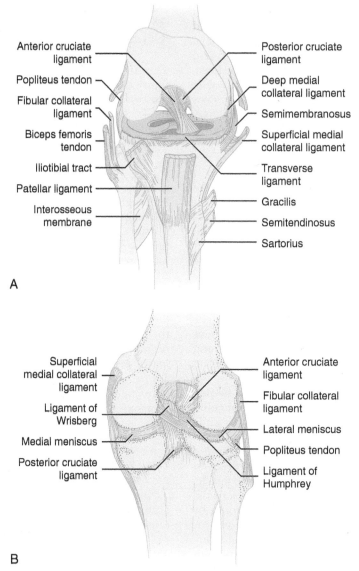

Anterior cruciate ligament
Popliteus tendon
Fibular collateral ligament
Biceps femoris tendon
Iliotibial tract
Patellar ligament
Interosseous membrane

Posterior cruciate ligament
Deep medial collateral ligament
Semimembranosus
Superficial medial collateral ligament
Transverse ligament
Gracilis
Semitendinosus
Sartorius

A

Superficial medial collateral ligament
Ligament of Wrisberg
Medial meniscus
Posterior cruciate ligament

Anterior cruciate ligament
Fibular collateral ligament
Lateral meniscus
Popliteus tendon
Ligament of Humphrey

B

Figure 9.5   The ligaments of the knee. **A,** Anterior view. **B,** Posterior view. (Adapted with permission from Scott WN, ed. *Ligament and Extensor Mechanism Injuries of the Knee.* St. Louis: Mosby; 1991.)

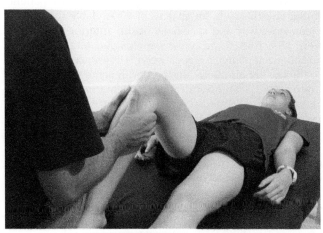

Figure 9.6   Anterior drawer test.

Falsely negative anterior drawer tests in instances of isolated ACL tears may occur secondary to protective spasm of the hamstring muscles and the anatomic configuration of the femoral condyle. Clinical practice shows that false-positive results may occur in the setting of PCL insufficiency in which posterior sagging of the tibia may result in a false sense of its neutral position, resulting in a false sense of excessive anterior translation, when in fact the tibia is moving from a posterior translated position into its normal neutral position.

Given the wide variation in reported sensitivities of the anterior drawer test, especially because performing examinations under general anesthesia is of somewhat limited utility in the clinical setting, examiners should be cautious to not rule out an acute ACL injury based solely on a negative anterior drawer test result. Conversely, because the specificity of the test is quite high, a positive anterior drawer test result would more strongly suggest the presence of ACL pathology.

Table 9.1 Anterior Cruciate Ligament Tests

Test	Review	Reliability/Validity Tests	Comments
Anterior drawer test	The subject is supine, hip flexed to 45 degrees and knee flexed to 90 degrees. The examiner sits on the subject's foot, with hands behind the proximal tibia and thumbs on the tibial plateau. Anterior force is applied to the proximal tibia. Hamstring tendons are palpated with index fingers to ensure relaxation. Increased tibial displacement compared with the opposite side is indicative of an ACL tear.	Harilainen 1987[8] Sensitivity: 41% Sensitivity (under anesthesia): 86% Katz and Fingeroth 1986[9] Sensitivity: 22.2% (acute) Sensitivity: 53.8% (chronic) Specificity: >95% (acute + chronic) Jonsson et al. 1982[10] Sensitivity: 33% (acute) Sensitivity: 95% (chronic) Donaldson et al. 1985[11] Sensitivity: 70% (acute) Sensitivity: 91% (under anesthesia) Specificity: Not reported Mitsou and Vallianatos 1988[12] Sensitivity: 40% (acute) Sensitivity: 95.2% (chronic) Specificity: Not reported Kim and Kim 1995[13] Sensitivity (under anesthesia): 79.6% Specificity: Not reported	Prospective study of 350 acute knees evaluated with 79 arthroscopically confirmed acute ACL injuries. *Testing performed only under anesthesia.* Retrospective study of limited sample size: 9 acute ACL injuries and 12 chronic. All 107 patients had documented acute or chronic ACL ruptures. Specificity was not assessed since only positive ACL ruptures were included. A retrospective study that was not designed to evaluate specificity since it was a review of only positive cases. Of 144 knees, 60 had acute injuries all assessed within 3 days of injury. In the group of 80 chronic injuries, the 4 false-negative drawer tests were associated with bucket-handle tears. *Testing performed only under anesthesia.* Retrospective study. All ACL injuries were chronic.
Lachman test	The patient lies supine. The knee is held between full extension and 15 degrees of flexion. The femur is stabilized with one hand while firm pressure is applied to the posterior aspect of the proximal tibia in an attempt to translate it anteriorly.	Torg et al. 1976[14] Sensitivity: 95% Specificity: Not reported Donaldson et al. 1985[11] Sensitivity: 99% Specificity: Not reported Katz and Fingeroth 1986[9] Sensitivity (under anesthesia): 84.6% Specificity (under anesthesia): 95% Kim and Kim 1995[13] Sensitivity (under anesthesia): 98.6% Specificity: Not reported Mitsou and Vallianatos 1988[12] Sensitivity: 80% (acute) Sensitivity: 98.8% (chronic) Jonsson et al. 1982[10] Sensitivity: 87% (acute) Sensitivity: 94% (chronic)	A study of 93 knees with combined tears of the ACL and median meniscus. All 5 false negatives were associated with bucket-handle tears of the meniscus. A retrospective study that was not designed to evaluate specificity since it was a review of only positive cases. *Testing performed only under anesthesia.* A retrospective study of limited sample size: 9 acute and 12 chronic ACL injuries. *Testing performed only under anesthesia.* Retrospective review study of ACL injuries all of which were chronic. Of 144 knees, 60 had acute injuries all assessed within 3 days of injury. All 107 patients had acute or chronic ACL injuries. Specificity was not assessed since only positive ACL ruptures were included.
Pivot shift test	The leg is picked up at the ankle. The knee is flexed by placing the heel of the hand behind the fibula. As the knee is extended, the tibia is supported on the lateral side with a slight valgus strain. A strong valgus force is placed on the knee by the upper hand. At approximately 30 degrees of flexion, the displaced tibia will suddenly reduce, indicating a positive pivot shift test result.	Lucie et al. 1984[15] Sensitivity: 95% Specificity: 100%* Katz and Fingeroth 1986[9] Sensitivity: 98.4% Specificity: >98% Donaldson et al. 1985[11] Sensitivity: 35% Sensitivity (under anesthesia): 98% Specificity: not reported	Fifty knees were tested. *There was not an adequate sample of intact ACLs to determine specificity. *Testing performed only under anesthesia.* A retrospective study of limited sample size: 9 acute and 12 chronic ACL injuries. A retrospective study that was not designed to evaluate specificity since it was a review of positive cases.

Continued on following page

Table 9.1   Anterior Cruciate Ligament Tests (Continued)

Test	Review	Reliability/Validity Tests	Comments
Lever Sign test	The patient is placed supine with the knees fully extended. The examiner places a closed fist under the proximal third of the calf. Moderate downward force to the distal third of the quadriceps is applied with the other hand. In the intact ACL, the heel rises up off of the table. With a partially or completely ruptured ACL, the heel is pulled down to the exam table.	Lelli et al. 2014[16] Reported 100% agreement with MRI findings of complete or partial rupture.	A single case series of 400 knees.

ACL, anterior cruciate ligament; *MRI,* magnetic resonance imaging.

LACHMAN TEST (Video 9-2)

The Lachman test was described by Joseph Torg,[14] who trained under Dr. Lachman at Temple University. Interestingly, Hans Paessler[17] traced descriptions of what we now call the Lachman test as far back as 1875, when it was described in a thesis by George Noulis in Paris. Despite these very early descriptions, the test was not widely recognized or used until Torg's classic description in 1976 (Fig. 9.7)[14]:

> The examination is performed with the patient lying supine on the table with involved extremity on the side of the examiner. With the patient's knee held between full extension and 15 degrees of flexion, the femur is stabilized with one hand while firm pressure is applied to the posterior aspect of the proximal tibia in an attempt to translate it anteriorly. A positive test indicating disruption of the anterior cruciate ligament is one in which there is proprioceptive and/or visual anterior translation of the tibia in relation to the femur with a characteristic "mushy" or "soft" end point. This is in contrast to a definite "hard" end point elicited when the anterior cruciate ligament is intact.

Numerous studies have looked at the sensitivity and specificity of the Lachman test, and other studies have compared the accuracy of this test with the original anterior drawer. Torg originally reported that in 88 of 93 (95%) individuals with combined lesions involving the ACL and medial meniscus, the Lachman test result was positive.[14] The false-negative test results were attributed to incarcerated bucket-handle tears blocking forward translation of the tibia. Donaldson and associates[11] noted a sensitivity of greater than 99% for this test and found it to be relatively unaffected by associated ligamentous or meniscal injuries. This was in contrast to the significant variability with the anterior drawer test when tested in those with injury to the secondary restraints of the knee. In a meta-analysis of nine high-quality studies, the sensitivity of the Lachman test ranged from 63% to 93% with a mean value of 86% and a specificity range of 55% to 99% with a mean of 91%.[20] In experienced hands, the Lachman's test characteristics are relatively unchanged by anesthesia with a

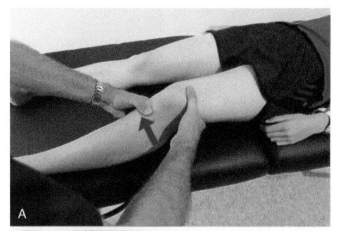

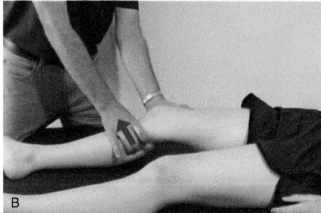

Figure 9.7 Lachman test.

sensitivity and specificity of 86% to 91% without and 85% to 95%, respectively, with general anesthesia.

Lachman testing exhibits impressive clinical predictive value. Compared with anterior drawer testing and composite testing, a positive Lachman test result showed a likelihood ratio (LR) of 25.0 (25-fold increased likelihood of ACL injury), while a negative Lachman test result yielded a negative likelihood ratio (−LR) of 0.1. Composite testing (Lachman plus anterior drawer) yielded virtually identical characteristics (+LR 25.0, –LR 0.04), again illustrating the superiority of the Lachman to the anterior drawer. While the pivot shift test (see subsequent section) has a higher composite specificity than the Lachman for ACL injury, these high sensitivities have only been demonstrated in anesthetized patients. In addition, the Lachman test yields consistently higher sensitivity than pivot shift testing in both awake and anesthetized patients. Hence, the Lachman test is the most clinically sensitive and specific test for diagnosis of ACL tear; however, there are certain limitations to the test. Draper and colleagues noted that the Lachman test is not easily performed when the patient has a large thigh girth or the examiner has small hands.[25] Various modifications of the Lachman have been propose including "prone," "drop leg," and "stabilized" Lachman tests.[26-28] Of these modified Lachman maneuvers, only the prone Lachman test has been described in more than a single publication. A handful of publications suggest that the prone Lachman test, originally described by Feagin in 1989,[27] has favorable test characteristics similar to that of the original supine test. The prone Lachman has a reported sensitivity of 71% and a specificity of 97%, with a +LR of 20 and a –LR of 0.[19,29] A single publication examining reliability of anterior instability tests suggests that the traditional Lachman has the highest intrarater reliability (Cohen's κ = 1.00), while the prone Lachman has the highest interrater reliability (Cohen's κ = 0.81).[30]

PIVOT SHIFT TEST (Video 9-3)

The pivot shift is both a clinical phenomenon that gives rise to the complaint of giving way of the knee and a physical sign that can be elicited upon examination of the injured knee (Fig. 9.8).[31] Hey Groves in 1920[32] and Palmer in 1938[33] both published photographs demonstrating patients voluntarily producing what is called the pivot shift phenomenon. The pivot shift phenomenon was characterized as an anterior subluxation of the lateral tibial plateau in relation to the femoral condyle when the knee approaches extension with reduction produced with knee flexion. The pivot shift phenomenon is enhanced by the convexity of the tibial plateau in the sagittal plane.[31,34,35] The pivot shift test was initially described as follows[31,36]:

> The leg is picked up at the ankle with one of the examiner's hands, and if the patient is holding the leg in extension, the knee is flexed by placing the heel of the other hand behind the fibula over the lateral head of the gastrocnemius. As the knee is extended, the tibia is supported on the lateral side with a slight valgus strain applied to it. In fact, this subluxation can be slightly increased by subtly internally rotating the tibia, with the hand that is cradling the foot and ankle. A strong valgus force is placed on the knee by the upper hand. This impinges the subluxed tibial plateau against the lateral femoral condyle, jamming the two joint surfaces together, preventing easy reduction as the tibia is flexed on the femur. At approximately 30 degrees of flexion, and occasionally more, the displaced tibial plateau will suddenly reduce in a dramatic fashion. At this point, the patient will jump and exclaim, "That's it!"

Recent meta-analysis of six available studies showed sensitivity ranging from 18% to 48% and an extremely high specificity of 97% to 99%.[20] However, the meta-analysis notes that because of relatively low study numbers and heteroge-

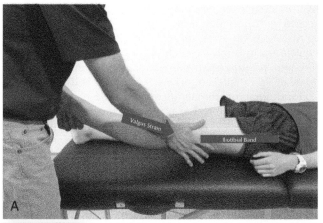

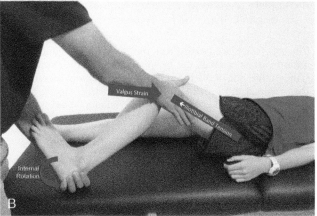

Figure 9.8 A and B, Pivot shift test.

neous methods (anesthesia vs awake), these studies were not appropriate for pooled meta-analysis. A more recent meta-analysis examining pivot shift testing in awake versus anesthetized patients found wide variations in sensitivity (38% awake, 63% anesthesia) and specificity (81% awake, 98% anesthesia).[21]

The pivot shift is a technically complicated test. Many authors have recommended various modifications on the classic pivot shift test for producing the pivot shift phenomenon, including the addition of hip abduction, knee flexion, and external tibial rotation.[34,36,37] Even mechanized pivot shift testing has been proposed in an effort to improve sensitivity and test mechanics.[38] In a recent review of 48 pivot shift testing articles, Arilla and colleagues[39] recommended that a 30-degree knee flexion angle be used along with a 10-Nm valgus torque and a 5-Nm internal rotation torque. Interestingly, Arilla and associates also found that robotic systems were used to interpret the pivot shift test in nearly one in four reported studies and that robotic systems were superior to human examiners in controlling forces during pivot shift testing and interpreting test results.[39] In summary, the bottom line remains the same: the pivot shift is marginally sensitive, especially in awake patients, but highly specific, especially when wielded by an experienced examiner.

Because the specificity is high, the presence of the pivot shift will usually be indicative of an ACL tear. Moreover, the presence of a positive pivot shift test result in a conscious patient may reflect an inability of the patient to protect the knee, which may suggest that these patients are less likely to succeed with nonoperative treatment. Additionally, following ACL reconstructive surgery, the pivot shift test has also been shown to be an excellent indicator of recurrent instability and postoperative outcomes. In a recent systematic review by Ayeni and coworkers,[40] the pivot shift test correlated with final functional outcomes in 85% of the included studies, demonstrating the pivot shift test to be a reliable evaluation of the success of a reconstructive surgery.

LEVER SIGN TEST

A newer test for either full or partial ACL tears is the lever sign or Lelli test. Developed in 2005 by Dr. Alessandro Lelli, the lever sign test is intended to be diagnostic of both partial and complete tears, as well as acute injuries. The lever sign test was originally described as follows[16]:

> The patient is placed supine with the knees fully extended on a hard surface such as the examining table. The examiner stands at the side of the patient and places a closed fist under the proximal third of the calf. This causes the knee to flex slightly. With his other hand, he applies moderate downward force to the distal third of the quadriceps. With this configuration, the patient's leg acts as a lever over a fulcrum—the clinician's fist. In an intact knee, the creation of a complete lever by the ACL allows the downward force on the quadriceps to more than offset the force of gravity, the knee joint rotates into full extension, and the heel rises up off of the examination table. With a partially or completely ruptured ACL, the ability to offset the force of gravity on the lower leg is compromised and the tibial plateau slides anteriorly with respect to the femoral condyles. In this case, the gravity pulls the heel down to the examination table.

In a single case-series of 400 patients with ACL tears, the Lever Sign test was shown to agree with magnetic resonance imaging (MRI) findings. The lever test result was negative for all uninjured, contralateral knees and positive for all injured knees.[16] This is the only published study on the Lever sign to date. No formal study has investigated the sensitivity and specificity of the test, and no studies have examined its predictive value in an undifferentiated primary care population. Thus, further work clearly is needed, but the lever sign test is quite simple and appears safe to perform on injured and uninjured patients.

POSTERIOR CRUCIATE TESTING

Three commonly used tests for the diagnosis of PCL injuries are the posterior sag sign, the posterior drawer test, and the quadriceps active test. Unlike the ACL, the PCL rupture does not have a definitive test, and the most accurate method of physical examination is still a matter of debate (Table 9.2).[23,41,42]

🎞 POSTERIOR SAG SIGN (Video 9-4)

Although it is unclear who coined the term *posterior sag sign*, Mayo Robson described this phenomenon in 1903.[41,49] A detailed description of the test as it is performed today follows (Fig. 9.9):

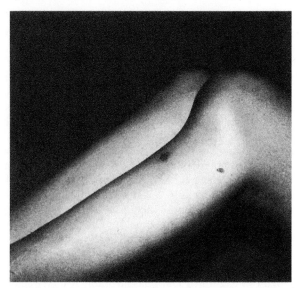

Figure 9.9 Posterior sag sign. (Reproduced with permission from Zarins B, Fish DN. Knee ligament injury. In: Nicholas J, Hershman E, eds. *The Lower Extremity and Spine in Sports Medicine.* 2nd ed. St Louis: Mosby; 1995:857.)

> The patient lies supine with the hip flexed to 45 degrees and the knee flexed to 90 degrees. In this position, the tibia 'rocks back,' or sags back, on the femur if the posterior cruciate ligament is torn. Normally, the medial tibial plateau extends 1 cm anteriorly beyond the femoral condyle when the knee is flexed 90 degrees. If this step off is lost, it is considered positive for a posterior cruciate tear.[50]

Few studies have been performed to establish the diagnostic sensitivity and specificity of the posterior sag sign in the diagnosis of PCL injuries. In a blinded, randomized, controlled study to assess the accuracy of the clinical examination in the setting of PCL injuries, Rubenstein and colleagues[43] reported a sensitivity of the posterior sag sign for detecting PCL injury of 79%, with a specificity of 100%. The overall sensitivity of the clinical exam for detecting PCL injury when all tests were utilized was 90%, with a specificity of 99%. In a nonrandomized, unblinded, uncontrolled study, Stäubli and Jakob[51] evaluated the accuracy of the "gravity sign near extension" in which the knee is maintained in near extension. They reported that the gravity sign near extension was detectable in 20 of 24 PCL-deficient knees, for a sensitivity of 83%.

Overall, the posterior sag sign appears to be a useful test for diagnosing PCL injuries, with a relatively high sensitivity and very high specificity when used in isolation. An important caveat is that all studies of PCL tests are small, with numbers of patients typically under 20, and they contain the experience of one or two examiners. Unlike ACL testing, no meta-analysis data are available for any PCL test, despite several attempts at systematic review.[23,42]

POSTERIOR DRAWER TEST (Video 9-5)

George Noulis accurately described the opposing forces of the ACL and PCL in his 1876 thesis.[17] In their historical review, Paessler and Michel[17] give the following

Table 9.2   Posterior Cruciate Ligament Tests

Test	Review	Reliability/Validity Tests	Comments
Posterior sag sign	The patient lies supine with the hip flexed to 45 degrees and the knee flexed to 90 degrees. In this position, the tibia rocks back, or sags back, on the femur if the PCL is torn. Normally, the tibial plateau extends 1 cm beyond the femoral condyle when the knee is flexed to 90 degrees. If this step off is lost, this step-off test result is considered positive.	Rubinstein et al. 1994[43] Sensitivity: 79% Specificity: 100%	Double-blinded, randomized, controlled study of 39 subjects (75 knees for analysis). Only included patients with chronic PCL tears. Examiners all fellowship trained in sports medicine with at least 5 years' experience.
Posterior drawer test	The subject is supine with the test hip flexed to 45 degrees, knee flexed to 90 degrees, and foot in neutral position. The examiner sits on the subject's foot with both hands behind the subject's proximal tibia and thumbs on the tibial plateau. A posterior force is applied to the proximal tibia. Increased posterior tibial displacement as compared with the uninvolved side is indicative of a partial or complete PCL tear.	Rubinstein et al. 1994[43] Sensitivity: 90% Specificity: 99% Loos et al. 1981[44] Sensitivity: 51% Specificity: Not reported Moore and Larson 1980[45] Sensitivity: 67% Specificity: Not reported Hughston et al. 1976[19,46] Sensitivity: 55.5% Specificity: Not reported Clendenin et al. 1980[47] Sensitivity 100% Specificity: Not reported Harilainen 1987[8] Sensitivity: 90% Specificity: Not reported	See text discussion of drawer test Compilation study from registry of knee surgeries in the US and Australia; it included 102 PCL injuries. Multiple examiners at different sites, without indication that study was randomized or controlled. Retrospective study of 20 patients. All false negatives were found to have both ACL and PCL injuries at surgery. Review of 54 acute PCL tears studied over a 10-year period. Posterior drawer test was performed under anesthesia. Retrospective study of only 10 patients Prospective study that included only 9 patients with arthroscopically confirmed PCL tears.
Quadriceps active test	The subject is supine with the knee flexed to 90 degrees in the drawer test position. The foot is stabilized by the examiner, and the subject is asked to slide the foot gently down the table. Contraction of the quadriceps muscle in the PCL deficient knee results in an anterior shift of the tibia of 2 mm or more. The test is qualitative.	Daniel et al. 1988[48] Sensitivity: 98% Specificity: 100% Rubinstein et al. 1994[43] Sensitivity: 54% Specificity: 97%	Study included 92 subjects, 25 with no history of knee injury. Study was not blinded or randomized because the examiners were told which knee was the index knee. Double-blinded, randomized, controlled study of 39 subjects (75 knees for analysis). Examiners all fellowship trained in sports medicine with at least 5 years' experience. Only included patients with chronic PCL tears.

ACL, anterior cruciate ligament; *PCL,* posterior cruciate ligament.

account of Noulis's description from the French text of his thesis:

When the leg was then moved forward and backward, it was found that the tibia will slide anteriorly and posteriorly. Noulis observed much movement of the tibia when both cruciates had been severed. When only the ACL was severed, movement of the tibia could be demonstrated when the knee was "barely flexed." However, when the posterior cruciate ligament had been divided, it took about 110 degrees of flexion to produce this movement of the tibia.

Paessler and Michel[17] clarify that Noulis's 110 degrees of flexion would translate into 70 degrees of flexion today because at that time they used 180 degrees as full extension. A more detailed and contemporary description of the posterior drawer test as it is commonly performed follows[52] (Fig. 9.10):

The subject is supine with the test hip flexed to 45 degrees, knee flexed to 90 degrees, and foot in neutral position. The examiner is sitting on the subject's foot with both hands behind the subject's proximal tibia and thumbs on the tibial plateau. Apply a posterior force to the proximal tibia. Increased posterior tibial displacement as compared to the uninvolved side is indicative of a partial or complete tear of the PCL.

Numerous individual studies and several systematic reviews report on the accuracy of the posterior drawer test for identifying injuries to the PCL.[23,41-43,51-53] As with the posterior sag sign, most studies of the posterior drawer lack adequate sample sizes or have other methodologic flaws, rendering interpretation of their results difficult and incompatible with combined meta-analysis. Rubenstein and coworkers[43] reported that the posterior drawer test was the

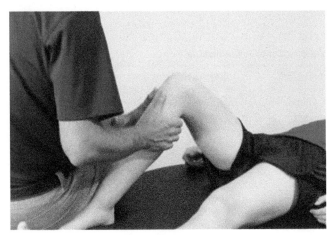

Figure 9.10   Posterior drawer test.

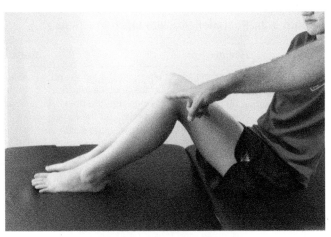

Figure 9.11   Quadriceps active test.

most accurate test for identifying PCL injuries, with a sensitivity of 90% and a specificity of 99%. In general, when all of the clinical tests for PCL injuries were analyzed based on the grade of PCL tear, the examination sensitivity for grade I sprains was only 70% with a 99% specificity, whereas the sensitivity of grade II and III sprains was 97%, with 100% specificity. The study included only patients with chronic PCL tears, so the accuracy of the posterior drawer test in the setting of acute PCL injuries cannot be inferred.

Loos and associates[44] identified 102 PCL injuries in 13,316 knee operations performed in the United States and Australia. In this study, the sensitivity of the posterior drawer test was 51%. The study was not designed to evaluate specificity, since only patients with surgically documented PCL injuries were included, and no control group was reported.

Hughston[52] reported a sensitivity of 55.5% when the posterior drawer test was performed under anesthesia. The large number of false-negative results was explained by a lack of injury to the posteriorly situated arcuate complex. Studies of patients under anesthesia by Clendenin and others[47] and Harilainen[8] noted positive posterior drawer test results in spite of intact posterior capsules.

In summary, while individual studies are limited, available systematic reviews[23,42] indicate that the posterior drawer test has a high sensitivity and specificity but that the highest diagnostic accuracy is obtained when results are combined with other tests for posterior instability, such as the posterior sag sign.

QUADRICEPS ACTIVE TEST (Video 9-6)

The quadriceps active test was described by Daniel and others[48] as follows (Fig. 9.11):

> With the subject supine, the relaxed limb is supported with the knee flexed to 90 degrees in the drawer-test position. The subject should execute a gentle quadriceps contraction to shift the tibia without extending the knee. At this 90-degree angle, the patellar ligament in the normal knee is oriented slightly posterior and contraction of the quadriceps does not result in an anterior shift of the tibia although there may be a slight posterior shift. If the posterior cruciate ligament is ruptured, the tibia sags into posterior subluxation and the

patellar ligament is then directed anteriorly. Contraction of the quadriceps muscle in the posterior cruciate-ligament deficient knee results in an anterior shift of the tibia of 2 mm or more. The test is qualitative.

In an unblinded, nonrandomized study, Daniel and others[48] reported a positive quadriceps active test in 41 of 42 knees that had a rupture of the PCL for a sensitivity of 98%. He reported a negative quadriceps active test result in all the normal knees and knees with only ACL disruptions but intact PCLs, for a specificity of 100%. Rubenstein and associates[43] reported a sensitivity for the quadriceps active test of 54% and a specificity of 97%. This compares with findings of 79% sensitivity and 90% sensitivity for the posterior sag sign and posterior drawer test, respectively, with 99% or greater specificity for both tests.

Significantly different sensitivities for the quadriceps active test may be a reflection of study methodology and slightly different patient populations. The blinded, randomized, and controlled study by Rubenstein and others[43] did not find the quadriceps active test to be as sensitive for detecting PCL disruption as other tests.

COLLATERAL LIGAMENT TESTS

The MCL is one of the most frequently injured ligaments in the knee. Valgus stress testing is the primary method used to diagnose MCL injury, but few studies have evaluated its accuracy or interexaminer reliability. Injuries of the LCL are rare, and there are even fewer studies evaluating the accuracy of the varus stress test in the diagnosis of this injury (Table 9.3).

VALGUS AND VARUS STRESS TESTS
(Videos 9-7 and 9-8)

Although the originator of the valgus and varus stress tests for detecting ligament laxity is unclear, in 1938, Palmer described "abduction and adduction rocking" of the knee to determine the integrity of the collateral ligaments, an early reference to the valgus and varus stress tests used

Table 9.3   Collateral Ligament Tests

Test	Review	Reliability/Validity Tests	Comments
Valgus stress test	The patient is supine on the exam table. Flex the knee to 30 degrees over the side of the table, place one hand about the lateral aspect of the knee, and grasp the ankle with the other hand. Apply abduction (valgus) stress to the knee. The test must also be performed in full extension.	Harilainen 1987[8] Sensitivity: 86% Specificity: Not reported	Study of 72 patients with MCL stress tears confirmed on arthroscopy. Valgus stress testing was performed in 20 degrees of flexion, and testing in extension was not done. Clinical exam performed in the ED under unknown conditions, and no indication is given regarding the number of examiners or their training. There is also no documentation of the elapsed time between ED evaluation and arthroscopic evaluation.
		Garvin et al. 1993[54] Sensitivity: 96% Specificity: Not reported	Retrospective study of 23 patients who had undergone surgery for MCL tears. Nonstandardized clinical examination of the MCL was used, sometimes under anesthesia, sometimes performed before anesthesia.
		McClure et al. 1989[55] Interrater reliability in extension: 68% Interrater reliability in 30 degrees flexion: 56% Sensitivity: Not reported Specificity: Not reported	Physicians did not perform testing in this study, and the physical therapist's experience was varied. Standardized examination techniques among the examiners were not employed. Data variability of the categories was insufficient to allow for accurate determination of reliability values.
Varus stress test	The patient is supine on the exam table. Flex the knee to 30 degrees over the side of the table, place one hand about the medial aspect of the knee, and grasp the ankle with the other hand. Apply adduction (varus) stress to the knee. The test must also be performed in full extension.	Harilainen 1987[8] Sensitivity: 25% Specificity: Not reported	Only 4 patients studied with LCL tears confirmed on arthroscopy. Varus stress testing was performed in 20 degrees of flexion, and testing in extension was not done. Clinical exam performed in the ED under unknown conditions, and no indication is given regarding the number of examiners or their training. There is also no documentation of the elapsed time between ED evaluation and arthroscopic evaluation.

ED, emergency room; *LCL*, lateral collateral ligament: *MCL*, medial collateral ligament.

today.[33] A description of Palmer's test from his 1938 paper follows[33]:

> In order to demonstrate lateral rocking, it is of the greatest importance that the patient be made to relax his muscles. In many cases this can be done if the extremity is grasped so that it rests firmly and painlessly in the grip of the examiner. The best way is to hold the leg with the foot supported in the armpit with the calf resting against the forearm. The other hand supports the back of the knee. When it is felt that the muscles are relaxed, a surprise abduction movement is made. It is then felt how the articular surfaces snap apart and, when the muscles start to function as a reflex action, spring together again with a click which is clearly discernible to the hand supporting the back of the knee.

Modern varus and valgus testing is performed with slight abduction of the hip and 30 degrees of knee flexion (Fig. 9.12). Hughston and associates[19] concluded that a valgus stress test positive at 30 degrees and negative at 0 degrees indicates a tear limited to the medial-compartment ligaments (MCL ±posterior capsule), whereas a valgus stress test positive at 0 degrees indicates a tear of both the PCL and the medial-compartment ligaments. He did not find that the integrity of the ACL had any effect on the valgus stress test in extension. Marshall and Rubin[56] noted that the valgus stress test in extension implicates one or both cruciates in addition to the MCL and posterior capsule.

Injuries resulting in straight lateral instability are rare. Hughston and coworkers[44] reported on the operative findings of three patients with straight lateral instability demonstrated by positive varus stress testing in extension. Surgery revealed a torn PCL, lateral capsule, and arcuate ligaments, as well a torn ACL in two patients, among other findings. In their review of the subject, Marshall and Rubin[56] reported that a positive varus stress test result in flexion implicates the LCL, whereas a positive test result in extension denotes a combined injury of the LCL and popliteal and cruciate ligaments. Recent data using arthrometers to measure force-strain ratios across the medial joint line support these early findings that valgus strain at full extension stresses

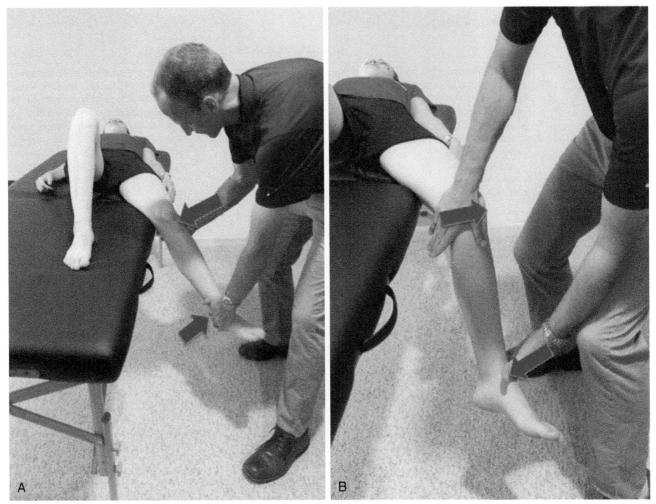

Figure 9.12   Valgus **(A)** and Varus **(B)** stress testing for collateral ligament injury.

different anatomic structures than valgus strain at 20 to 30 degrees of flexion.[57] Aronson and coworkers[57] conclude that clinical valgus stress testing should be done with the knee near full extension and repeated with the knee near 20 degrees of flexion to completely interrogate all medial stabilizers of the knee.

Little is known regarding the accuracy of valgus and varus stress testing. Harilainen[8] noted that of 72 patients with arthroscopically confirmed MCL tears, 62 were diagnosed on clinical examination for a sensitivity of 86%. Of four patients with a LCL tear confirmed on arthroscopy, one "instability" was diagnosed on clinical examination, for a sensitivity of 25%. The flawed design of this study significantly limits the overall clinical utility of the findings.

A few studies have been done comparing the clinical examination of collateral ligament injuries using varus–valgus stress testing with MRI imaging of the ligaments. Yao and colleagues[58] reported that the agreement between MRI and the clinical grade of injury was modest with a 65% correct classification. Mirowitz and Shu[59] reported a correlation coefficient between MRI diagnosis and clinical diagnosis of 0.73 for MCL injuries. In a retrospective study, Garvin and coworkers[54] reported that a tear of the MCL was predicted from the clinical examination in 22 of 23 patients, for a sensitivity of 96%. The retrospective design of the study

with inclusion of only serious injuries, along with the nonstandardized clinical exam primarily done under anesthesia, limits the clinical usefulness of this study. A more recent analysis combined traditional valgus stress testing with dynamic MRI and found that physical exam was accurate at identifying both injury and degree of injury when compared with discrete displacement measurements on MRI.[60] Finally, a single study comparing instrumented valgus testing with MRI showed agreement in 19 of 21 examined patients (kappa [κ] score, 0.83; standard error [SE], 0.10).[62]

McClure and colleagues[55] addressed the interexaminer reliability of the valgus stress test. Tests were performed by three physical therapists on 50 patients with unilateral knee problems. Interexaminer reliability was 0.6 with 68% agreement between examiners for the knee in extension and 0.16 with 56% agreement among examiners for the knee in 30 degrees of flexion. In a small, underpowered study examining the contribution of history and examination to diagnosis of medial collateral injury, both pain and laxity with valgus stress at 15 degrees of flexion were associated with injury ($P < 0.15$).[61] In the same study, an examination finding of pain with valgus stress at 15 degrees of flexion produced a +LR ratio for MCL injury of 2.3. This improved to a LR of 6.4 when both pain and laxity at 15 degrees were present.[61]

In summary, there is a lack of well-designed studies that evaluate the sensitivity and specificity of the varus–valgus stress test, the interexaminer reliability of the test, and the correlation with clinical diagnosis and grading of collateral ligament injuries.[53] While future studies could be educationally useful, they would be logistically challenging to design and of questionable clinical relevance. The majority of patients with collateral ligament injuries are successfully managed without the need for surgery and experience excellent outcomes. Therefore, the gold standard of arthroscopically identifying collateral ligament injuries would be hard to justify in terms of morbidity and mortality, and the adoption of a gold standard of MRI diagnosis would be technically challenging and also difficult to justify from a cost perspective.

PATELLOFEMORAL PAIN EXAMINATION

Anterior knee pain is among the most common overuse musculoskeletal complaints encountered by medical providers, with patellofemoral pain syndrome (PFS) specifically identified as accounting for nearly 25% of all sports-related knee injuries.[63] Principal pathologies encountered by medical providers include patellar instability, patellofemoral arthrosis, and PFS.[64] PFS is particularly challenging to manage because the etiology is thought to be multifactorial with no "gold standard" diagnostic criteria, with the reliability of most clinical tests low or untested.[65] Most authorities, however, believe that the principal pathology that underlies PFS is malalignment of the extensor mechanism with subsequent overload of the retinaculum and subchondral bone.[63,66] Physical examination tests that are commonly utilized to diagnose patellofemoral disorders attempt to either directly reproduce or provoke the pain of PFS and instability (the patellar compression or "grinding" test and the patellar apprehension test) or assess patellar mobility (the patellar tilt test and the patellar glide test [PGT]). In addition, functional testing is emerging as a viable tool to assist in diagnosing and managing PFS; the lateral step-down test is commonly used and is reviewed (Table 9.4).

Table 9.4   Patellofemoral Tests

Test	Description	Reliability/Validity Studies	Comments
Patellar grind test	The subject is supine with the knees extended. The examiner stands next to the involved side and places the web space of the thumb on the superior border of the patella. The subject is asked to contract the quadriceps muscle, while the examiner provides downward pressure on the patella. Pain with movement of the patella or an inability to complete the test is indicative of patellofemoral dysfunction.	No studies were found that document the sensitivity or specificity of the patellofemoral grinding test in the diagnosis of PFS.	The diagnosis of PFS is based on clinical exam, including the patella compression test. The lack of another gold standard (eg, border arthroscopy) in the diagnosis of PFS makes any determination of sensitivity or specificity of specific clinical tests for this condition problematic.
		O'Shea 1996[67] Sensitivity: 37%	Prospective study of patients with suspected chondromalacia patella.
Clarke sign	The subject is lying supine with the knees extended. The examiner stands next to the involved side and places the web space of the thumb on the superior border of the patella. The subject is asked to contract the quadriceps muscle, while the examiner applies downward and inferior pressure on the patella. Pain with movement of the patella or an inability to complete the test is indicative of patellofemoral dysfunction.	Doberstein 2008[68] Sensitivity: 39% Specificity: 67%	A single examiner tested 106 patients awaiting knee arthroscopy for reasons unrelated to the patellofemoral joint. There are no data examining the predictive value of the Clarke test in patients with suspected PFS.
Patellar apprehension test	This test is carried out by pressing on the medial aspect of the patella with the knee flexed 30 degrees with the quadriceps relaxed. It requires the thumbs of both hands pressing on the medial patella to exert the laterally directed pressure. Often the finding is surprising to the patient, who becomes uncomfortable and apprehensive as the patella reaches the point of maximum passive displacement, with the result that the patient begins to resist and attempts to straighten the knee, thus pulling the affected patella back into a relatively normal position.	Sallay et al. 1996[69] Sensitivity: 39% Specificity: Not reported	In this study, 19 patients underwent arthroscopic evaluation for patella dislocation, and all 19 exhibited gross lateral laxity of the patellofemoral articulation under anesthesia. This laxity was most prominent at 70–80 degrees of flexion.

Continued on following page

Table 9.4   Patellofemoral Tests (Continued)

Test	Description	Reliability/Validity Studies	Comments
Passive patellar tilt test	This test is performed with the knee extended and the quadriceps relaxed. Standing at the foot of the examination table, the examiner lifts the lateral edge of the patella from the lateral femoral condyle. The patella should remain in the trochlea and should not be allowed lateral subluxation. An excessively tight lateral retinacular restraint is demonstrated by a neutral or negative angle to the horizontal.	No studies were found that identified the accuracy of this specific test.	
Patellar glide test		No studies were found that identified the accuracy of this specific test.	
Step-down test	The subject is asked to stand in single-limb support with the hands on the waist, the knee straight, and the foot positioned close to the edge of a 20-cm-high step. The contralateral leg is positioned over the floor adjacent to the step and is maintained with the knee in extension. The subject then bends the tested knee until the contralateral leg gently contacts the floor and then re-extends to the start position. This maneuver is repeated five times. The examiner faces the subject and scores the test based on five criteria: (1) Arm strategy: If the subject uses an arm strategy in an attempt to recover balance, 1 point is added; (2) Trunk movement: If the trunk leans to any side, 1 point is added; (3) Pelvis plane: If pelvis rotates or elevates one side compared with the other, 1 point is added; (4) Knee position: If the knee deviates medially and the tibial tuberosity crosses an imaginary vertical line over the second toe, add 1 point, or if the knee deviates medially and the tibial tuberosity crosses an imaginary vertical line over the medial border of the foot, add 2 points; and (5) Maintain steady unilateral stance: If the subject steps down on the nontested side or if the subject's tested limb becomes unsteady (ie, wavers from side to side on the tested side), add 1 point. Total score of 0 or 1 is classified as good quality of movement, total score of 2 or 3 is classified as medium quality, and total score of 4 or more is classified as poor quality of movement.	No studies were found that identified the accuracy of this specific test.	

PFS, patellofemoral pain syndrome.

PATELLOFEMORAL GRINDING TEST (Video 9-9)

The term "chondromalacia patellae" did not appear in published form until 1924.[70] Budinger is credited with first clinically recognizing the disorder as "fissures in the patellar cartilage" in 1906, although the first mention of chondromalacia in the English language was in 1933 by Kulowski.[71] In 1936, Owre[72] published the results of a clinical and pathologic investigation of the patella. The complete description of the patellofemoral grinding test by Owre[72] follows:

Pressure-pain over the patella is tested by clasping the patella with the thumb and index finger of each hand with the remaining fingers resting against the thigh and leg. While the patient lies with the leg relaxed and extended the patella is pressed against the medial and lateral femoral condyles. By moving the patella in an upward and downward direction, the greater part of the surface cartilage may be examined in this manner. In some cases pain is elicited on the slightest pressure of the patella against the condyle; at other times considerable pressure must be exerted to obtain a positive response of an unpleasant sensation.

Owre considered a positive test result as indicated by pain to be predictive of pathologic changes to the retropatellar cartilage, or chondromalacia patella. In current use, a positive test result may or may not be associated with the pathologic diagnosis of chondromalacia patella as determined by direct arthroscopic visualization and probing. There are no studies that document either the sensitivity or specificity of the patellofemoral grinding test in the diagnosis of patellofemoral syndrome. There are several studies over the past 20 years, however, that do show a generally poor correlation between retropatellar pain and articular cartilage damage.[73-77] O'Shea and others[67] reported on the diagnostic accuracy of clinical examination of the knee in patients with arthroscopically documented knee pathology, including chondromalacia patella. They reported that only 11 of 29 patients were correctly diagnosed with having the pathologic findings of chondromalacia patella based on the history, physical exam, and standard radiographs, for a sensitivity of 37%.

PATELLAR COMPRESSION TEST (CLARKE SIGN [Video 9-10])

A more contemporary description of the test is as follows[23] (Fig. 9.13):

> The subject is lying supine with the knees extended. The examiner stands next to the involved side and places the web space of the thumb on the superior border of the patella. The subject is asked to contract the quadriceps muscle, while the examiner applies downward and inferior pressure on the patella. Pain with movement of the patella or an inability to complete the test is indicative of patellofemoral dysfunction.

Complicating the issue of Clarke sign testing is that many examiners routinely perform the Clarke maneuver at the end of a patellar grind test. Thus, the patellar grind test and Clarke sign are sometimes used synonymously in the literature and sometimes refer to two distinct maneuvers in patellofemoral testing. Additionally, there is debate in the literature regarding what constitutes a positive test result.[68] The Clarke maneuver is inherently disquieting, and the distinction between "positive discomfort" and "normal discomfort" is very subjective. The test characteristics of the Clarke sign in isolation from patellar grind testing have been evaluated in a single study of 106 patients awaiting knee arthroscopy for reasons unrelated to the patellofemoral joint.[68] A single examiner performed the Clarke test, and then chondromalacia was assessed arthroscopically and correlated with Clarke test outcomes. As might be expected in this situation, test characteristics were very poor with a sensitivity of 39%, a specificity of 67%, a +LR of 1.18, and a −LR of 0.91. There are no data examining the predictive value of Clarke test in patients with suspected PFS.

PATELLAR APPREHENSION TEST (Video 9-11)

Patellar instability, as previously identified, can either present as its own clinical entity with clinical episodes of

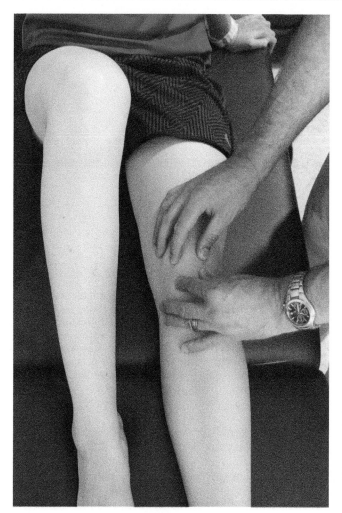

Figure 9.13 Patellofemoral grind test.

instability or frank recurrent dislocation or complicate patellofemoral tracking disorders. Patellar instability is commonly assessed by the patellar apprehension test. This test was first described by Fairbank in 1935, and the test is often referred to as Fairbank's apprehension test. His description follows[78]:

> While examining cases of suspected recurrent dislocation of the patella, I have been struck by the marked apprehension often displayed by the patient when the patella is pushed outwards in testing the stability of this bone. Not uncommonly, the patient will seize the examiner's hands to check the manipulation, which she finds uncomfortable and regards as distinctly dangerous. This sign, when present, I regard as strong evidence in favour of a diagnosis of slipping patella.

A more detailed and more recent description of the apprehension test for subluxation of the patella was given by Hughston.[79] His description of the apprehension test follows (Fig. 9.14):

> This test is carried out by pressing on the medial side of the patella with the knee flexed about 30 degrees and with the quadriceps relaxed. It requires the thumbs of both hands pressing on the medial side of the patella to exert the laterally directed pressure. Accordingly the leg with muscles relaxed is allowed to project over the side of the examining table and

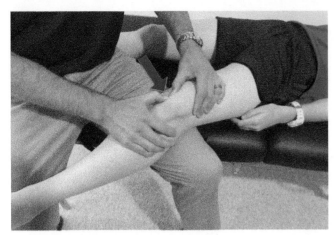

Figure 9.14 Patellar apprehension sign.

is supported with the knee at 30 degrees of flexion by resting the leg on the thigh of the examiner who is sitting on a stool. In this position the examiner can almost dislocate the patella over the lateral femoral condyle. Often the finding is surprising to the patient and he becomes uncomfortable and apprehensive as the patella reaches the point of maximum passive displacement, with the result that he begins to resist and attempts to straighten the knee, thus pulling the affected patella back into a relatively normal position.

In their 1996 study, Sallay and coworkers[69] reported on the characteristic clinical and arthroscopically determined pathologic findings associated with patellar dislocations. Only 39% of patients with a history of dislocation were noted to have a positive apprehension sign. In contrast, 83% exhibited a moderate to large effusion, and 70% of patients had significant tenderness over the posterior medial soft tissues. MRI revealed a moderate to large effusion on all scans. Increased signal adjacent to the adductor tubercle was seen in 96%, tearing of the medial patellofemoral ligament (MPFL) was found in 87%, and increased signal was noted in the vastus medialis oblique (VMO) muscle in 78% of cases. Upon arthroscopic evaluation, gross lateral laxity of the patellofemoral articulation of all subjects was most prominent at 70 to 80 degrees of flexion. This degree of flexion is significantly higher than the 30 degrees classically recommended for the apprehension sign and may explain the low sensitivity of this test in the diagnosis of patella dislocation.

PASSIVE PATELLAR TILT TEST

One of the principal "culprits" cited in the literature contributing to patellofemoral dysfunction and malalignment is that of a tight lateral retinacular restraint. Boden and associates[64] postulated that excessive lateral patellar tilt can contribute to lateral facet compression syndrome by leading to decreased patellar mobility and higher patellofemoral joint reaction forces between the lateral patellar facet and the lateral trochlea of the femur. Kolowich and coworkers[80] specifically studied the role of a tight lateral retinaculum by correlating preoperative physical examination findings with results after an isolated lateral retinacular release procedure for managing PFS. Patients were divided into two groups;

group I contained patients (n = 74) who were entirely satisfied with the procedure, and group II included patients (n = 43) for whom the procedure was a complete failure. Results indicated that the most predictable criterion for success was a negative passive patellar tilt; secondary criteria included a medial and lateral patellar glide of two quadrants or less. Patients had less predictable results after an isolated lateral release with a positive (>5 degrees) passive patellar tilt and a three-quadrant or greater medial and lateral patellar glide. Kolowich's description of the patellar tilt test follows[80]:

This test is performed with the knee extended and the quadriceps relaxed. Standing at the foot of the examination table, the examiner lifts the lateral edge of the patella from the lateral femoral condyle. The patella should remain in the trochlea and should not be allowed lateral subluxation. An excessively tight lateral retinacular restraint is demonstrated by a neutral or negative angle to the horizontal.

PATELLAR GLIDE TEST

The PGT, similar to the passive patellar tilt test, is one of several tests that attempt to measure passive patellar mediolateral range of motion. The PGT is actually a modification of the passive lateral hypermobility test, previously described by Hughston[79]; Kolowich's description of the PGT follows[80]:

The test is performed with the knee flexed 20 to 30 degrees and the quadriceps relaxed. The patella is divided into four imaginary longitudinal quadrants. The examiner then attempts to displace in a lateral to medial direction, and then a medial to lateral direction using the index finger and thumb. Medial mobility of one quadrant or less is consistent with a tight lateral restraint; three quadrants or more is consistent with a hypermobile patella.

Several authors have postulated the role of tightness of the lateral retinacular restraints limiting medial glide and their association to PFS. Puniello[81] studied 17 consecutive patients with PFS and found that more than 70% demonstrated tightness in the iliotibial band as well as limited patellar medial glide. Despite this association, others have recognized the difficulty in quantitatively assessing patellar mobility, citing the reliability of measurements as low. Skalley and co workers[82] assessed a calibrated handheld device (Patella Pusher) to exert a fixed force to accurately record patellar displacement in 67 high school students during routine preparticipation examinations. The authors concluded that clinical assessment of the passive limits of patellar motion should include examination at knee flexion angles of 0 degree and 35 degrees. Interestingly, however, the manually produced displacement was found to be more reproducible than displacement by the Patella Pusher ($P < 0.05$). Sweitzer and associates[83] assessed the reliability of 4 individual patellar mobility tests in 98 patients with anterior knee pain; the interrater reliability for the 4 individual patellar mobility tests was moderately strong, with diminished medial-lateral patellar mobility demonstrating the strongest reliability (κ score, 0.59; 95% confidence interval [CI], 0.42 to 0.72). Medial-lateral patellar mobility was second in diagnostic accuracy (sensitivity, 54%; specificity, 69%; LR ± 1.8; 95% CI, 0.9 to 3.6).

LATERAL STEP-DOWN TEST

In addition to static testing of the patellofemoral joint, several authors have suggested that dynamic testing may be of value in both diagnosis and management. Researchers in this area have identified that hip abductor weakness has an association with PFS.[65,84] The current thinking is that these muscles help to maintain pelvic stability by eccentrically controlling femoral internal rotation during weight-bearing activities. Weakness may result in increased medial femoral rotation and valgus knee moments, augmenting compressive forces on the patellofemoral joint and contributing to PFS.[65,85] Altered movement patterns may be recognized during physical examination testing as movements performed with poor quality. One of the more common tests used to assess functional movements of the extensor mechanism is the lateral step-down test, developed by Piva and associates,[86] and described as follows:

> Quality of movement during the lateral step down test was assessed using a scale designed for this purpose. The subject was asked to stand in single limb support with the hands on the waist, the knee straight, and the foot positioned close to the edge of a 20-cm-high step. The contralateral leg was positioned over the floor adjacent to the step and was maintained with the knee in extension. The subject then bent the tested knee until the contralateral leg gently contacted the floor and then re-extended the knee to the start position. This maneuver was repeated for 5 repetitions. The examiner faced the subject and scored the test based on 5 criteria: (1) Arm strategy. If subject used an arm strategy in an attempt to recover balance, 1 point was added; (2) Trunk movement. If the trunk leaned to any side, 1 point was added; (3) Pelvis plane. If pelvis rotated or elevated one side compared with the other, 1 point was added; (4) Knee position. If the knee deviated medially and the tibial tuberosity crossed an imaginary vertical line over the second toe, add 1 point, or, if the knee deviated medially and the tibial tuberosity crossed an imaginary vertical line over the medial border of the foot, add 2 points; and (5) Maintain steady unilateral stance. If the subject stepped down on the non-tested side, or if the subject tested limb became unsteady (i.e. wavered from side to side on the tested side), add 1 point. Total score of 0 or 1 was classified as good quality of movement, total score of 2 or 3 was classified as medium quality, and total score of 4 or above was classified as poor quality of movement.

In a study of 30 patients with PFS, Piva and colleagues[86] demonstrated a reliability coefficient of 0.67, which is consistent with good reliability. However, in a subsequent study of six clinical tests used to assess core stability, Weir[87] found an intraclass coefficient of only 0.39, demonstrating poor interobserver reliability. Weir[87] concluded that there is a clear need to develop more reliable clinical tests for evaluating core stability. In a study involving 55 Israeli military recruits, Rabin and associates[88] subsequently demonstrated an association of decreased ankle dorsiflexion ROM with poorer quality of movement among healthy male participants during the lateral step-down test. This observation implies that an abnormality detected during functional screening with tests such as the lateral step-down test requires further analysis into potential culprits.

MENISCAL TEARS

Meniscal tears occur commonly, but their clinical diagnosis is often difficult even for an experienced clinician (Table 9.5). Because the menisci are avascular and have no nerve supply on their inner two thirds, an injury to the meniscus can result in little or no pain or swelling, which makes accurate diagnosis even more challenging. Moreover, our evolving understanding of meniscal pathology clearly shows that not all meniscus tears require surgical intervention. Clinically then, the question has evolved beyond, "Is the meniscus torn or not?" to the more important issue of, "Does the patient have a meniscal tear that is likely to require surgery?"

In 1803, William Hey[96] described "internal derangement of the knee," and since that time there has been significant literature on the clinical diagnosis of meniscal tears. In evaluating the subsequent evidence, it is important to keep in mind that the age of arthroscopy and MRI has revolutionized detection and treatment of meniscal injury. In turn, the age of evidence-based medicine and patient-oriented outcomes has pushed back on the clinical relevance of many radiographic or arthroscopic meniscus "tears."

JOINT LINE TENDERNESS (Video 9-12)

Joint line palpation is one of the most basic maneuvers, yet it often provides more useful information than the provocative maneuvers designed to detect meniscal tears. Flexion of the knee enhances palpation of the anterior half of each meniscus. The medial edge of the medial meniscus becomes more prominent with internal rotation of the tibia, allowing for easier palpation. Alternatively, external rotation allows improved palpation of the lateral meniscus.

A systematic review in 2001 summarized four articles reporting on the finding of joint line tenderness. Sensitivity ranged from 55% to 85% with a mean value of 79%. Specificity was much lower, ranging from 11% to 43% with a mean calculated value of 15%.[23] As expected with such low specificity, the likelihood ratio of a positive joint line tenderness test was 0.9 (95% CI, 0.8 to 1.0) and of a negative test result was 1.1 (95% CI, 1.0 to 1.3). Thus, while joint line tenderness is likely to be present in those with meniscal tears, it is also likely to be present in many other knee conditions and is not useful in isolation in the diagnosis of meniscal injury.

McMURRAY TEST (Video 9-13)

The McMurray test is one of the primary clinical tests to evaluate for the presence of a meniscal tear (Fig. 9.15). T. P. McMurray first described the test in 1940.[33,93] The original description of the test follows[33]:

> In carrying out the manipulation with patient lying flat, the knee is first fully flexed until the heel approaches the buttock; the foot is then held by grasping the heel and using the forearm as a lever. The knee being now steadied by the surgeon's other hand, the leg is rotated on the thigh with the knee still in full flexion. During this movement the posterior section of the cartilage is rotated with the head of the tibia, and if the whole cartilage, or any fragment of the posterior

Table 9.5   Meniscal Tests

Test	Review	Reliability/Validity Tests	Comments
Joint line tenderness	Flexion of the knee enhances palpation of the anterior half of each meniscus. The medial edge of the medial meniscus becomes more prominent with internal rotation of the tibia, allowing for easier palpation. Additionally, external rotation allows improved palpation of the lateral meniscus.	Kurosaka et al. 1999[89] Sensitivity: 55% Specificity: 67%	Prospective blinded study of 160 patients with meniscal tears that were arthroscopically identified. Acute injuries were excluded.
		Fowler and Lubliner 1989[90] Sensitivity: 85% Specificity: 29.4%	Prospective study of 160 patients (161 knees) with meniscal tears that were arthroscopically identified.
		Anderson and Lipscomb 1986[91] Sensitivity: 77% Specificity: Not reported	Prospective evaluation of 100 patients by one examiner.
		Solomon 2001[23] Sensitivity: 55%–85% (mean 79%) Specificity: 11%–43% (mean 16%)	Systematic review on four articles reporting the findings of joint line tenderness.
		Konan 2009[92] Medial meniscus Sensitivity: 83% Specificity: 76% Lateral meniscus Sensitivity: 68% Specificity: 98%	Study of 109 patients with suspected meniscal injuries awaiting arthroscopy.
McMurray test	With the patient lying flat, the knee is first fully flexed; the foot is held by grasping the heel. The leg is rotated on the thigh with the knee still in full flexion. By altering the position of flexion, the whole of the posterior segment of the cartilages can be examined from the middle to their posterior attachment. Bring the leg from its position of acute flexion to a right angle, while the foot is retained first in full IR and then in full ER. When the click occurs (in association with a torn meniscus), the patient is able to state that the sensation is the same as experienced when the knee gave way previously.	Evans et al. 1993[93] Sensitivity: 16% Specificity: 98%	Prospective study of 104 patients. Interexaminer reliability between the two examiners of the study was only fair.
		Fowler and Lubliner 1989[90] Sensitivity: 29% Specificity: 95%	Prospective study of 160 patients (161 knees) with meniscal tears that were arthroscopically identified.
		Kurosaka et al. 1999[89] Sensitivity: 37% Specificity: 77%	Prospective blinded study of 160 patients with meniscal tears that were arthroscopically identified. Acute injuries were excluded.
		Anderson and Lapscomb 1986[91] Sensitivity: 58% Specificity: not reported	Prospective evaluation of 100 patients by one examiner.
		Solomon 2001[23] Sensitivity: 53% Specificity: 59%	Systematic review on four classic studies.
		Konan 2009[92] Medial meniscus Sensitivity: 50% Specificity: 77% Lateral meniscus Sensitivity: 68% Specificity: 97%	Study of 109 patients with suspected meniscal injuries awaiting arthroscopy.

Table 9.5   Meniscal Tests (Continued)

Test	Review	Reliability/Validity Tests	Comments

Thessaly test	The clinician supports the patient by holding his or her outstretched hands while the patient stands flat footed. The patient then rotates his or her knee and body, internally and externally three times, while keeping the knee flexed at 20 degrees of flexion. The patient is asked to describe and localize pain created by this maneuver. Pain localized to the joint line (medial or lateral) is a positive test result.	Karachalios et al. 2005[94]
		  Sensitivity: 80%–92%
		  Specificity: 91%–97%
		Harrison et al. 2009[95]
		  Sensitivity: 90%
		  Specificity: 98%
		
		Konan 2009[92]
		  Medial meniscus
		    Sensitivity: 59%
		    Specificity: 67%
		  Lateral meniscus
		    Sensitivity: 32%
		    Specificity: 95%
		Goossens[5]
		  Sensitivity: 64%
		  Specificity: 53%
			Prospective study of 410 symptomatic and asymptomatic patients
			Retrospective cohort study of 116 patients awaiting arthroscopy for suspected meniscal pathology.
			Study of 109 patients with suspected meniscal injuries awaiting arthroscopy.
			
			Study of 593 patients with suspected meniscal tears.

Apley grind test	The patient is prone. The surgeon grasps one foot in each hand, externally rotates as far as possible and then flexes both knees together to their limit. The feet are then rotated inward and knees extended. The surgeon then applies his or her left knee to the back of the patient's thigh. The foot is grasped in both hands, the knee is bent to a right angle, and powerful external rotation is applied. Next, the patient's leg is strongly pulled up, with the femur being prevented from rising off the couch. In this position of distraction, external rotation is repeated. The surgeon leans over the patient and compresses the tibia downward. Again he or she rotates powerfully and if addition of compression has produced an increase of pain, this grinding test result is positive and meniscal damage is diagnosed.	Fowler and Lubliner 1989[90]
		  Sensitivity: 16%
		  Specificity: 80%
		
		Kurosaka et al. 1999[89]
		  Sensitivity: 13%
		  Specificity: 90%
			Prospective study of 160 patients (161 knees) with meniscal tears that were arthroscopically identified.
			Prospective blinded study of 160 patients with meniscal tears that were arthroscopically identified. Acute injuries were excluded.

Bounce home test	The test is performed with the patient supine with the patient's foot cupped in the examiner's hand. With the patient's knee completely flexed, the knee is passively allowed to extend. The knee should extend completely, or bounce home into extension with a sharp end point. If extension is not complete or has a rubbery end feel, there is probably a torn meniscus, or some other blockage present.	No studies were found that identified the accuracy of this specific test.	N/A

ER, external rotation; *IR*, internal rotation; *N/A*, not applicable.

section is loose, this movement produces an appreciable snap in the joint. By external rotation of the leg the internal cartilage is tested, and by internal rotation any abnormality of the posterior part of the external cartilage can be appreciated. By altering the position of flexion of the joint, the whole of the posterior segment of the cartilages can be examined from the middle to their posterior attachment. Probably the simplest routine is to bring the leg from its position of acute flexion to a right angle, whilst the foot is retained first in full internal, and then in full external rotation. When the click occurs with a normal but lax cartilage, the patient experiences no pain or discomfort, but when produced by a broken cartilage,

which has already given trouble, the patient is able to state that the sensation is the same as he experienced when the knee gave way previously.

Several studies have been performed to determine the clinical accuracy of the McMurray test in predicting meniscal pathology. Four classic studies evaluate the McMurray test as it was originally described. A systematic analysis of these studies shows a mean sensitivity of 53%, a mean specificity of 59%, a +LR of 1.3 (95% CI, 0.9 to 1.7), and a −LR of 0.8 (95% CI, 0.6 to 1.1).[23]

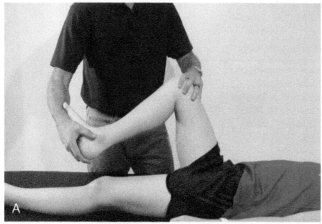

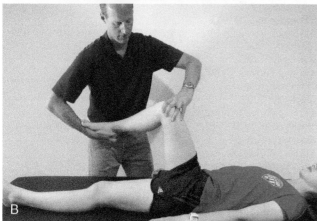

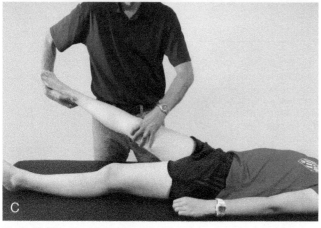

Figure 9.15. The McMurray test. **(A)** Starting position for McMurray; **(B)** Tibia is internally rotated; **(C)** Knee is extended with a valgus stress placed on the knee. Steps B through C are repeated with external rotation and varus stress.

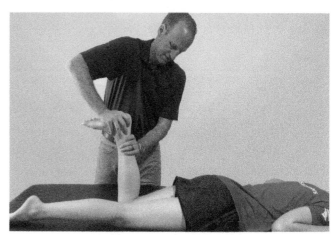

Figure 9.16 The Apley grind test.

when negative or positive, given its low diagnostic likelihood ratios.

APLEY GRIND TEST

The Apley grind test was described by A. G. Apley in 1947. The original description of the test follows (Fig. 9.16)[97]:

> For this examination the patient lies on his face. He should be on a couch not more than two feet high, or the tests become difficult, and he must be well over to the edge of the couch nearest the surgeon. To start the examination, the surgeon grasps one foot in each hand, externally rotates as far as possible, and then flexes both knees together to their limit. When this limit has been reached, he changes his grasp, rotates the feet inward, and extends the knees together again. The surgeon then applies his left knee to the back of the patient's thigh. It is important to observe that in this position his weight fixes one of the levers absolutely. The foot is grasped in both hands, the knee is bent to a right angle, and the powerful external rotation is applied. This test determines whether simple rotation produces pain. Next, without changing the position of the hands, the patient's leg is strongly pulled upward, while the surgeon's weight prevents the femur from rising off the couch. In this position of distraction, the powerful external rotation is repeated. Two things can be determined: (1) whether or not the maneuver produces pain and (2), still more important, whether the pain is greater than in rotation alone without the distraction. If the pain is greater, the distraction test is positive, and a rotation sprain may be diagnosed.
>
> Then the surgeon leans well over the patient and, with his whole body weight, compresses the tibia downward onto the couch. Again he rotates powerfully, and if addition of compression had produced an increase of pain, this grinding test is positive, and meniscal damage is diagnosed.

Given the wide variation in the reported sensitivities (16% to 63%) and specificities (13% to 100%) of the McMurray test for detecting meniscal tears, the findings of Evans and co workers,[93] indicating low agreement between examiners, are not surprising.

Overall, these findings indicate that the McMurray test is best used in combination with other physical exam tests and in patients with a history suggestive of meniscal involvement. The test should not be overly emphasized

In their report of five clinical signs for meniscal pathology, Fowler and Lubliner[90] prospectively evaluated the accuracy of the Apley grind test. They reported an overall sensitivity of 16%, even in this population in which all patients were known to have a meniscus injury. Kurosaka and others[89] noted a sensitivity of 13% and a specificity of 90%, with an overall accuracy of 28% for the Apley grind. The results of these prospective studies demonstrate the limited predictive value of the Apley grind test for the diagnosis of meniscal injuries.

BOUNCE-HOME TEST (Video 9-14)

The bounce-home test is designed to evaluate a lack of full extension in the knee, which may indicate a torn meniscus or other pathology such as a loose body or a joint effusion. The test is performed with the patient supine with the patient's foot cupped in the examiner's hand. With the patient's knee completely flexed, the knee is passively allowed to extend. The knee should extend completely, or bounce home into extension with a sharp end point. If extension is not complete or has a rubbery end feel, there is probably a torn meniscus or some other blockage present.[98]

Oni[99] described a modification of the bounce-home test, which he labeled the "knee jerk test," in which the knee is forcibly extended in one quick jerk and pain occurs in the region of tissue injury. Shybut and McGinty[100] described the forced hyperextension test of the knee that in contrast to the bounce-home test and the jerk test involves forced hyperextension of an already extended knee.[100] A block to full extension indicates a positive test result and may indicate a meniscal tear. In their study on the predictive value of five clinical tests for meniscal pathology, Fowler and Lubliner[90] reported a sensitivity of 44% and a specificity of 95% for the forced hyperextension of the knee test.

THESSALY TEST (Video 9-15)

The Thessaly test is performed by having the clinician support the patient by holding his or her outstretched hands while the patient stands flat footed. The patient then rotates the knee and body, internally and externally three times, while keeping their knee flexed at 20 degrees of flexion. The patient is asked to describe and localize pain created by this maneuver. Pain localized to the joint line (medial or lateral) is a positive test result.[95]

As is common with many special tests, initial reports on the Thessaly test were exceptionally positive. Karachalios[94] reported that in a series of 410 patients including asymptomatic and symptomatic individuals, the Thessaly test at 20 degrees of knee flexion had a diagnostic accuracy of 94% for medial meniscus tears and 96% for lateral meniscus tears. Harrison and associates[95] showed similar results in a series of 116 patients awaiting arthroscopy. In this population, the Thessaly test was 90% sensitive and 98% specific and had a positive predictive value of 98.5%. However, in other populations, the Thessaly test has not performed nearly as well. In a cohort of middle-aged adults (mean age, 39 years) the Thessaly had a diagnostic accuracy of 61% for medial meniscus tears and 80% for lateral meniscus tears. This was roughly equivalent to McMurray's test, whose accuracy was 57% for medial meniscus tears and 77% for lateral meniscus tears.[92] In a recent and large cohort study, Goossens and associates[5] evaluated 593 patients of whom 493 (83%) had a meniscal tear, as determined by the arthroscopic examination. Thessaly testing had a sensitivity of 64%, specificity of 53%, positive predictive value of 87%, negative predictive value of 23%, and positive and negative likelihood ratios of 1.37 (95% CI: 1.10, 1.70) and 0.68 (95% CI: 0.59, 0.78), respectively. Furthermore, in this analysis, the combination of positive Thessaly and McMurray test results showed a sensitivity of 53% and specificity of 62%.

The recent history of Thessaly testing illustrates several key points germane to many special tests. To an inexperienced practitioner, special tests offer the allure of making a scintillating diagnosis in a single deft maneuver. Unfortunately, experience and evidence show that special tests are at best important adjuncts to a complete history and physical exam. At worst, special tests can provide no additional or confounding information in the quest for the correct diagnosis. Caution is advised when interpreting any new physical exam maneuver. Initial reports tend to overestimate true sensitivity and specificity parameters, probably because of physician experience and population discrepancies.[5,94] While the conventional wisdom is to use special tests in thematic combinations[20,23,92] (ie, McMurray, joint line tenderness, and Thessaly for suspected meniscus; anterior drawer, Lachman, and pivot shift to interrogate the ACL), there is no substitute for experience and knowing the literature (as presented previously) regarding pitfalls and limitations for these common physical exam maneuvers. With this knowledge, a thoughtful clinician is better able to plan both diagnostic and treatment strategies for the painful knee.

AUTHOR'S APPROACH

The knee exam is unique in that special tests are numerous, and if you're not careful, you could take all day to examine your patient. To avoid spending all day, it's important to determine if the patient has an acute, traumatic injury or a chronic overuse injury.* Every knee exam should start with basic inspection. You should examine the knee for erythema, effusion, ecchymosis, and other visible abnormalities. Have the patient walk (if able to bear weight) so you can examine the gait and also how the knee interacts with the rest of the kinetic chain. Then perform manual tests for effusion because the presence of effusion can greatly change the focus of your examination.

Next have the patient lie supine with the foot on the bed and the knee flexed to approximately 90 degrees. Palpation starts with the knee in this flexed position. First palpate the joint lines, then the lateral femoral condyle for iliotibial band pain, and then the pes anserine area. Following this, extend the patient's knee and palpate the extensor mechanism: tibial tubercle, patella, and patellar tendon, including retropatellar tenderness. During palpation, you should also briefly check distal pulses and sensation.

The final step in the basic exam is ROM testing, which should be performed with the patient supine. Have the patient bring his or her heel as far toward his or her buttock as possible on the unaffected leg and then repeat on the injured leg. Next, have the patient fully extend the knee and instruct the patient to kick the palm of your hand held approximately 18 inches over the toes. If the patient can toe kick your palm, a significant quad or patellar tendon tear is quite unlikely. Having assessed strength as part of the

---

*It's also possible for the patient to have an acute nontraumatic condition, such as an infection or gout, or secondary Lyme disease. But that is outside the scope of this musculoskeletal textbook.

observed gait exam, you are now ready to move on to special tests. Special tests will help rule in or rule out suspected diagnoses; perform only those applicable, rather than trying to perform every special test on every patient.

SPECIAL TESTS FOR TRAUMATIC INJURY

For acute traumatic injuries whether contact or noncontact, the major concerns are ligaments, menisci, and patellar dislocations. Palpation along with varus–valgus testing is most helpful to diagnose MCL and LCL injuries. The collateral ligaments are usually, blissfully straightforward. To evaluate for an ACL tear, the Lachman exam is always the initial test performed because it has been clearly shown to be the best. If the Lachman exam result is positive, you should do a drawer test (looking for both posterior and anterior translocation); try a Lever sign since this is a relatively new test and might prove useful. A pivot shift test is challenging for a first-time, acute ACL tear. I find it more useful to do a pivot shift when looking for ACL re injury or for chronic ACL tears. For PCL injuries, history of a direct blow to the tibial tubercle will see me from performing the sag, the posterior drawer, the quad active test, and other tests looking at rotary stability of the posterior lateral corner. Absent this history, the sag test (performed as part of the inspection and palpation sequence when the patient is supine with the knee at 90 degrees) is the only test I routinely do for PCL injury unless there is a traumatic history or history of instability.

To interrogate the meniscus, you should use joint line tenderness (supine), the McMurray test (supine), and the Thessaly test (standing). During any knee examination, the patient will be supine and standing quite a lot, so these are handy tests. Apley compression requires the prone position and isn't very predictive, so it is less likely to be useful.

Patellar stability can be observed first during active range of motion of the knee, looking for abnormal lateral tracking of the patella during knee extension (the "J-sign"). The patellar apprehension test and tenderness to palpation of the medial patella (over the MPFL) is very helpful to assess for subluxation/dislocation mechanics.

SPECIAL TESTS FOR OVERUSE INJURIES

In overuse injury, the list of special tests is shorter, but the possible culprits are much more numerous than for an acute injury. Given this, accurate palpation is key. Patellofemoral testing is much more extensive, with careful attention to retropatellar tenderness, the Clarke sign, and patellar glide testing. The Clarke maneuver often gives useful information about patellofemoral irritation, whereas the grind test just seems to hurt everyone indiscriminately, so it is less useful in my hands.

The key to successful treatment of overuse injury is the identification of culprits, weak links, or otherwise offending structures that are causing injury to the primary victims. So finding patellofemoral irritation will prompt the Ober test for iliotibial band tightness and assessment of core strength. Finding pes anserine or iliotibial band tenderness to palpation will also trigger the Ober test, Noble test, and core strength assessment. As a general rule, overuse injuries should *not* cause a knee effusion, with the possible excep-

tions of a degenerative meniscus tear or a patellofemoral chondral fragment from severe patellofemoral pain. Remembering this rule can be very helpful in ensuring that patients with acute injury are not accidently misdiagnosed with overuse pathology.

REFERENCES

1. Hoppenfeld S. *Physical Examination of the Spine and Extremities.* Norwalk, CT: Appleton-Century-Crofts; 1976.
2. Griffith CJ, LaPrade RF, Johansen S, et al. Medial knee injury: Part 1, static function of the individual components of the main medial knee structures. *Am J Sports Med.* 2009;37:1762-1770.
3. Liu F, Yue B, Gadikota HR, et al. Morphology of the medial collateral ligament of the knee. *J Orthop Surg Res.* 2010;5:69.
4. Yan J, Takeda S, Fujino K, et al. Anatomical reconsideration of the lateral collateral ligament in the human knee: anatomical observation and literature review. *Surg Sci.* 2012;3:484-488.
5. Goossens P, Keijsers E, van Geenen RJ, et al. Validity of the Thessaly test in evaluating meniscal tears compared with arthroscopy: a diagnostic accuracy study. *J Orthop Sports Phys Ther.* 2015;45:18-24, B11.
6. Medina O, Arom GA, Yeranosian MG, et al. Vascular and nerve injury after knee dislocation: a systematic review. *Clin Orthop Relat Res.* 2014;472:2621-2629.
7. Natsuhara KM, Yeranosian MG, Cohen JR, et al. What is the frequency of vascular injury after knee dislocation? *Clin Orthop Relat Res.* 2014;472:2615-2620.
8. Harilainen A. Evaluation of knee instability in acute ligamentous injuries. *Ann Chir Gynaecol.* 1987;76:269-273.
9. Katz JW, Fingeroth RJ. The diagnostic accuracy of ruptures of the anterior cruciate ligament comparing the Lachman test, the anterior drawer sign, and the pivot shift test in acute and chronic knee injuries. *Am J Sports Med.* 1986;14:88-91.
10. Jonsson T, Althoff B, Peterson L, et al. Clinical diagnosis of ruptures of the anterior cruciate ligament: a comparative study of the Lachman test and the anterior drawer sign. *Am J Sports Med.* 1982;10:100-102.
11. Donaldson WF 3rd, Warren RF, Wickiewicz T. A comparison of acute anterior cruciate ligament examinations. Initial versus examination under anesthesia. *Am J Sports Med.* 1985;13:5-10.
12. Mitsou A, Vallianatos P. Clinical diagnosis of ruptures of the anterior cruciate ligament: a comparison between the Lachman test and the anterior drawer sign. *Injury.* 1988;19:427-428.
13. Kim SJ, Kim HK. Reliability of the anterior drawer test, the pivot shift test, and the Lachman test. *Clin Orthop Relat Res.* 1995;317:237-242.
14. Torg JS, Conrad W, Kalen V. Clinical diagnosis of anterior cruciate ligament instability in the athlete. *Am J Sports Med.* 1976;4:84-93.
15. Lucie RS, Wiedel JD, Messner DG. The acute pivot shift: clinical correlation. *Am J Sports Med.* 1984;12:189-191.
16. Lelli A, Di Turi RP, Spenciner DB, et al. The "Lever Sign": a new clinical test for the diagnosis of anterior cruciate ligament rupture. *Knee Surg Sports Traumatol Arthrosc.* 2014 [Epub ahead of print].
17. Paessler HH, Michel D. How new is the Lachman test? *Am J Sports Med.* 1992;20:95-98.
18. Strobel M, Stetfeld HW. *Diagnostic Evaluation of the Knee.* New York: Springer-Verlag; 1990.
19. Hughston JC, Andrews JR, Cross MJ, et al. Classification of knee ligament instabilities. Part I. The medial compartment and cruciate ligaments. *J Bone Joint Surg Am.* 1976;58:159-172.
20. Ostrowski JA. Accuracy of 3 diagnostic tests for anterior cruciate ligament tears. *J Athl Train.* 2006;41:120-121.
21. van Eck CF, van den Bekerom MP, Fu FH, et al. Methods to diagnose acute anterior cruciate ligament rupture: a meta-analysis of physical examinations with and without anaesthesia. *Knee Surg Sports Traumatol Arthrosc.* 2013;21:1895-1903.
22. Konin JG. *Special Tests for Orthopedic Examination.* Thorofare, NJ: Stack; 1997.
23. Solomon DH, Simel DL, Bates DW, et al. The rational clinical examination. Does this patient have a torn meniscus or ligament of the knee? Value of the physical examination. *JAMA.* 2001;286:1610-1620.

24. Peeler J, Leiter J, MacDonald P. Accuracy and reliability of anterior cruciate ligament clinical examination in a multidisciplinary sports medicine setting. *Clin J Sport Med.* 2010;20:80-85.
25. Draper DO, Schulthies SS. Examiner proficiency in performing the anterior drawer and Lachman tests. *J Orthop Sports Phys Ther.* 1995;22:263-266.
26. Adler GG, Hoekman RA, Beach DM. Drop leg Lachman test. A new test of anterior knee laxity. *Am J Sports Med.* 1995;23: 320-323.
27. Feagin JA, Cooke TD. Prone examination for anterior cruciate ligament insufficiency. *J Bone Joint Surg Br.* 1989;71:863.
28. Wroble RR, Lindenfeld TN. The stabilized Lachman test. *Clin Orthop Relat Res.* 1988;237:209-212.
29. Mulligan EP, Harwell JL, Robertson WJ. Reliability and diagnostic accuracy of the Lachman test performed in a prone position. *J Orthop Sports Phys Ther.* 2011;41:749-757.
30. Lange T, Freiberg A, Droge P, et al. The reliability of physical examination tests for the diagnosis of anterior cruciate ligament rupture—a systematic review. *Man Ther.* 2015;20: 402-411.
31. Galway HR, MacIntosh DL. The lateral pivot shift: a symptom and sign of anterior cruciate ligament insufficiency. *Clin Orthop Relat Res.* 1980;147:45-50.
32. Hey Groves EW. The crucial ligaments of the knee joint: their function, rupture and the operative treatment of the same. *Br J Surg.* 1920;7:505-515.
33. Palmer I. On the injuries to the ligaments of the knee joint: a clinical study. 1938. *Clin Orthop Relat Res.* 2007;454:17-22, discussion 14.
34. Kujala UM, Nelimarkka O, Koskinen SK. Relationship between the pivot shift and the configuration of the lateral tibial plateau. *Arch Orthop Trauma Surg.* 1992;111(4):228-229.
35. Larson RL. Physical examination in the diagnosis of rotatory instability. *Clin Orthop Relat Res.* 1983;172:38-44.
36. Noyes FR, Grood ES, Cummings JF, et al. An analysis of the pivot shift phenomenon. The knee motions and subluxations induced by different examiners. *Am J Sports Med.* 1991;19:148-155.
37. Bach BR Jr, Warren RF, Wickiewicz TL. The pivot shift phenomenon: results and description of a modified clinical test for anterior cruciate ligament insufficiency. *Am J Sports Med.* 1988; 16:571-576.
38. Musahl V, Voos J, O'Loughlin PF, et al. Mechanized pivot shift test achieves greater accuracy than manual pivot shift test. *Knee Surg Sports Traumatol Arthrosc.* 2010;18:1208-1213.
39. Arilla FV, Yeung M, Bell K, et al. Experimental execution of the simulated pivot-shift test: a systematic review of techniques. *Arthroscopy.* 2015;31:2445-2454.
40. Ayeni OR, Chahal M, Tran MN, et al. Pivot shift as an outcome measure for ACL reconstruction: a systematic review. *Knee Surg Sports Traumatol Arthrosc.* 2012;20:767-777.
41. Barton TM, Torg JS, Das M. Posterior cruciate ligament insufficiency. A review of the literature. *Sports Med.* 1984;1:419-430.
42. Kopkow C, Freiberg A, Kirschner S, et al. Physical examination tests for the diagnosis of posterior cruciate ligament rupture: a systematic review. *J Orthop Sports Phys Ther.* 2013;43:804-813.
43. Rubinstein RA Jr, Shelbourne KD, McCarroll JR, et al. The accuracy of the clinical examination in the setting of posterior cruciate ligament injuries. *Am J Sports Med.* 1994;22:550-557.
44. Loos WC, Fox JM, Blazina ME, et al. Acute posterior cruciate ligament injuries. *Am J Sports Med.* 1981;9:86-92.
45. Moore HA, Larson RL. Posterior cruciate ligament injuries. Results of early surgical repair. *Am J Sports Med.* 1980;8: 68-78.
46. Hughston JC, Andrews JR, Cross MJ, et al. Classification of knee ligament instabilities. Part II. The lateral compartment. *J Bone Joint Surg Am.* 1976;58:173-179.
47. Clendenin MB, DeLee JC, Heckman JD. Interstitial tears of the posterior cruciate ligament of the knee. *Orthopedics.* 1980;3(8): 764-772.
48. Daniel DM, Stone ML, Barnett P, et al. Use of the quadriceps active test to diagnose posterior cruciate-ligament disruption and measure posterior laxity of the knee. *J Bone Joint Surg Am.* 1988;70:386-391.
49. Mayo Robson AW. Ruptured cruciate ligaments and their repair by operation. *Ann Surg.* 1903;37:716-718.
50. Hawkins RJ. *Musculoskeletal Examination.* St. Louis: Mosby; 1993.
51. Stäubli HU, Jakob RP. Posterior instability of the knee near extension. A clinical and stress radiographic analysis of acute injuries of the posterior cruciate ligament. *J Bone Joint Surg Br.* 1990;72:225-230.
52. Hughston JC. The absent posterior drawer test in some acute posterior cruciate ligament tears of the knee. *Am J Sports Med.* 1988;16:39-43.
53. Malanga GA, Andrus S, Nadler SF, et al. Physical examination of the knee: a review of the original test description and scientific validity of common orthopedic tests. *Arch Phys Med Rehabil.* 2003;84:592-603.
54. Garvin GJ, Munk PL, Vellet AD. Tears of the medial collateral ligament: magnetic resonance imaging findings and associated injuries. *Can Assoc Radiol J.* 1993;44:199-204.
55. McClure PW, Rothstein JM, Riddle DL. Intertester reliability of clinical judgments of medial knee ligament integrity. *Phys Ther.* 1989;69:268-275.
56. Marshall JL, Rubin RM. Knee ligament injuries—a diagnostic and therapeutic approach. *Orthop Clin North Am.* 1977;8:641-668.
57. Aronson PA, Gieck JH, Hertel J, et al. Tibiofemoral joint positioning for the valgus stress test. *J Athl Train.* 2010;45:357-363.
58. Yao L, Dungan D, Seeger LL. MR imaging of tibial collateral ligament injury: comparison with clinical examination. *Skeletal Radiol.* 1994;23(7):521-524.
59. Mirowitz SA, Shu HH. MR imaging evaluation of knee collateral ligaments and related injuries. Comparison of T1-weighted, T2-weighted, and fat-saturated T2-weighted sequences—correlation with clinical findings. *J Magn Reson Imaging.* 1994;4: 725-732.
60. Studler U, White LM, Deslandes M, et al. Feasibility study of simultaneous physical examination and dynamic MR imaging of medial collateral ligament knee injuries in a 1.5-T large-bore magnet. *Skeletal Radiol.* 2011;40:335-343.
61. Kastelein M, Wagemakers HP, Luijsterburg PA, et al. Assessing medial collateral ligament knee lesions in general practice. *Am J Med.* 2008;121:982-988.
62. Rasenberg EI, Lemmens JA, van Kampen A, et al. Grading medial collateral ligament injury: comparison of MR imaging and instrumented valgus-varus laxity test-device. A prospective double-blind patient study. *Eur J Radiol.* 1995;21:18-24.
63. Fulkerson JP. Diagnosis and treatment of patients with patellofemoral pain. *Am J Sports Med.* 2002;30:447-456.
64. Boden BP, Pearsall AW, Garrett WE Jr, et al. Patellofemoral instability: evaluation and management. *J Am Acad Orthop Surg.* 1997;5:47-57.
65. Fredericson M, Yoon K. Physical examination and patellofemoral pain syndrome. *Am J Phys Med Rehabil.* 2006;85:234-243.
66. Pal S, Besier TF, Beaupre GS, et al. Patellar maltracking is prevalent among patellofemoral pain subjects with patella alta: an upright, weightbearing MRI study. *J Orthop Res.* 2013;31:448-457.
67. O'Shea KJ, Murphy KP, Heekin RD, et al. The diagnostic accuracy of history, physical examination, and radiographs in the evaluation of traumatic knee disorders. *Am J Sports Med.* 1996;24: 164-167.
68. Doberstein ST, Romeyn RL, Reineke DM. The diagnostic value of the Clarke sign in assessing chondromalacia patella. *J Athl Train.* 2008;43(2):190-196.
69. Sallay PI, Poggi J, Speer KP, et al. Acute dislocation of the patella. A correlative pathoanatomic study. *Am J Sports Med.* 1996;24:52-60.
70. Dugdale TW, Barnett PR. Historical background: patellofemoral pain in young people. *Orthop Clin North Am.* 1986;17:211-219.
71. Kulowski J. Chondromalacia of the patella; fissurel cartilage degeneration; traumatic chondropathy; report of three cases. *JAMA.* 1933;100:1837-1840.
72. Owre A. Chondromalcia patellae. *Acta Chir Scand.* 1936;77(suppl 41):1-159.
73. Abernethy P, Wilson G, Logan P. Strength and power assessment. Issues, controversies and challenges. *Sports Med.* 1995;19:401-417.
74. Darracott J, Vernon-Roberts B. The bony changes in "chondromalacia patellae." *Rheumatol Phys Med.* 1971;11:175-179.
75. Dehaven KE, Dolan WA, Mayer PJ. Chondromalacia patellae in athletes. Clinical presentation and conservative management. *Am J Sports Med.* 1979;7:5-11.

76. Leslie IJ, Bentley G. Arthroscopy in the diagnosis of chondromalacia patellae. *Ann Rheum Dis.* 1978;37:540-547.

77. Tria AJ Jr, Palumbo RC, Alicea JA. Conservative care for patellofemoral pain. *Orthop Clin North Am.* 1992;23:545-554.

78. Fairbank HA. Internal Derangement of the Knee in Children and Adolescents: (Section of Orthopaedics). *Proc R Soc Med.* 1937;30:427-432.

79. Hughston JC. Subluxation of the patella. *J Bone Joint Surg Am.* 1968;50:1003-1026.

80. Kolowich PA, Paulos LE, Rosenberg TD, et al. Lateral release of the patella: indications and contraindications. *Am J Sports Med.* 1990;18:359-365.

81. Puniello MS. Iliotibial band tightness and medial patellar glide in patients with patellofemoral dysfunction. *J Orthop Sports Phys Ther.* 1993;17(3):144-148.

82. Skalley TC, Terry GC, Teitge RA. The quantitative measurement of normal passive medial and lateral patellar motion limits. *Am J Sports Med.* 1993;21:728-732.

83. Sweitzer BA, Cook C, Steadman JR, et al. The inter-rater reliability and diagnostic accuracy of patellar mobility tests in patients with anterior knee pain. *Phys Sportsmed.* 2010;38:90-96.

84. Ireland ML, Willson JD, Ballantyne BT, et al. Hip strength in females with and without patellofemoral pain. *J Orthop Sports Phys Ther.* 2003;33:671-676.

85. Tyler TF, Nicholas SJ, Mullaney MJ, et al. The role of hip muscle function in the treatment of patellofemoral pain syndrome. *Am J Sports Med.* 2006;34:630-636.

86. Piva SR, Fitzgerald K, Irrgang JJ, et al. Reliability of measures of impairments associated with patellofemoral pain syndrome. *BMC Musculoskelet Disord.* 2006;7:33.

87. Weir A, Darby J, Inklaar H, et al. Core stability: inter- and intraobserver reliability of 6 clinical tests. *Clin J Sport Med.* 2010;20:34-38.

88. Rabin A, Kozol Z, Spitzer E, et al. Ankle dorsiflexion among healthy men with different qualities of lower extremity movement. *J Athl Train.* 2014;49(5):617-623.

89. Kurosaka M, Yagi M, Yoshiya S, et al. Efficacy of the axially loaded pivot shift test for the diagnosis of a meniscal tear. *Int Orthop.* 1999;23:271-274.

90. Fowler PJ, Lubliner JA. The predictive value of five clinical signs in the evaluation of meniscal pathology. *Arthroscopy.* 1989;5:184-186.

91. Anderson AF, Lipscomb AB. Clinical diagnosis of meniscal tears. Description of a new manipulative test. *Am J Sports Med.* 1986;14:291-293.

92. Konan S, Rayan F, Haddad FS. Do physical diagnostic tests accurately detect meniscal tears? *Knee Surg Sports Traumatol Arthrosc.* 2009;17:806-811.

93. Evans PJ, Bell GD, Frank C. Prospective evaluation of the McMurray test. *Am J Sports Med.* 1993;21:604-608.

94. Karachalios T, Hantes M, Zibis AH, et al. Diagnostic accuracy of a new clinical test (the Thessaly test) for early detection of meniscal tears. *J Bone Joint Surg Am.* 2005;87:955-962.

95. Harrison BK, Abell BE, Gibson TW. The Thessaly test for detection of meniscal tears: validation of a new physical examination technique for primary care medicine. *Clin J Sport Med.* 2009;19:9-12.

96. Hey W. *Practical Observations in Surgery.* Philadelphia: James Humphreys; 1805.

97. Gould JD, Dabies GJ. *Orthopaedic and Sports Physical Therapy.* Toronto: Mosby; 1985.

98. Magee DJ. *Orthopedic Physical Assessment.* 3rd ed. Philadelphia: W.B. Saunders; 1997:506-598.

99. Oni AO. The knee jerk test for diagnosis of torn meniscus [letter]. *Clin Orthop.* 1985;193:309.

100. Shybut GT, McGinty JB. The office evaluation of the knee. *Orthop Clin North Am.* 1982;13:497-509.

Physical Examination of the Foot and Ankle

10

Lt Col Ross A. Schumer, MD | Mederic M. Hall, MD |
Annunziato Amendola, MD

INTRODUCTION

This chapter provides a review of foot and ankle anatomy and examination followed by an evidence-based discussion of the major provocative tests employed to diagnose ankle and foot injuries. Epidemiologically, foot and ankle complaints are the third most common musculoskeletal reason for adult patients to present in a primary care setting, ranking only behind back and knee pain.[1] In the pediatric population, foot pain is the most common musculoskeletal complaint in patients under 15 years of age.[1] We review anatomy, discuss basic principles of examination related to the foot and ankle, and focus on specific testing for common clinical scenarios. Our goal is to provide the clinician with an understanding of the science (or lack thereof) that guides our examination and its subsequent interpretation.

GENERAL DEFINITIONS

Before discussing the specifics of examination, it is necessary to have a fundamental understanding of anatomic terminology to effectively communicate the general alignment and movement of the foot. Complex multiplanar joint movements and joint-to-joint interactions generate the motions we simplify in our clinical exam. There is a lack of consistency complicated by the fact that we use terms to describe relationships to both the body and the foot itself. Varus and valgus use the midsagittal plane of the body as a reference point. However, abduction and adduction reference the longitudinal axis of the foot. As opposed to the hand, which uses the third ray, the longitudinal axis of the foot is described as a line from the center of the heel through the second metatarsal shaft. For example, hallux valgus (Fig. 10.1) uses the midsagittal axis of the body, whereas abduction of the hallux is deviation of the great toe away from the foot and actually toward the body. This can be even more confusing when considering terms such as metatarsus adductus (Fig. 10.2), which again, references the position of the metatarsals in relation to the body.

Tibiotalar, talocalcaneal, and transverse tarsal motions are complex, interdependent, and not confined to one plane.[2,3] For this reason, we will clarify our use of the following terms: *dorsiflexion* and *plantar flexion* refer to tibiotalar joint motion, while *calcaneus* and *equinus* define the ankle's static position; *inversion* and *eversion* delineate talocalcaneal (subtalar) joint movement; *internal rotation* and *external rotation* of the ankle refer to combined tibiotalar and talocalcaneal motion; and *pronation* and *supination* are composite movements involving the midfoot and forefoot.[3] *Pronation* is characterized by external rotation and abduction of the forefoot relative to the tibia combined with hindfoot eversion, thus plantarflexing the medial column. *Supination* elevates the medial column through internal rotation and adduction of the foot on the tibia combined with hindfoot inversion.[4]

ANATOMY AND PHYSICAL EXAMINATION

INSPECTION

Assessment of the foot and ankle begins with observation of a patient's gait pattern and static standing posture and the style and wear pattern of the shoes. Shoes, particularly well-worn shoes, can provide evidence about foot position and

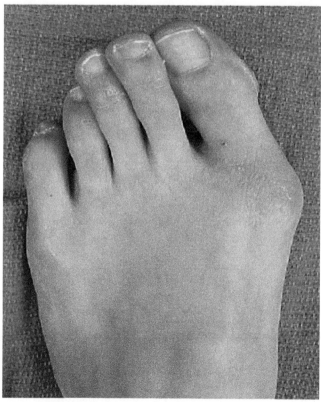

Figure 10.1 Clinical photograph of hallux valgus.

199

Table 10.1   Racial Differences in Foot Type

	Total Sample n = 1691	African Americans n = 528 (31.2%)	Whites n = 1163 (68.8%)	Unadjusted OR (95% CI)	Adjusted OR (95% CI)*
Pes planus	391 (23.1%)	202 (38.8%)	189 (16.3%)	3.19 (2.53–4.04)	2.94 (2.31–3.75)
Pes cavus	79 (4.7%)	8 (1.5%)	71 (6.1%)	0.24 (0.11–0.50)	0.28 (0.13–0.59)

*Adjusted for age, sex, body mass index, and education; reference = white.
CI, Confidence interval; *OR*, odds ratio.
Adapted from Golightly YM, Hannan MT, Dufour AB, et al. Racial differences in foot disorders and foot type. Arthritis Care Res. 2012;64:1756-1769.

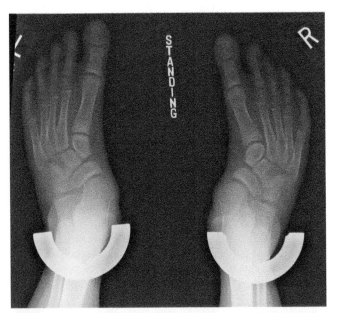

Figure 10.2 Radiograph of a skeletally immature patient with skew-foot, a complex condition with metatarsus adductus, midfoot abductus, and hindfoot valgus.

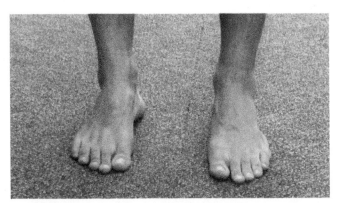

Figure 10.3 Cavovarus foot (right) with "peek-a-boo" heel.

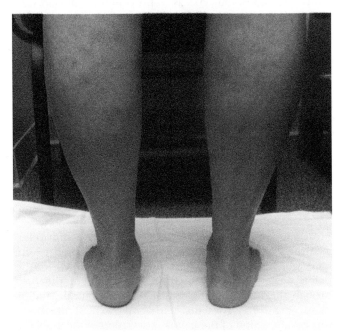

Figure 10.4 Hindfoot valgus (left) with "too many toes."

gait patterns. Wear on the lateral heel is associated with a varus hindfoot, while significant medial wear is typically seen in pes planus.

Particular attention must be given to careful skin inspection of dorsal, plantar, and interdigital regions of all feet, but especially the neuropathic foot (eg, patients with diabetes with peripheral polyneuropathies), to examine for bruising, erythema, pressure sores, nail abnormalities, blisters, and calluses. Be observant of any pigmented melanotic areas because melanoma of the foot accounts for 1.5% to 7% of cutaneous melanomas in a predominantly white population and up to 72% in darker skinned populations.[5-10] As skin pigment increases, the overall incidence of cutaneous melanoma decreases, but the rate of acral lentiginous melanoma seems to stay the same. These lesions are often not identified or are misdiagnosed as benign lesions at initial presentation, which can result in a delay in diagnosis and treatment and subsequent negative effect on patient outcome.[11]

The weight-bearing posture should be observed with both shoes and socks removed. In general, alignment can be classified as neutral, cavovarus (Fig. 10.3), or planovalgus (Fig. 10.4). Although there are numerous variations, most feet

fall into one of these categories. The Johnston County Osteoarthritis Project reported on 1691 adult patients (age = 68.0 ± 9.1 years) who were evaluated for racial differences in foot disorders and alignment type[12] (Table 10.1). *Pes cavovarus* is defined as a high medial arch and varus heel. It can be associated with numerous complaints, including lateral ankle instability, peroneal tendon pathology, ankle arthritis, and lateral foot overload.[13] Although originally used to describe the appearance of the foot due to post-compartment syndrome muscle contractures, the "peek-a-boo" heel sign (see Fig. 10.3) has become a valuable clinical exam tool for the "subtle cavovarus foot."[14] The peek-a-boo heel sign is viewed from the front with the patients' feet pointing straight ahead. If the examiner can identify the medial border of the plantar fat pad, there is some component of varus hindfoot alignment. Although the peek-a-boo heel sign is commonly referenced in the literature, to our knowledge, there has not been a study to evaluate the diagnostic accuracy of this test. A cavus foot can be the result of a plantar flexed first ray elevating the arch and tipping the hindfoot into varus, from rigid hindfoot varus, or a combination of the two. The Coleman block test can be used to determine the flexibility of the hindfoot deformity and assess for forefoot driven hindfoot varus.[15] The Coleman block test is performed by placing a block under the lateral column of the foot and unloading the first metatarsal by allowing it to hang over the edge. If the hindfoot is flexible and corrects into valgus, then it is said to be forefoot-driven hindfoot varus. If the hindfoot remains in varus, then the etiology may be secondary to abnormal morphology or pathology of the talus, calcaneus, or subtalar joint.

Contrary to the "peek-a-boo heel" sign, the "too-many-toes" sign is a clinical tool for evaluating pes planovalgus.[16] The examiner observes the patient from behind and looks for exposed toes on the lateral aspect of the tibia. The number of toes visualized can be used to quantify the severity of forefoot abduction associated with hindfoot valgus (see Fig. 10.4).

Inspection of the patient's stance and gait is important. Normally, the foot passively pronates during the initial ground contact in the early stance phase. This subtalar eversion unlocks the transverse tarsal joint to allow for force dissipation. The foot should not remain pronated during heel rise and lift off. As the body transfers over the foot, inversion of the subtalar joint stiffens up the transverse tarsal joint in preparation for toe-off. Failure to initiate heel inversion may be associated with tibialis posterior tendon insufficiency. The foot should contact the ground with the heel first, and the heel should begin to rise at 35% of the gait cycle. Early heel rise may occur as a result of tightness of the gastroc–soleus complex or anterior ankle impingement. Late heel rise may be secondary to weakness of the gastro-soleus musculature.[17]

PALPATION

BONES AND JOINTS

The ankle mortise consists of two joints: the distal tibiofibular joint (tibiofibular syndesmosis) and the talocrural articulation (ankle mortise). The talocrural joint involves articulation of the talus with both the tibia and fibula. The foot can be divided into sections: hindfoot, midfoot, and forefoot (Fig. 10.5). The hindfoot consists of the talus and calcaneus. The midfoot includes the navicular, cuboid, and cuneiforms. The metatarsals and phalanges make up the forefoot.

Palpation of the ankle should include the medial and lateral gutters, the tibiotalar plafond, the talar dome, and the syndesmosis. Proximally at the ankle, the medial malleolus of the tibia and the lateral malleolus of the fibula are prominent and should always be palpable. Note that the

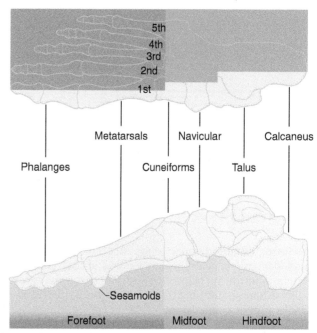

Figure 10.5 Anatomic zones of the foot. (Adapted with permission from Starkey C, Ryan JL. *Evaluation of Orthopedic and Athletic Injuries.* Philadelphia: FA Davis; 2001:48.)

lateral malleolus of the fibula extends farther distally than does the medial tibial malleolus. When an ankle injury is in question, one should palpate the tibial and fibular shafts several centimeters proximal to the malleoli looking for gross deformity or tenderness. Syndesmotic ankle injuries can be associated with fractures of the proximal fibula (Maisonneuve fracture). This follows the general tenet of orthopedic physical examinations that one should always examine the joints above and below an injury.

In 1992, Stiell and others[18] published a set of guidelines to aid in clinical decision making for the use of radiography in acute ankle injuries. These guidelines became known as the "Ottawa ankle rules" (Fig. 10.6). These "rules" suggest that ankle radiographs are indicated if there is pain in the malleolar zone and bony tenderness at area A or B, or the inability to take 4 complete steps both immediately after the injury and in the ER. Foot radiographs are indicated if there is pain in the midfoot zone and bony tenderness at area C or D, or the inability to take 4 complete steps both immediately and in the ER. Numerous studies have looked at the utility of these guidelines. Bachmann and colleagues[19] performed a systematic review and meta-analysis on 27 studies reporting on 15,581 patients. Their data analysis supports the Ottawa ankle rules as a screening tool with approximately 98% sensitivity and median specificity of 31.5%. They concluded that routine use should reduce the number of unnecessary radiographs by 30% to 40%.[19]

In the setting of a rotational ankle injury with distal fibula fracture or syndesmotic disruption, careful examination of the medial soft tissues is critical. If there is clinical concern for a deltoid ligament injury, stress radiographs should be obtained because numerous studies have shown stress-view radiographs to be more sensitive and specific than physical exam alone.[20-24] Gravity stress views are as sensitive and generally more comfortable for the patient than manual stressing.[24-27]

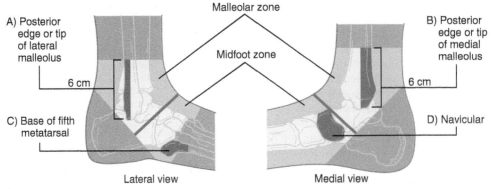

Figure 10.6 Ottawa ankle rules. (From Stiell IG, McKnight RD, Greenberg GH et al: Implementation of the Ottawa ankle rules. *JAMA.* 1994;16;271(11):827-832.)

Moving distally, the next joints encountered are the talonavicular and talocalcaneal (subtalar) joints. The talonavicular joint can be palpated dorsally between the extensor hallucis longus and tibialis anterior tendons, medial to the tibialis anterior and laterally, just lateral to the extensor digitorum longus tendons. Gentle lateral and medial rocking of the talocalcaneal and transverse tarsal joints by gripping the calcaneus in the opposite hand while pressing in this location will make the talonavicular joint more readily appreciated. Anterior and slightly distal to the lateral malleolus, a depression between the talus and calcaneus, termed the *sinus tarsi*, is accessible. Tenderness and swelling at the sinus tarsi may be noted after ankle sprains, which may indicate a subtalar injury component. In addition, it is important to palpate the lateral process of the talus because fractures here, also known as a "snowboarder's fractures," are commonly misdiagnosed as an "ankle sprain."[28,29] Subacute or chronic pain in the setting of pes planus may indicate subfibular impingement. Once thought to be a benign anatomic variant, the accessory anterolateral talar facet has been shown by several authors to be a potential source of pain in both adult and pediatric flat-footed patients.[30-32]

The calcaneus has several bony prominences, which can be palpated. The anterior process of the calcaneus and the calcaneocuboid joint should be palpated and any tenderness noted. Posteriorly, the Achilles tendon inserts on the calcaneal tuberosity. Pain and swelling in this region may be related to tendinopathy, enthesopathy, superficial tendoachilles ("pump bump"), or retrocalcaneal bursitis (Fig. 10.7). In pediatric or adolescent patients calcaneal apophysitis (Sever disease) can occur in this region. Medially, the sustentaculum tali is the prominence just distal to the medial malleolus and functions as the insertion site for the calcaneal attachment of the deltoid and spring ligaments as well as the roof of the fibro-osseous tunnel for the flexor hallucis longus (FHL) tendon. Immediately inferior and distal to the lateral malleolus lies the peroneal trochlea, which divides the peroneus brevis (dorsal to the trochlea) and the peroneus longus (plantar to the trochlea).

Other bony landmarks and structures of clinical importance include the navicular tuberosity medially and the styloid process of the fifth metatarsal laterally. The metatarsal shafts are appreciated on the dorsum of the foot while the metatarsal heads are typically more accessible to palpation on the plantar surface.

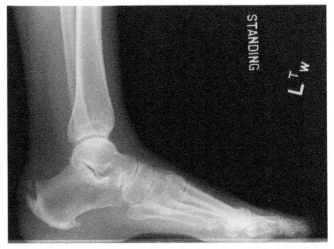

Figure 10.7 Lateral ankle radiograph with enlarged Haglund deformity and Achilles enthesopathy.

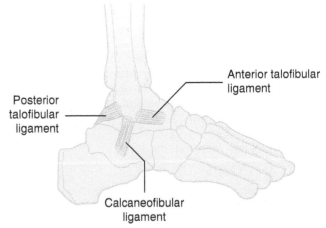

Figure 10.8 The lateral ankle ligaments. (Adapted with permission from Starkey C, Ryan JL. *Evaluation of Orthopedic and Athletic Injuries.* Philadelphia: FA Davis; 2001:89.)

SOFT TISSUE STRUCTURES

The medial and lateral collateral ligaments of the ankle are composed of the anterior talofibular ligament (ATFL), posterior talofibular ligament (PTFL), and calcaneofibular ligament (CFL) laterally (Fig. 10.8), and the deltoid ligament complex medially (Fig. 10.9). The ATFL, PTFL, and CFL should each be palpated from their origin on the lateral malleolus to their insertion points. Lateral ankle sprains are the most common sports injuries.[8,33] Among a series of 321 consecutive acute ankle sprains, Broström[34] described a prevalence of complete ligament rupture in 75% of cases. Of these, isolated rupture of the ATFL occurred in about 65% of cases, combined ATFL–CFL tears in about 20%, and isolated tibiofibular (syndesmosis) rupture in about 10%.

The ATFL is actually an extension of the anterior joint capsule and is in the order of 20 mm long, 10 mm wide, and 2 to 5 mm thick. It originates from the anterior border of the lateral malleolus and inserts distally on the body of the talus just anterior to the articular facet. Its fibers are oriented approximately 75 degrees to the floor. The ligament is most taut and positioned essentially in line with the long axis of the tibia in the plantar flexed ankle.[35] It requires the least load to failure of any of the lateral ligaments.[36,37] Rupture of this ligament is associated with tearing the anterior joint capsule,[19] and bony avulsion of the fibular malleolus is also relatively common.[37,38]

The CFL is extracapsular, crosses both the tibiotalar and talocalcaneal joints, and measures on average 2 cm long, 5 mm wide, and 3 mm thick.[39] It is most taut with the ankle in neutral or slight dorsiflexion, when its fibers are positioned in line with the long axis of the tibia.[35] The origin of this ligament, which is 2.5 times stronger than the ATFL,[36,40]

is from the distal pole of the fibular malleolus, and the insertion is into a small posterolateral tubercle on the calcaneus. The CFL constitutes the medial wall of the peroneal tendon sheath as the tendons pass under the lateral malleolus. Broström[41] noted intraoperatively that the ruptures of the CFL were associated with tears of the medial wall of this tendon sheath. Rubin and Witten[42] found the CFL to be lax in weight bearing, and this supports the fact that ankle stability during axial loading derives primarily from the tibiotalar and talocalcaneal joint articulations.[43,44]

The PTFL, similar to the ATFL, is confluent with the ankle joint capsule. It traverses from its origin on the posterior fibular malleolus to a lateral tubercle on the posterior talus. Its fibers are oriented nearly horizontal. The PTFL is the strongest of the lateral ligaments and is taut only at the extremes of dorsiflexion with avulsion of the lateral malleolus occurring before PTFL disruption.[33,37,45]

The deltoid ligament courses from the medial malleolus, dividing into four parts: the anterior and posterior tibiotalar ligaments, the tibiocalcaneal ligament, and the tibionavicular ligament. It has both superficial and deep portions and is stronger than any of the lateral ankle ligaments.

The distal tibiofibular syndesmosis is important because it is involved in many moderate to severe ankle sprains, often termed *high ankle sprains*. There are four ligaments that make up the distal tibiofibular syndesmosis: the anterior tibiofibular, posterior tibiofibular, transverse tibiofibular, and interosseous ligaments. The anterior tibiofibular ligament is palpable at the anterolateral ankle. Although its proximity to the ATFL may limit the specificity of diagnosing a syndesmotic versus lateral ankle sprain, pain with palpation of this structure seems to be the most sensitive screening test[46,47] (Table 10.2).

Spanning the sole of the foot from the calcaneus to the bases of the proximal phalanges is the plantar aponeurosis or plantar fascia, which is often tender at its medial calcaneal origin when inflamed. The plantar fascia is easier to palpate when tensioned through the windlass mechanism by extension of the metatarsophalangeal (MTP) joints.

THE GREAT TOE

First MTP joint pain can be divided into inflammatory, degenerative, and traumatic. Hallux rigidus (degenerative arthritis of the first MTP joint) presents with pain and/or stiffness. Osteophytes can often be palpated along the dorsal aspect of both the metatarsal head and base of the proximal phalanx. Patients may have pain throughout range of motion (ROM) or only at the extremes of flexion and

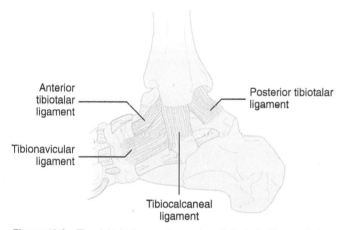

Anterior tibiotalar ligament

Posterior tibiotalar ligament

Tibionavicular ligament

Tibiocalcaneal ligament

Figure 10.9 The deltoid ligament complex. (Adapted with permission from Starkey C, Ryan JL. *Evaluation of Orthopedic and Athletic Injuries.* Philadelphia: FA Davis; 2001:89.)

Table 10.2 Summary of Three Common Clinical Tests for Syndesmotic Injury

Test	Sensitivity (%) Ryan[a] et al.[48]	Sensitivity (%) Sman[b] et al.[47]	Specificity (%) Ryan[a] et al.[48]	Specificity (%) Sman[b] et al.[47]
Pain with palpation	83	92	63	29
Squeeze test	36	26	89	88
External rotation stress test	68	71	83	63

[a]Ryan et al.[48] used arthroscopy as the gold standard.
[b]Sman et al.[47] used magnetic resonance imaging as the gold standard.

extension. The diagnosis is confirmed with radiographs, and treatment is typically conservative with pressure relief over the dorsal aspect of the joint and using a carbon fiber or steel insert to limit motion through the joint with walking.[49,50] Pain at the plantar aspect of the first MTP joint may be seen with a plantar plate injury (ie, "turf toe") or injury to one of the two sesamoid bones that buttress the FHL tendon just proximal to the MTP joint (ie, sesamoiditis, osteonecrosis, fracture). The sesamoids can typically be palpated, and the point of maximal pain should be noted. Varus and valgus stressing is performed to evaluate the collateral ligaments, and drawer testing is performed to evaluate the integrity of the plantar plate. Plain radiographs are the initial imaging modality of choice looking for fracture, sclerosis, or proximal migration of the sesamoids. Please note that 2.7% to 14.3% of the population will have incidental finding of a bipartite sesamoid.[51,52]

THE LESSER TOES

The differential diagnosis of pain around the lesser MTP joints includes synovitis, metatarsal stress fracture, Freiberg's infraction, degenerative arthritis, inflammatory arthritis, plantar plate injury/capsular degeneration, and interdigital neuroma.[53] Plantar plate injuries can result in pain and progressive deformity of the MTP joints. Drawer testing is performed to assess for MTP joint instability. It involves grasping the metatarsal shaft in one hand and the proximal phalanx in the other. The MTP of the involved toe should be dorsiflexed 25 degrees before applying a dorsally directed force on the proximal phalanx.[53] Increased translation indicates a positive test result. It is helpful when this is compared with other uninvolved toes. Klein and associates reported on the diagnostic statistics of common physical examination techniques compared with intraoperative findings of a plantar plate abnormality as the reference standard.[54,55] Pain at the second metatarsal head (98%), edema at the second metatarsal head (95.8%), and a positive drawer sign (80.6%) are the most sensitive physical examination tests for a plantar plate injury.[54] The drawer sign is far more specific (99.8%) compared with pain (11.1%) and edema (11.1%).[54] When evaluating the ability for a drawer test to differentiate between high-grade and low-grade plantar plate tears, Klein and others reported the drawer test maintained a high specificity at 91.5%, but the sensitivity dropped to 22%.[55] If there is clinical concern, both magnetic resonance imaging (MRI) and ultrasound are extremely sensitive in identifying plantar plate injuries.[56-58]

TENDONS

At the medial aspect of the ankle, behind the medial malleolus, pass three tendons along with the posterior tibial artery and nerve through the flexor retinaculum. A useful mnemonic for remembering these structures is "Tom, Dick, and very nervous Harry," which stands for the posterior tibialis, the flexor digitorum longus, vessels (posterior tibial artery), posterior tibial nerve, and the flexor hallucis longus. Passing just anterior to the medial malleolus is the anterior tibialis tendon, which is recognized prominently during ankle dorsiflexion. The extensor hallucis longus tendon can also be palpated as it crosses the dorsomedial ankle and foot on its way to insertion at the great toe.

Posterior to the lateral malleolus pass the peroneus longus and brevis, while the peroneus tertius crosses the ankle anterior to the lateral malleolus just lateral to the extensor digitorum longus. Asking the patient to evert the ankle should allow one to distinguish the peroneus tertius from the extensor digitorum longus (Fig. 10.10). The peroneal tendons should be palpated for tenderness and stability. Peroneal tendon instability can cause painful clicking or snapping over the lateral ankle and is best assessed through resisted eversion in a dorsiflexed position.

VASCULAR EXAMINATION

The pulses of the posterior tibial and dorsalis pedis arteries are both palpable in normal individuals. The posterior tibial pulsation can be found just posterior to the medial malleolus as it runs alongside the tendons of the posterior tibialis, flexor digitorum longus (FDL), and FHL contained by the flexor retinaculum. The pulse of the dorsalis pedis is readily appreciated in the interspace between the proximal aspect of the first and second metatarsals. Pulses should be palpated and documented in every clinical encounter. Despite popular opinion, there is no universally accepted standard grading of pulses. Scales range from a 3- to 5-point grading system. Although a 4-point score seems to be most common (0 = no palpable pulse; 1+ is diminished, but detectable pulse; 2+ is normal; 3+ is bounding), we find descriptive terms to be more clinically valuable. If no pulses are palpable, describe the temperature, color, and capillary refill of the feet and toes to provide a clinical picture of the general vascular status. Perform Doppler ultrasound if available.

BIOMECHANICS

TIBIOTALAR JOINT

Ankle plantar flexion and dorsiflexion are sagittal plane motions that occur primarily at the tibiotalar joint. Dorsiflexion involves cephalad tilting of the foot toward the tibial shaft, with a normal range of 20 degrees. Downward pointing of the foot occurs with plantar flexion, with the normal range of 50 degrees. Interestingly, Siegler and associates[3] showed in vitro that up to 20% of dorsiflexion or plantar flexion motion is generated at the subtalar joint. Limitations of joint motion may be due to any combination of osseous, cartilaginous, ligamentous, musculotendinous, or fibrous restrictions. Ligamentous laxity is common and may contribute to individual differences in the ankle ROM of healthy subjects.[42,59] In a cohort of 18 healthy subjects who underwent a biomechanical analysis of ankle ROM, Siegler and colleagues[60] found no significant side-to-side differences.

Dorsiflexion is the position of stability for the tibiotalar joint. Rubin and Witten[42] noted that, in a dorsiflexed ankle, the broader anterior part of the talus is in firm contact with the malleoli and resists talar tilt. In dorsiflexion, the fibular malleolus is displaced 2 to 3 mm laterally. The main function of the lateral ankle ligaments is to stabilize the joint near its neutral position, while at extremes of ROM bone-to-bone contact provides stability.[61] Furthermore, several researchers

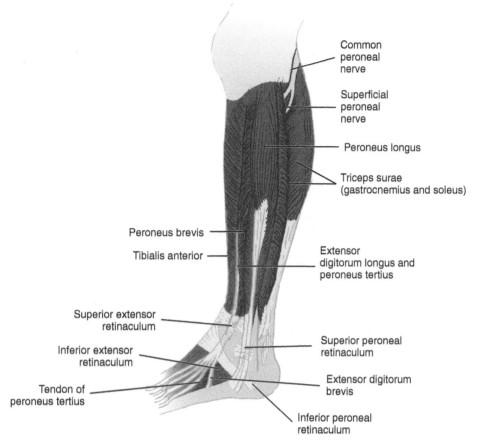

Figure 10.10 Lateral soft tissue anatomy. (Reproduced with permission from Bachner EJ, Friedman MJ. Injuries to the leg. In: Nicholas J, Hershman E, eds. *The Lower Extremity and Spine in Sports Medicine,* 2nd ed. St. Louis: Mosby; 1995:527.)

have demonstrated that the ankle articulation is inherently stable under loaded conditions.[43,44,62,63] Boardman and Liu[64] added that the integrity of the anterolateral joint capsule also contributes significantly to ankle stability.

Range of motion of the ankle should be performed with the knee both flexed and extended utilizing the Silfverskiöld test. The foot is dorsiflexed with the knee flexed and then repeated with the knee extended to document the maximum dorsiflexion in both positions. Because the gastrocnemius muscle originates on the posterior femur, the muscle–tendon unit is placed on maximum stretch by extending the knee. By testing with the knee flexed, the proximal gastrocnemius muscle is relaxed. A normal ankle has dorsiflexion of at least 10 degrees with the knee extended and should improve another 10 degrees with knee flexion. Normal dorsiflexion with the knee flexed, which significantly decreases with knee extension, indicates primary gastrocnemius contracture, whereas a contracture that does not improve with knee flexion can represent a capsular contracture, combined gastroc-soleus contracture, or bony impingement.

TALOCALCANEAL JOINT

Hindfoot inversion and eversion occur primarily at the subtalar or talocalcaneal articulation. While some advocate that subtalar motion should be measured with the tibiotalar

joint held in neutral dorsiflexion to ensure that the talus is firmly grasped in the mortise, others have noted good joint congruence throughout the range of talocalcaneal motion.[65] Inman[66] noted a large variability in subtalar motion, from 20 to 60 degrees, due to variation in subtalar axis and anatomy, kinematic coupling with the ankle joint, and maintenance of true subtalar neutral positioning. Siegler and coworkers[3] showed that, at extremes of motion, the tibiotalar joint can also contribute to inversion and eversion.

Talocalcaneal motion is assessed with the patient sitting, holding the calcaneus in one hand and the forefoot in the other. The examiner subsequently can move the subtalar joint into inversion and eversion. There is usually twice as much inversion as eversion and a lack of subtalar motion may indicate abnormalities such as arthritis, peroneal spastic flat foot, or tarsal coalition. Excessive inversion may be noted after injury to the lateral ankle ligaments.[17]

TRANSVERSE TARSAL JOINT (CHOPART JOINT)

The talonavicular and calcaneocuboid articulations together comprise the transverse tarsal joint. Forefoot supination and pronation occur at this collective joint and should be tested with the hindfoot maintained in subtalar neutral because motion at the transverse tarsal joint is affected by talocalcaneal inversion and eversion. As with the talocalcaneal joint, side-to-side comparison is helpful in determining unilateral restrictions. Decreased transverse tarsal motion may be seen in chronic tibialis posterior tendon insufficiency and arthrosis involving the transverse tarsal joint. Midfoot amputation at this level is commonly called a Chopart amputation.

TARSOMETATARSAL JOINT (LISFRANC JOINT)

The cuboid and three cuneiforms adjoin the five metatarsal bones to form the collective tarsometatarsal joint, or Lisfranc joint. Tenderness at the interval between the first and second metatarsal bases may indicate rupture of the Lisfranc ligament and should trigger advanced imaging such as stress-view x-rays or MRI to evaluate for ligamentous injury. Ross and Cronin[67] reported the "plantar ecchymosis sign" as a clinical finding to aid in the diagnosis of Lisfranc injuries.

EXTRINSIC MUSCLES OF THE ANKLE AND FOOT

PLANTAR FLEXION

The triceps surae or gastrocnemius–soleus complex contains the prime plantar flexors of the ankle (Fig. 10.11). The gastrocnemius has medial and lateral heads originating from the medial and lateral femoral condyles, respectively. Their obliquely oriented fibers adjoin into a common Achilles tendon that is also shared by the soleus muscle and inserts into the calcaneal tuberosity. The posterior tibialis, peroneus longus, FDL, and FHL, and to a lesser extent, the plantaris muscle, comprise the accessory plantar flexors of the ankle and foot.[65]

DORSIFLEXION

The most important ankle dorsiflexors of the ankle and foot are the tibialis anterior and the extensor digitorum longus. The peroneus tertius and extensor hallucis longus serve as supplemental dorsiflexors.

INVERSION AND SUPINATION

The main invertors are the tibialis anterior and tibialis posterior muscles, which also contribute to forefoot supination. The FDL and FHL can serve as auxiliary forefoot supinators as well. In a neutral hindfoot, the triceps surae produce calcaneal inversion. However, in a valgus hindfoot, the moment arm of the Achilles actually moves lateral to the axis of the subtalar joint and functions as an evertor.

EVERSION AND PRONATION

The peroneus longus, peroneus brevis, and peroneus tertius act in concert to evert the forefoot. The lateral portion of the extensor digitorum longus can aid in this function.

INTRINSIC MUSCLES OF THE FOOT

INTERPHALANGEAL AND METATARSOPHALANGEAL FLEXION

The FDL and flexor digitorum brevis (FDB), the FHL, and the quadratus plantae all serve as interphalangeal joint flexors. The MTP joints are flexed by the FDL, FDB, FHL, flexor hallucis brevis and flexor digiti minimi brevis, abductor hallucis and abductor digiti minimi, and all the lumbricals and interossei.

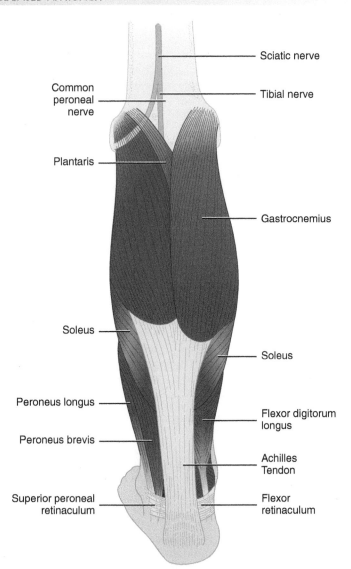

Figure 10.11   The posterior soft tissue anatomy. (Adapted with permission from Bachner EJ, Friedman MJ. Injuries to the leg. In: Nicholas J, Hershman E, eds. *The Lower Extremity and Spine in Sports Medicine.* 2nd ed. St Louis: Mosby; 1995:526.)

METATARSOPHALANGEAL EXTENSION

The extensor digitorum longus and brevis, and the extensor hallucis longus and brevis all contribute to MTP extension.

NEUROLOGIC EXAMINATION

The tibial nerve enters the ankle and foot region coursing behind the medial malleolus and subsequently dividing into medial and lateral plantar branches. The tibial nerve supplies the ankle plantar flexors, invertors, and extrinsic toe flexors in the leg and then divides into the medial and lateral plantar branches that are analogous to the median and ulnar nerves in the hand. The medial plantar nerve innervates the abductor hallucis, FDB, flexor hallucis brevis, and first two lumbricals and provides cutaneous sensation to the medial three and a half digits. The lateral plantar nerve supplies the quadratus plantae, flexor digiti quinti brevis, abductor digiti quinti, the lateral three lumbricals, the interossei, and cutaneous sensation to the lateral plantar aspect of the foot. The first branch of the lateral plantar nerve (Baxter's nerve) can become entrapped between the fascia of the abductor hallucis and the medial aspect of the quadratus plantae or the calcaneus itself. The point of maximal tenderness is typically more dorsal than that associated with plantar fasciitis, and pressure in this area can cause radiation of pain into the lateral foot.

While the peripheral nerves innervating the structures of the ankle and foot are not typically palpable, the examiner should be aware of interdigital neuromas (eg, Morton's neuroma) (Fig. 10.12) and nerve entrapments, including tarsal tunnel syndrome (entrapment of the tibial nerve as it crosses the ankle through the flexor retinaculum), as sources of foot pain (Fig. 10.13).

The examination for interdigital neuroma includes squeezing the affected interspace and compressing the metatarsals as well as looking for a "Mulder's click." This is performed by placing plantar pressure at the interspace and squeezing the distal metatarsals together combined with translation in a superior/inferior direction.[68] A "click"

is often felt or heard when a neuroma is present. This is due to the distal metatarsals contacting the thickened soft tissue mass, causing it to be rapidly displaced. The thumb-index finger squeeze test (web space tenderness test) is performed by squeezing the involved intermetatarsal space at the level of the metatarsal heads.[40,69] The associated toes should splay apart, and the test result is considered positive if the test produces pain. Mahadevan and others[40] evaluated the diagnostic accuracy of seven physical examination tests for the diagnosis of an interdigital neuroma using ultrasound confirmation as the standard measurement (Table 10.3). Claassen and associates[70] reported on 71 patients who underwent operative treatment of an interdigital neuroma and found clinical assessment to be more accurate than MRI in predicting the presence of neuroma at the time of surgery (Table 10.4).

Tarsal tunnel syndrome is a compression neuropathy of the posterior tibial nerve and its branches as it passes behind the medial malleolus. Several tests have been described to

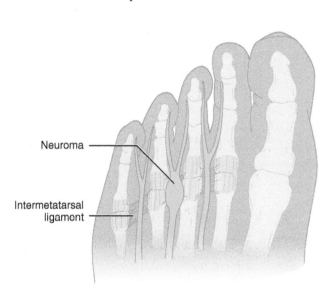

Figure 10.12 Morton's neuroma. (Adapted with permission from Mann RA. Entrapment neuropathies of the foot. In: DeLee JC, Drez D, eds. *Orthopedic Sports Medicine Principles and Practice.* Philadelphia: WB Saunders; 1994:1838.)

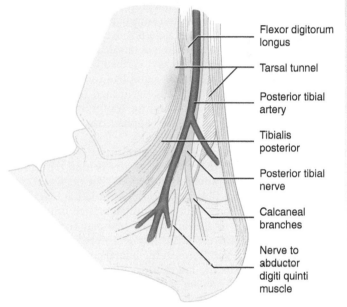

Figure 10.13 The tarsal tunnel. (Adapted with permission from Mann RA. Entrapment neuropathies of the foot. In: DeLee JC, Drez D, eds. *Orthopedic Sports Medicine Principles and Practice.* Philadelphia: WB Saunders; 1994:1832.)

Table 10.3   Diagnostic Statistics of Seven Tests for Interdigital Neuroma Compared with Ultrasonography

Test	Positive Test (*n*) (%)	Sensitivity (%)	Specificity (%)	PPV (%)	NPV (%)	Accuracy (%)
Thumb-index finger squeeze	51 (96)	96	100	100	33	96
Mulder's click	34 (64)	62	100	100	0	61
Foot squeeze	23 (43)	41	0	95	0	41
Plantar percussion	19 (36)	36	100	100	3	37
Dorsal percussion	17 (32)	26	100	100	3	33
Abnormal light touch	13 (25)	25	100	100	2	26
Abnormal pin prick	13 (25)	25	100	100	2	26

Adapted from Mahadevan D, Venkatesan M, Bhatt R, et al. Diagnostic accuracy of clinical tests for Morton's neuroma compared with ultrasonography. J Foot Ankle Surg. 2015;54:549-553.

Table 10.4   Clinical Assessment vs Magnetic Resonance Imaging in Diagnosis of Interdigital Neuroma

Test	Sensitivity (%)	Specificity (%)	PPV (%)	NPV (%)
Clinical Assessment	94	33	97	20
MRI	84	33	97	8

NPV, Negative predictive value; *PPV,* positive predictive value.
From Claassen L, Bock K, Ettinger M, et al. Role of MRI in detection of morton's neuroma. Foot Ankle Int. 2014;35:1002-1005.

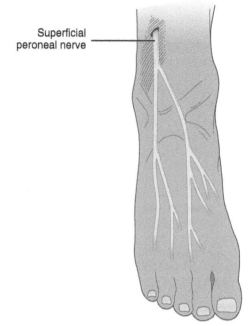

Figure 10.14   The superficial peroneal nerve. (Adapted with permission from Mann RA. Entrapment neuropathies of the foot. In: DeLee JC, Drez D, eds. *Orthopedic Sports Medicine Principles and Practice.* Philadelphia: WB Saunders; 1994:1837.)

help identify tarsal tunnel syndrome. Kinoshita and colleagues[71] described the dorsiflexion-eversion test in which the foot is maximally everted and dorsiflexed with the MTP joints extended and held in that position for 5 to 10 seconds. This compresses the nerve as it runs beneath the flexor retinaculum. Pain, numbness, and a positive Tinel's sign at the tarsal tunnel support a diagnosis of tarsal tunnel syndrome.[71] The triple compression test, as described by Abouelela and Zohiery,[72] is essentially the complete opposite of the dorsiflexion-eversion test. It is performed by placing the ankle in full planter flexion and the foot in inversion, with even, constant digital pressure applied over the posterior tibial nerve for up to 30 seconds.[72] Pain, tingling, and burning all indicate a positive test result.

The common peroneal nerve divides behind the fibular head into deep and superficial portions. The deep peroneal nerve supplies the tibialis anterior, extrinsic toe extensors, and peroneus tertius, while its terminal branch brings cutaneous sensation to the interspace between the first and second toes. The superficial peroneal nerve supplies the peroneus longus and brevis in the lateral compartment and then typically exits the fascia 10 to 12 cm proximal to the tip of the lateral malleolus to become subcutaneous to provide cutaneous sensation to the anterolateral lower leg and dorsum of the foot (Fig. 10.14).

The sural nerve is formed from branches of the tibial and common peroneal nerves and supplies sensation to the lateral dorsum and heel of the foot (Fig. 10.15). The joint capsules and collateral ligaments of the ankle are richly innervated with pain and proprioceptive fibers.

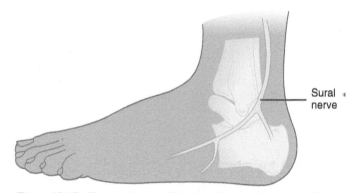

Figure 10.15   The sural nerve. (Adapted with permission from Mann RA. Entrapment neuropathies of the foot. In: DeLee JC, Drez D, eds. *Orthopedic Sports Medicine Principles and Practice.* Philadelphia: WB Saunders; 1994:1835.)

SPECIAL TESTS FOR THE ANKLE AND FOOT

ANKLE STABILITY TESTING

See Table 10.5.

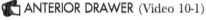 ANTERIOR DRAWER (Video 10-1)

Anterior drawer testing is performed to assess the integrity of the lateral ankle ligaments and, in particular, the ATFL (Fig. 10.16). Isolated ATFL tears constitute between one third and two thirds of all lateral ligament injuries, and

tears are usually complete and involve the anterior joint capsule.[41,76]

In 1968, Landeros and colleagues[77] described the maneuver as follows:

With the patient relaxed, the knee flexed and the ankle at right angles, the ankle is grasped on the tibial side by one hand, whose index finger is placed on the posteromedial part of the talus and whose middle finger lies on the posterior tibial malleolus. The heel of this hand braces the anterior distal leg. On pulling the heel forward with the other hand, relative anteroposterior motion between the 2 fingers (and thus between talus and tibia) is easily palpated and is also visible to both patient and examiner.

Table 10.5 Summary of Physical Examination Tests for Instability

Test	Description	Reliability/Validity	Comments
Anterior drawer test	Grasp the tibia with one hand and the heel with the other. Pull forward on the heel, attempting to draw the talus forward.	Lindstrand 1976[73] Sensitivity: 95% Specificity: 84% Van Dijk et al. 1996[74] Sensitivity: 80% Specificity: 74%	Must compare to contralateral side because there is significant variability among individuals.
Anterolateral drawer test	Grasp the tibia with one hand and the heel with the other. Place the thumb of the lower hand on the lateral gutter. Provide anterior and internal rotation force while feeling for displacement of lateral talus from fibula.	Phisitkul et al. 2009[75] Sensitivity: 100% Specificity: 100%	Studied in cadaveric specimens only. No clinical reports. Used 3 mm or more of displacement as threshold to diagnose lateral ligament rupture.
External rotation or Kleiger test	The patient is seated with knee flexed 90 degrees. Grasp the leg with one hand and place an external rotation force on the forefoot with the other. Pain over the syndesmosis is a positive test result.	Ryan[a] et al. 2014[48] Sensitivity: 68% Specificity: 83% Sman[b] et al. 2015[47] Sensitivity: 71% Specificity: 63%	Medial pain may indicate a deltoid ligament injury.
Syndesmotic ligament palpation test	Palpate the area of the anterior tibiofibular ligament and the region of the syndesmosis just proximal to that.	Ryan[a] et al. 2014[48] Sensitivity: 83% Specificity: 63% Sman[b] et al. 2015[47] Sensitivity: 92% Specificity: 29%	Be precise because the anterior talofibular ligament is close, and pain with palpation of this structure may result in a false positive.
Syndesmotic squeeze test	Manually compress the fibula to the tibia above the level of the syndesmosis. Pain at level of syndesmosis is a positive test result.	Ryan[a] et al. 2014[48] Sensitivity: 39% Specificity: 89% Sman[b] et al. 2015[47] Sensitivity: 29% Specificity: 88%	
Talar tilt	Grasp the tibia with one hand and the heel with the other. Invert heel to feel for displacement of the talus	NA	Routine use (with or without imaging) is not supported by literature.

[a]Ryan et al.[48] used arthroscopy as the gold standard.
[b]Sman et al.[47] used magnetic resonance imaging as the gold standard.
NA, Not available.

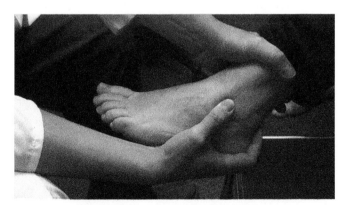

Figure 10.16 The anterior drawer test.

In 1976, Frost and Hanson[78] devoted a short article to further describing the technique, noting several pearls. Excerpts follow:

The anterior and posterior muscles which actuate the ankle joint must be relaxed. ... The ankle must be positioned at 90 degrees to the leg. ... Place the heel of the right hand over the anterior ankle distal tibia just proximal to the ankle joint. Extend the fingers around the medial side of the tibia, and place the index finger on the posterior prominence of the astragalus (i.e., talus), the third finger on the posterior tibial malleolus on its medial aspect. These fingers serve as "sensors" to detect any relative anteroposterior displacement of the talus on the tibia. Curve the left hand around the foot, the palm on the underside of the heel; the fingers curled around the posterior aspect of the tuber os calcis. ... Pull forward on the heel with the left hand, and push posteriorly on the distal tibia with the right hand, thereby attempting to draw the talus anteriorly in the mortise.

Tohyama and colleagues[79] showed that a relatively low anterior load (30 N) during the anterior drawer test was more sensitive than a higher load (60 N) in distinguishing a significant difference between injured to normal anterior displacement. The greater anterior load tends to elicit a protective muscle contraction, which may mask the anterior talar displacement. The validity, sensitivity, and specificity of such manual stress testing as the anterior drawer maneuver has been studied, and the results are conflicting. Lindstrand[73] consecutively examined 100 skiers with acute ankle sprains with a modified anterior drawer maneuver, the results of which were compared with findings at surgery. Eighty of 100 persons had a positive drawer sign, 9 of which were only observed under local anesthesia. Overall, the sensitivity of the anterior drawer sign was 95%, specificity was 84.2%, and the positive predictive value (PPV) of the test was 96.25%, while the negative predictive value (NPV) was 80%.[73]

Funder and others[80] examined 444 patients with acute lateral ankle sprains for direct and indirect ligament tenderness, manually elicited anterior drawer (at 30 degrees of plantar flexion), and talar tilt (ankle flexion angle not specified) tests without local anesthesia. Findings were compared with arthrography as the gold standard. There were 209 arthrographically confirmed ligament ruptures. Of the 35 cases with a positive anterior drawer sign, 71% of these had arthrographically proven ligament tears. Of the 53 positive talar tilt test results, 68% of those had arthrographically demonstrated ligament rupture. Arthrography could not distinguish between or confirm which ligaments had ruptured. Swelling over the lateral malleolus 4 cm or greater in diameter proved to be the single most valuable diagnostic sign; 70% with this sign had ligament rupture. If such swelling was present in conjunction with direct and indirect tenderness of the lateral ligaments, there was a 91% probability of ligament rupture.

Caution must be exercised in assessing the anterior drawer in those with ligamentous laxity because false-positive findings may be seen in up to 19% of uninjured ankles in those with such laxity.[76] Always compare with the unaffected ankle.

Van Dijk and coworkers[74] compared physical examination delayed 5 days after ankle sprain with arthrography and surgical findings in 160 consecutive patients. Of these 160 patients, 135 patients went on to have surgery, and of those, 122 ligament tears were confirmed. The anterior drawer test was found to have a sensitivity of 80%, specificity of 74%, PPV of 91%, and NPV of 52%. The combination of pain on lateral ligament palpation, hematoma formation at the lateral ankle, and a positive anterior drawer test diagnosed a lateral ligament lesion correctly in 95% of cases.

More recently, several authors have questioned the clinical validity of anterior drawer testing.[81-84] There is significant variation in "normal", and even when performed with ultrasound quantification, the ability to detect clinically relevant laxity seems limited.[82] Croy and coworkers[82] summarize it best by stating, "The ADT provides limited ability to detect excessive anterior talocrural joint laxity; however, it may provide useful information when used in side-to-side ankle comparisons and in conjunction with other physical exam procedures, such as palpation."

ANTEROLATERAL DRAWER TEST

Phisitkul[75] and Vaseenon[83] described an anterolateral drawer test (ALDT) and reported increased accuracy (sensitivity 100% and specificity 100%) when compared with traditional anterior drawer testing (sensitivity, 75%, and specificity, 50%) in a cadaveric study. The ALDT uses the principle that the intact medial deltoid ligament acts as a hinge for internal rotation in the setting of a deficient ATFL. The test is performed with the foot in 10 to 15 degrees of resting equinus. The thumb of the hand holding

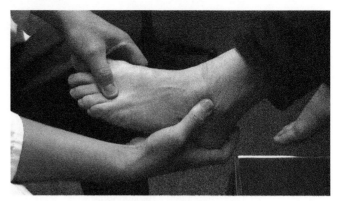

Figure 10.17 The talar tilt test.

the hindfoot is placed over the lateral joint line while the other hand stabilizes the tibia. A combined anterior displacement and internal rotation force is applied, and the separation of the lateral talus from the distal fibula is recorded and compared with the contralateral side. This helps both quantify the amount of translation and eliminate subtalar motion from the assessment. Although this technique shows promising results in cadaveric specimens, it has not been studied in vivo.

TALAR TILT (Video 10-2)

By definition, the talar tilt angle is the angle formed by the opposing articular surfaces of the tibia and talus when these surfaces are separated laterally by a supination force applied to the hind part of the foot (Fig. 10.17).

In 1944, Bonnin[59] stated that 4% to 5% of ankles without a history of injury had a significant tilt up to 25 degrees. Rubin and Witten[42] reported that normal talar tilt could range from 0 to 23 degrees. Broström[34] described 239 cases of arthrographically confirmed lateral ligament rupture. He found that talar tilt instability was frequently seen in the contralateral uninjured ankle, so he concurred with Rubin and Witten who asserted the talar tilt test is not a reliable indicator of ligament injury.[34,42]

Frost and Amendola[85] additionally found that talar tilt x-rays were not reliable in diagnosing lateral ligament injury. In the most methodologically sound studies reviewed, there still was a significant degree of variability in the values defining a normal talar tilt; they included 7 degrees, 10 degrees, 11 degrees, and 3 mm as the upper limits of normal, utilizing both manual and mechanical devices to induce stress (Telos radiographic ankle stress apparatus, Telos Medical, Fallston, MD, USA). Overall, the literature does not support the use of the talar tilt test either with or without radiography.

SYNDESMOSIS INJURIES

The distal tibiofibular syndesmosis consists of four stabilizing ligaments, termed the *anterior, posterior, transverse,* and *interosseous tibiofibular ligaments* (Fig. 10.18). Maisonneuve[86] first described how an external rotation of the talus in the ankle mortise could result in fractures at the ankle and proximal fibula and could be associated with damage to the tibiofibular ligaments. Sprains of the distal tibiofibular

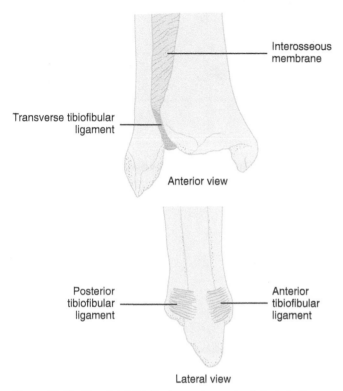

Figure 10.18 The distal tibiofibular syndesmosis. (Adapted with permission from Starkey C, Ryan JL. *Evaluation of Orthopedic and Athletic Injuries.* Philadelphia: FA Davis: 2001:90.)

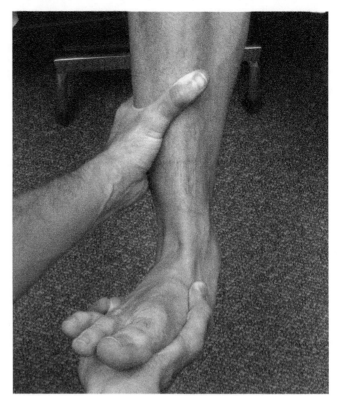

Figure 10.19 The external rotation test.

syndesmosis occur in between 1% and 11% of all ankle injuries and are thought to be the result of a strong external rotation force at the ankle.[87,88] Recovery times for syndesmotic ankle sprains may be extended up to twice as long as for patients with complete lateral ligament injuries.[87-90] Syndesmosis ligament injury is difficult to detect using standard radiographs because minor disruption of the ligaments may be missed, especially in the acute setting.[91-92] MRI is the most sensitive and is also quite specific in both acute and chronic settings, but its expense limits its use as a screening test. Delayed radiography several weeks after syndesmosis injury may reveal heterotopic ossification of the interosseous membrane in 50% or more of those with a partial rupture.[88,90] Three well-described exam maneuvers are used to detect syndesmosis injury: the external rotation test (Fig. 10.19), syndesmosis ligament palpation (Fig. 10.20), and the squeeze test (Fig. 10.21). Two independent studies have reported tenderness with palpation over the anterior syndesmosis to be the most sensitive (83% to 92%) and a positive squeeze test to be the most specific (88% to 89%) physical exam findings compared with MRI or arthroscopy[47,48] (see Table 10.5). External rotation stressing seems to be neither sensitive nor specific, but it can be useful in conjunction with other physical examination maneuvers.

EXTERNAL ROTATION OR KLEIGER TEST (Video 10-3)

In 1954, Barnard Kleiger was the first to explain the external rotation test, or Kleiger test, to identify syndesmotic injury[93] (see Fig. 10.19). The patient is seated with the knee hanging over the edge of the examination table. The examiner stabilizes the tibia with one hand and applies a small force on the medial border of the foot with the other, rotating it laterally. The rotation causes the talus to press against the lateral malleolus, resulting in tibiofibular joint widening. The patient will have pain anterolaterally over the syndesmosis when the test result is positive. The examiner may also feel the talus displace from the medial malleolus, which would suggest a deltoid ligament tear and significant instability.

Boytim and associates[87] analyzed the records of 15 professional football players with syndesmosis sprains and compared them with others with lateral ankle injuries. The diagnosis was made based on tenderness over the anterior and/or posterior tibiofibular and interosseous ligaments and increased pain on external rotation stress. Acute radiographs showed an avulsion of the posterior tibial tubercle in 2 of 13 players, and no abnormalities of the mortise were seen. Follow-up radiographs 1 month later demonstrated calcification of the interosseous membrane in 6 of 8 players. The 15 players with syndesmosis sprains missed significantly more games and practices and required more physical therapy than those with lateral ankle sprains.

Alonso and coworkers[91] investigated the interrater reliability of various tests for syndesmotic injury but failed to describe the gold standard by which syndesmotic injury was identified. They concluded that the external rotation test has the best interrater reliability. Stricker and others[94] compared the findings of a standardized history and physical examination with radiography among 74 patients with acute ankle injuries to determine factors significantly associated with fractures and syndesmosis injuries. Two examiners performed the external rotation stress test, direct syndesmosis

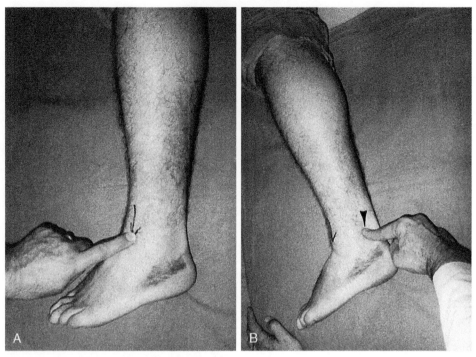

Figure 10.20   The syndesmosis ligament palpation test. **A,** Over the anterior tibiofibular ligament. **B,** Over the posterior tibiofibular ligament.

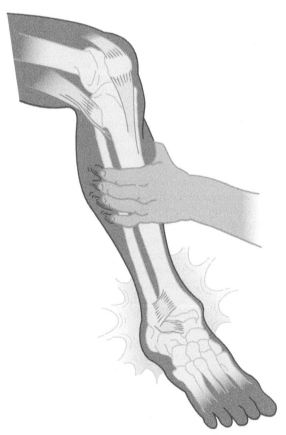

Figure 10.21   The syndesmosis squeeze test.

palpation, and mid-calf squeeze test for syndesmotic injuries. They found that external rotation stress was the only test that showed significant association with an abnormal mortise or fracture. The possibility of a fracture or abnormal mortise was 5.1 times greater in those with syndesmosis pain during the external rotation test.

SYNDESMOTIC LIGAMENT PALPATION TEST
(Video 10-4)

The palpation test involves palpation over the area of the ATFL and proximal to the anterior talofibular ligament, with a positive test result indicated by the report of tenderness in this area (see Fig. 10.20).[87,91]

Variation in the area palpated can increase the rate of false positives. The ATFL is located close to the more commonly injured lateral ligaments, specifically the anterior talofibular ligament. A varying amount of pressure applied by each examiner can lead to different findings.

SYNDESMOSIS SQUEEZE TEST (Video 10-5)

The squeeze test is performed by manually compressing the fibula to the tibia above the midpoint of the calf (see Fig. 10.21).[88,95] A positive test result produces pain over the area of the syndesmotic ligaments.

ANKLE SYNOVITIS AND IMPINGEMENT SYNDROMES

Plantarflexion of the ankle allows palpation of the talar dome. Focal tenderness or crepitus in the proper clinical setting may be indicative of impingement, synovitis, or an osteochondral lesion.[96,97] Anterolateral impingement (ALI) of the ankle causes pain secondary to mechanical impingement of abnormal soft tissues. Acute or repetitive trauma, typically inversion type sprains, can lead to scarring, fibrosis, and hypertrophy in the anterolateral soft tissues.[97] Liu and

Table 10.6   Summary of Achilles Tendon Rupture Tests

Test	Description	Reliability/Validity (Maffulli 1998[100])	Comments
Matles test	In the prone position, with the foot over the end of the table, the patient actively flexes the knee to 90 degrees. If the foot falls into neutral or any dorsiflexion, the test result is positive.	Sensitivity: 0.88 Specificity: 0.85	Our preference is to place the patient prone, flex the knee to 90 degrees and compare the resting equinus posture with the uninjured side.
O'Brien test	Place a 25-gauge needle into Achilles and passively move one ankle.	Sensitivity: 0.80 Specificity: ?	Included for historical purposes. Rarely indicated.
Palpation test	Palpate the course of the Achilles tendon for a depression or sulcus.	Sensitivity: 0.73 Specificity: 0.89	Surprisingly well tolerated even in the acute setting.
Thompson test	The patient is prone. Squeeze the calf over the proximal gastrocnemius muscle belly. Lack of passive plantar flexion indicates Achilles rupture.	Sensitivity: 0.96 Specificity: 0.93	May have a partial response in subacute or chronic ruptures. Always compare with the contralateral side.

coworkers[96] reported overall sensitivity of 94% and specificity of 75% for clinical examination alone in predicting ALI when using arthroscopic findings as the reference standard. Their clinical criteria for diagnosing ALI were having at least five of the following six clinical findings: (1) anterolateral ankle joint tenderness, (2) anterolateral joint swelling, (3) pain with forced dorsiflexion and eversion, (4) pain with single-leg squat, (5) pain with activities, and (6) absence of ankle instability.[96] McCarthy and colleagues[97] demonstrated ultrasound to be accurate in confirmation of clinically suspected ALI.

Posterior impingement testing is performed by placing the ankle in a position of maximum passive plantar flexion. Pain in the posterior ankle is considered a positive test result and should be further evaluated with a lateral radiograph looking for a large lateral talar tubercle, "Stieda's process," or os trigonum. This area can also be palpated in the interval between the Achilles tendon and peroneal tendons. The posteromedial ankle should be evaluated because tenosynovitis of the FHL tendon often coexists.[98,99] Palpation of the FHL between the Achilles tendon and medial malleolus with both active and passive ROM of the great toe may elicit pain or triggering.

ACHILLES TENDON RUPTURE (TABLE 10.6)

Achilles tendon rupture can occur in a relatively healthy tendon or in one that is scarred from repetitive trauma.[101] The most common mechanisms of Achilles rupture are pushing off with the weight-bearing forefoot while extending the knee, sudden unexpected dorsiflexion of the ankle, or violent dorsiflexion of the plantar flexed foot as in a fall from a height.[102,103] Disruption also can occur from a direct blow to the contracted tendon or from a laceration.

THOMPSON TEST (SIMMONDS–THOMPSON OR SQUEEZE TEST) (Video 10-6)

There is controversy over whom to credit with first identifying the squeeze test (Fig. 10.22). As described by Thompson and Doherty in 1962,[104] it is performed in the following manner: The patient is placed in a prone position with the foot extending over the end of the table. The calf muscles

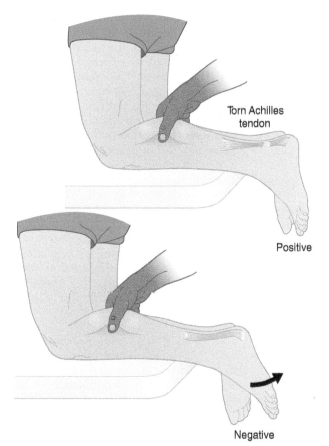

Figure 10.22 Thompson's test for Achilles tendon rupture. (Reproduced with permission from The athletic heel. *Foot Ankle Clin.* 1999:867.)

are squeezed in the middle third below the place of the widest girth. Passive plantar movement of the foot is seen in a normal reaction. A positive reaction is seen when there is no plantar movement of the foot and indicates a rupture of the heel cord.

In 1957, Simmonds[105] first published a description of the calf squeeze test for rupture of the calcaneal tendon (see Table 10.3). Five years later, Thompson[106] published his description of the test and explained that he had observed the effects of this examination in 1955, 2 years before Simmonds. They both noted that when examining a patient with heel cord rupture, no motion of the foot occurred when squeezing the calf of the affected leg. However, when squeezing the calf of the unaffected leg, the foot responded by being passively plantar flexed.

In 1962, Thompson and Doherty[104] noted (and Scott and others[107] later confirmed) that plantar flexion of the foot with a squeeze of the calf requires an intact soleus musculotendinous unit. When performed on cadavers, if 90% of the soleus tendon was cut, the foot responded less strongly. When the tendon was completely cut, the foot remained in neutral position on the squeeze test.

Maffulli[100] studied 174 patients with complete Achilles tendon tears using all four provocative tests described in Table 10.6, with and without the influence of anesthesia. The calf squeeze test was found to have a sensitivity of 0.96, a specificity of 0.93, and a PPV of 0.98.

MATLES TEST

The Matles test was first described in 1975 by Arthur Matles.[108] In the prone position, with the foot over the end of the table, the patient is asked to actively flex the knee through 90 degrees. The position of the foot is observed throughout the arc, and if the foot falls into neutral or the slightest position of dorsiflexion, the test result positive. In normal patients, the foot is held in plantar flexion. The test cannot be used if the patient has an associated knee injury preventing knee flexion. Active flexion of the knee causes shortening of the Achilles tendon because the gastrocnemius is a two-joint muscle and crosses the knee.

The knee may be passively flexed as well. Whether the test is performed with active or passive knee flexion, the position of the ankle and foot is carefully observed during flexion of the knee. If the foot on the affected side falls into neutral or into dorsiflexion, an Achilles tendon tear is diagnosed. On the uninjured side, the foot remains in slight plantar flexion when the knee is 90 degrees. Maffulli[100] studied the Matles test and noted a sensitivity of 0.88 and a PPV of 0.92. The specificity was 0.85.

PALPATION TEST

As described by Maffulli: "The examiner gently palpates the course of the tendon. The gap is classified as present or absent."[100] The palpation test may be uncomfortable in the setting of acute injury, but it is generally well tolerated by most patients in our experience. The palpation test was found to be the least sensitive at 0.73 in the study by Maffulli.[100] The specificity was noted to be 0.89.

SUMMARY

Maffulli[100] concluded that each of the four tests described could diagnose an Achilles tendon tear with a high degree of certainty. These tests may also be used to correctly determine when the Achilles tendon is not torn. When two or more of those tests indicate an Achilles tendon tear, the diagnosis is established. The sensitivity of the tests increased under anesthesia, but the differences did not reach statistical significance. The sensitivity of the squeeze and Matles tests approached 0.90, and both tests were significantly more sensitive than the other maneuvers.

AUTHORS' PREFERRED APPROACH

After obtaining an appropriate history, the patient should be observed in a standing position with both shoes and socks removed. Evaluate the standing alignment from the front and then ask the patient to turn around so you may view the hindfoot from the back. Have the patient do double- and single-limb heel raises to assess the function of the tibialis posterior tendon and strength of the gastroc–soleus complex. Look for the initiation of hindfoot inversion before the heel rise. Tibialis posterior deficiency may result in pain or weakness. The patient should then sit on an elevated examination table. Dorsalis pedis and posterior tibial pulses are palpated. The skin is inspected, and locations of erythema, breakdown, and hypertrophic calluses are noted. Prior surgical incisions are noted and palpated for potential hypersensitivity. Sensation to light touch is assessed in the sural, saphenous, deep, and superficial peroneal nerves and medial and lateral plantar nerve distributions. A straight-leg raise should be performed if there is any concern for lumbar radiculopathy. Manual motor testing of the tibialis anterior, tibialis posterior, peroneals, extensor hallucis longus and gastroc–soleus muscles is performed and compared with the contralateral side. Although it is often difficult, we attempt to differentiate true weakness from pain inhibition. The ankle is placed through full passive ROM, and the mortise is thoroughly palpated for focal tenderness or impingement. With the subtalar joint held in a neutral position, a Silfverskiöld test is performed to evaluate for ankle ROM.

After a thorough generalized evaluation of the lower extremity, we move into a more focused examination based on the patient's chief complaint and history and our preliminary findings.

ACHILLES TENDON

For the diagnosis of acute tears of the Achilles tendon, we prefer to examine the patient prone and perform a combination of palpation of the tendon (which often reveals a palpable defect) followed by a modified Matles test and Thompson squeeze test. These tests are typically well tolerated by an awake patient and are generally diagnostic of a complete rupture. We prefer to report a description of each test rather than using a positive versus negative result to eliminate errors in communication. For example, "Thompson squeeze test of the calf demonstrates no passive plantar flexion," rather than "Thompson test is positive". Plain radiographs are obtained to evaluate for any bony abnormality or soft tissue calcifications. Ultrasound and MRI are typically not needed in the setting of an acute rupture and are reserved for rare instances when the diagnosis is inconclusive with physical examination alone.

INSTABILITY

Any instability examination should include careful evaluation for hindfoot varus because this can be a key contributing factor to recurrent lateral ankle instability. Thorough palpation of the ankle mortise, medial and lateral malleoli, lateral talar process, subtalar joint, anterior process of the calcaneus and base of the 5fifth metatarsal is followed by examination of the peroneal tendons. Peroneal tendons should be palpated and manual motor testing performed to assess both strength and stability. The peroneal tendons should stay behind the fibula throughout circumduction and resisted eversion. We prefer to perform the anterior lateral drawer test by placing a thumb of the distal hand on the lateral talar dome. We also perform a modified talar tilt test using a similar technique by palpating the lateral talar process as it displaces from the lateral malleolus.

CONCLUSION

Injuries of the ankle and foot are commonly seen in clinical practice. Not only must the practitioner understand anatomy and biomechanics, but should also be knowledgeable of the routinely used physical exam maneuvers. In this chapter, we have provided the original description of selected commonly used special tests of the ankle and foot and outlined the validity of these special tests as substantiated by the current literature.

REFERENCES

1. Jordan KP, Kadam UT, Hayward R, et al. Annual consultation prevalence of regional musculoskeletal problems in primary care: an observational study. *BMC Musculoskelet Disord.* 2010;11:144.
2. Manter JT. Movements of the subtalar and transverse tarsal joints. *Anat Record.* 1941;80:397410.
3. Siegler S, Chen J, Schneck CD. The three-dimensional kinematics and flexibility characteristics of the human ankle and subtalar joints. I: Kinematics. *J Biomech Eng.* 1988;110:364-373.
4. Stiehl JB. Biomechanics of the ankle joint. In: Stiehl JB, ed. *Inman's Joints of the Ankle.* 2nd ed. Baltimore: Williams & Wilkins; 1991:39-63.
5. Bennett DR, Wasson D, MacArthur JD, et al. The effect of misdiagnosis and delay in diagnosis on clinical outcome in melanomas of the foot. *J Am Coll Surg.* 1994;179:279-284.
6. Bulliard JL, De Weck D, Fisch T, et al. Detailed site distribution of melanoma and sunlight exposure: aetiological patterns from a Swiss series. *Ann Oncol.* 2007;18:789-794.
7. Dwyer PK, MacKie RM, Watt DC, et al. Plantar malignant melanoma in a white Caucasian population. *Br J Dermatol.* 1993;128:115-120.
8. Garsaud P, Boisseau-Garsaud AM, Ossondo M, et al. Epidemiology of cutaneous melanoma in the French West Indies (Martinique). *Am J Epidemiol.* 1998;147:66-68.
9. Green A, MacLennan R, Youl P, et al. Site distribution of cutaneous melanoma in Queensland. *Int J Cancer.* 1993;53:232-236.
10. Krishnamurthy S, Yeole B, Joshi S, et al. The descriptive epidemiology and trends in incidence of nonocular malignant melanoma in Bombay and India. *Indian J Cancer.* 1994;31:64-71.
11. Gray RJ, Pockaj BA, Vega ML, et al. Diagnosis and treatment of malignant melanoma of the foot. *Foot Ankle Int.* 2006;27:696-705.
12. Golightly YM, Hannan MT, Dufour AB, et al. Racial differences in foot disorders and foot type. *Arthritis Care Res.* 2012;64:1756-1769.
13. Chilvers M, Manoli A 2nd. The subtle cavus foot and association with ankle instability and lateral foot overload. *Foot Ankle Clin.* 2008;13:315-324.
14. Beals TC, Manoli A. The "peek-a-boo" heel sign in the evaluation of hindfoot varus. *Foot.* 1996;6:205-206.
15. Coleman SS, Chesnut WJ. A simple test for hindfoot flexibility in the cavovarus foot. *Clin Orthop Relat Res.* 1977;123:60-62.
16. Johnson KA. Tibialis posterior tendon rupture. *Clin Orthop Relat Res.* 1983;177:140-147.
17. Mann RA. Principles of examination of the foot and ankle. In: Mann RA, Coughlin MJ, eds. *Surgery of the Foot and Ankle.* St. Louis: Mosby; 1993.
18. Stiell IG, Greenberg GH, McKnight RD, et al. A study to develop clinical decision rules for the use of radiography in acute ankle injuries. *Ann Emerg Med.* 1992;21:384-390.
19. Bachmann LM, Kolb E, Koller MT, et al. Accuracy of Ottawa ankle rules to exclude fractures of the ankle and mid-foot:systematic review. *BMJ.* 2003;326:417-423.
20. DeAngelis NA, Eskander MS, French BG. Does medial tenderness predict deep deltoid ligament incompetence in supination-external rotation type ankle fractures? *J Orthop Trauma.* 2007;21:244-247.
21. Egol KA, Amirtharajah M, Tejwani NC, et al. Ankle stress test for predicting the need for surgical fixation of isolated fibular fractures. *J Bone Joint Surg Am.* 2004;86-A:2393-2398.
22. McConnell T, Creevy W, Tornetta P III. Stress examination of supination external rotation-type fibular fractures. *J Bone Joint Surg Am.* 2004;86-A:2171-2178.
23. Park SS, Kubiak EN, Egol KA, et al. Stress radiographs after ankle fracture: the effect of ankle position and deltoid ligament status on medial clear space measurements. *J Orthop Trauma.* 2006;20:11-18.
24. Stufkens SA, van den Bekerom MP, Knupp M, et al. The diagnosis and treatment of deltoid ligament lesions in supination-external rotation ankle fractures: a review. *Strategies Trauma Limb Reconstr.* 2012;7:73-85.
25. Gill JB, Risko T, Raducan V, et al. Comparison of manual and gravity stress radiographs for the evaluation of supination-external rotation fibular fractures. *J Bone Joint Surg Am.* 2007;89:994-999.
26. Michelson JD, Varner KE, Checcone M. Diagnosing deltoid injury in ankle fractures: the gravity stress view. *Clin Orthop Relat Res.* 2001;387:178-182.
27. Schock HJ, Pinzur M, Manion L, et al. The use of gravity or manual-stress radiographsin the assessment of supination-external rotation fractures of the ankle. *J Bone Joint Surg Br.* 2007;89:1055-1059.
28. Langer P, DiGiovanni C. Incidence and pattern types of fractures of the lateral process of the talus. *Am J Orthop.* 2008;37:257-258.
29. Sharma S. Fracture of lateral process of the talus presenting as ankle pain. *Emerg Med J.* 2003;20:E2.
30. Martus JE, Femino JE, Caird MS, et al. Accessory anterolateral talar facet as an etiology of painful talocalcaneal impingement in the rigid flatfoot: a new diagnosis. *Iowa Orthop J.* 2008;28:1-8.
31. Martus JE, Femino JE, Caird MS, et al. Accessory anterolateral facet of the pediatric talus. An anatomic study. *J Bone Joint Surg Am.* 2008;90:2452-2459.
32. Niki H, Hirano T, Akiyama Y, et al. Accessory talar facet impingement in pathologic conditions of the peritalar region in adults. *Foot Ankle Int.* 2014;35:1006-1014.
33. Safran MR, Benedetti RS, Bartolozzi AR, et al. Lateral ankle sprains: a comprehensive review. I: Etiology, pathoanatomy, histopathogenesis, and diagnosis. *Med Sci Sport Exer.* 1999;31(suppl 7):S429-S437.
34. Broström L. Sprained ankles. III: Clinical observations in recent ligament ruptures. *Acta Chir Scand.* 1965;130:560-569.
35. Bulucu C, Thomas KA, Halvorson TL, et al. Biomechanical evaluation of the anterior drawer test: the contribution of the lateral ankle ligaments. *Foot Ankle.* 1991;11:389-393.
36. Attarian DE, McCrackin HJ, DeVito DP, et al. Biomechanical characteristics of human ankle ligaments. *Foot Ankle.* 1985;6:54-58.
37. Siegler S, Block J, Schneck CD. The mechanical characteristics of the collateral ligaments of the ankle joint. *Foot Ankle.* 1988;8:234-242.
38. Kumai T, Takakura Y, Rufai A, et al. The functional anatomy of the human anterior talofibular ligament in relation to the ankle sprains. *J Anat.* 2002;200:457-465.
39. Lassiter TE, Malone TR, Garrett WE. Injury to the lateral ligaments of the ankle. *Ortho Clin North Am.* 1989;20:629-640.
40. Mahadevan D, Venkatesan M, Bhatt R, et al. Diagnostic accuracy of clinical tests for Morton's neuroma compared with ultrasonography. *J Foot Ankle Surg.* 2015;54:549-553.
41. Broström L. Sprained ankles. I: Anatomic lesions in recent sprains. *Acta Chir Scand.* 1964;128:483-495.
42. Rubin G, Witten M. The talar-tilt angle and the fibular collateral ligaments: a method for determination of talar tilt. *J Bone Joint Surg.* 1960;42A:311-326.

43. Sammarco GJ, Burstein AH, Frankel VA. Biomechanics of the ankle: a kinematic study. *Orthop Clin North Am.* 1973;4:75-96.

44. Stormont DM, Morrey BF, An D, et al. Stability of the loaded ankle: relation between articular restraint and primary and secondary static restraints. *Am J Sport Med.* 1985;13:295-300.

45. Bonnin JG. Editorials and annotations: injury to the ligaments of the ankle. *J Bone Joint Surg.* 1965;47B:609-611.

46. Sman AD, Hiller CE, Refshauge KM. Diagnostic accuracy of clinical tests for diagnosis of ankle syndesmosis injury: a systematic review. *Br J Sports Med.* 2013;47:620-628.

47. Sman AD, Hiller CE, Rae K, et al. Diagnostic accuracy of clinical tests for ankle syndesmosis injury. *Br J Sports Med.* 2015;49:323-329.

48. Ryan LP, Hills MC, Chang J, et al. The lambda sign: a new radiographic indicator of latent syndesmosis instability. *Foot Ankle Int.* 2014;35:903-908.

49. Smith RW, Katchis SD, Ayson LC, et al. Outcomes in hallux rigidus patients treated nonoperatively: a long-term follow-up study. *Foot Ankle Int.* 2000;21:906-913.

50. Thompson JA, Jennings MB, Hodge W, et al. Orthotic therapy in the management of osteoarthritis. *J Am Podiatr Med Assoc.* 1992;82:136-139.

51. Coskun N, Yuksel M, Cevener M, et al. Incidence of accessory ossicles and sesamoid bones in the feet: a radiographic study of the Turkish subjects. *Surg Radiol Anat.* 2009;31:19-24.

52. Favinger JL, Porrino JA, Richardson ML, et al. Epidemiology and imaging appearance of the normal bi-/multipartite hallux sesamoid bone. *Foot Ankle Int.* 2015;36:197-202.

53. Coughlin MJ, Baumfeld DS, Nery C. Second MTP joint instability: grading of the deformity and description of surgical repair of capsular insufficiency. *Phys Sport Med.* 2011;39:132-140.

54. Klein EE, Weil L Jr, Weil LS Sr, et al. Clinical examination of plantar plate abnormality: a diagnostic perspective. *Foot Ankle Int.* 2013;34:800-804.

55. Klein EE, Weil L Jr, Weil LS Sr, et al. Positive drawer test combined with radiographic deviation of the third metatarsophalangeal joint suggests high grade tear of the second metatarsophalangeal joint plantar plate. *Foot Ankle Spec.* 2014;7:466-470.

56. Gregg J, Silberstein M, Schneider T, et al. Sonographic and MRI evaluation of the plantar plate: a prospective study. *Eur Radiol.* 2006;16:2661-2669.

57. Klein EE, Weil L Jr, Weil LS Sr, et al. Musculoskeletal ultrasound for preoperative imaging of the plantar plate: a prospective analysis. *Foot Ankle Spec.* 2013;6:196-200.

58. Sung W, Weil L Jr, Weil LS Sr, et al. Diagnosis of plantar plate injury by magnetic resonance imaging with reference to intraoperative findings. *J Foot Ankle Surg.* 2012;51:570-574.

59. Bonnin JG. The hypermobile ankle. *Proc R Soc Med.* 1944;37:282-286.

60. Siegler S, Wang D, Plasha E, et al. Technique for in-vivo measurement of the three-dimensional kinematics and laxity characteristics of the ankle joint complex. *J Orthop Res.* 1994;12:421-431.

61. Siegler S, Chen J, Schneck CD. The effect of damage to the lateral collateral ligaments on the mechanical characteristics of the ankle joint: an in-vitro study. *J Biomech Eng.* 1990;112:129-137.

62. Liu W, Maitland ME, Nigg BM. The effect of axial load on the in-vivo anterior drawer test of the ankle joint complex. *Foot Ankle Int.* 2000;21:420-426.

63. McCullough CJ, Burge PD. Rotatory stability of the load-bearing ankle: an experimental study. *J Bone Joint Surg.* 1980;62B:460-464.

64. Boardman DL, Liu SH. Contribution of the anterolateral joint capsule to the mechanical stability of the ankle. *Clin Orthop.* 1997;341:224-232.

65. Rosse C, Gaddum-Rosse P. The free lower limb: thigh, leg, and foot. In: Rosse C, Gaddum-Rosse P, eds. *Hollinshead's Textbook of Anatomy.* 5th ed. Philadelphia: Lippincott–Raven; 1997:337-418.

66. Inman VT. *The Joints of the Ankle.* Baltimore: Williams & Wilkins; 1976.

67. Rosse C, Cronin R, Hausenblas J, et al. Plantar ecchymosis sign: a clinical aid to diagnosis of occult Lisfranc tarsometatarsal injuries. *J Orthop Trauma.* 1996;10:119-122.

68. Mulder JD. The causative mechanism in Morton's metatarsalgia. *J Bone Joint Surg.* 1951;33B:94-95.

69. Owens R, Gougoulias N, Guthrie H, et al. Morton's neuroma: Clinical testing and imaging in 76 feet, compared to a control group. *Foot Ankle Surg.* 2011;17:197-200.

70. Claassen L, Bock K, Ettinger M, et al. Role of MRI in detection of morton's neuroma. *Foot Ankle Int.* 2014;35:1002-1005.

71. Kinoshita M, Okuda R, Morikawa J, et al. The dorsiflexion-eversion test for diagnosis of tarsal tunnel syndrome. *J Bone Joint Surg Am.* 2001;83-A:1835-1839.

72. Abouelela AA, Zohiery AK. The triple compression stress test for diagnosis of tarsal tunnel syndrome. *Foot (Edinb).* 2012;22:146-149.

73. Lindstrand A. New aspects in the diagnosis of lateral ankle sprains. *Ortho Clin North Am.* 1976;7:247-249.

74. van Dijk CN, Lim LSL, Bossuyt PMM, et al. Physical examination is sufficient for the diagnosis of sprained ankles. *J Bone Joint Surg Br.* 1996;78B:958-962.

75. Phisitkul P, Chaichankul C, Sripongsai R, et al. Accuracy of anterolateral drawer test in lateral ankle instability: a cadaveric study. *Foot Ankle Int.* 2009;30:690-695.

76. Kaikkonen A, Hyppanen E, Kannus P, et al. Long-term functional outcome after primary repair of the lateral ligaments of the ankle. *Am J Sports Med.* 1997;25:150-155.

77. Landeros O, Frost H, Higgins CC. Post-traumatic anterior ankle instability. *Clin Orthop Relat Res.* 1968;56:169-178.

78. Frost H, Hanson CA. Technique for testing the drawer sign in the ankle. *Clin Orthop.* 1977;123:49-51.

79. Tohyama H, Beynnon BD, Renstrom PA, et al. Biomechanical analysis of the ankle anterior drawer test for anterior talofibular ligament injuries. *J Ortho P. Res.* 1995;13:609-614.

80. Funder V, Jorgensen JP, Andersen A, et al. Ruptures of the lateral ligaments of the ankle: clinical diagnosis. *Acta Orthop Scand.* 1982;53:997-1000.

81. Becker HP, Komischke A, Danz B, et al. Stress diagnostics of the sprained ankle: evaluation of the anterior drawer test with and without anesthesia. *Foot Ankle.* 1993;14:459-464.

82. Croy T, Koppenhaver S, Saliba S, et al. Anterior talocrural joint laxity: diagnostic accuracy of the anterior drawer test of the ankle. *J Orthop Sports Phys Ther.* 2013;43:911-919.

83. Vaseenon T, Gao Y, Phisitkul P. Comparison of two manual tests for ankle laxity due to rupture of the lateral ankle ligaments. *Iowa Orthop J.* 2012;32:9-16.

84. Wiebking U, Pacha TO, Jagodzinski M. An accuracy evaluation of clinical, arthrometric, and stress-sonographic acute ankle instability examinations. *Foot Ankle Surg.* 2015;21:42-48.

85. Frost SC, Amendola A. Critical review. Is stress radiography necessary in the diagnosis of acute or chronic ankle instability? *Clin J Sport Med.* 1999;9:40-45.

86. Maisonneuve JG. Recherches sur la fracture du péroné. *Arch Gen Med.* 1840;165:433.

87. Boytim MJ, Fischer DA, Neumann L. Syndesmotic ankle sprains. *Am J Sports Med.* 1991;19:294-298.

88. Hopkinson WJ, St Pierre P, Ryan JB, et al. Syndesmotic sprains of the ankle. *Foot Ankle.* 1990;10:325-330.

89. Mullins JF, Sallis JG. Recurrent sprain of the ankle joint with diastasis. *J Bone Joint Surg.* 1958;40B:270-273.

90. Taylor DC, Englehardt DL, Bassett FH. Syndesmosis sprains of the ankle: the influence of heterotopic ossification. *Am J Sports Med.* 1992;20:146-150.

91. Alonso A, Khoury L, Adams R. Clinical test for ankle syndesmosis injury: reliability and prediction of return of function. *J Orthop Sports Phys Ther.* 1998;27:276-284.

92. Monk CJE. Injuries to the tibio-fibular ligaments. *J Bone Joint Surg.* 1969;51B:330-337.

93. Kleiger B. The diagnosis and treatment of traumatic lateral ankle instability. *NY State J Med.* 1954;54:2573-2577.

94. Stricker PR, Spindler KP, Gautier KB. Prospective evaluation of history and physical examination: variables to determine radiography in acute ankle injuries. *Clin J Sport Med.* 1998;8:209-214.

95. Teitz CC, Harrington RM. A biochemical analysis of the squeeze test for sprains of the syndesmotic ligaments of the ankle. *Foot Ankle Int.* 1998;19:489-492.

96. Liu SH, Nuccion SL, Finerman G. Diagnosis of anterolateral ankle impingement: comparison between MRI and clinical examination. *Am J Sports Med.* 1997;25:389-393.

97. McCarthy CL, Wilson DJ, Coltman TP. Anterolateral ankle impingement: findings and diagnostic accuracy with ultrasound imaging. *Skeletal Radiol.* 2008;37:209-216.

98. Brodsky AE, Khalil MA. Talar compression syndrome. *Foot Ankle.* 1987;7:338-344.

99. Uzel M, Cetinus E, Bilgic E, et al. Bilateral os trigonum syndrome associated with bilateral tenosynovitis of the flexor hallucis longus muscle. *Foot Ankle Int.* 2005;26:894-898.

100. Maffulli N. The clinical diagnosis of subcutaneous tear of the Achilles tendon: a prospective study in 174 patients. *Am J Sports Med.* 1998;26:266-270.

101. Cook J, Khan K, Purdam C. Achilles tendinopathy. *Man Ther.* 2002;7:121-130.

102. Mazzone MF, McCue T. Common conditions of the Achilles tendon. *Am Fam Physician.* 2002;65:1805-1810.

103. Title CI, Katchis SD. Traumatic foot and ankle injuries in the athlete: acute athletic trauma. *Orthop Clin N Am.* 2002;33:587-598.

104. Thompson TC, Doherty JH. Spontaneous rupture of tendon of Achilles: a new clinical diagnostic test. *J Trauma.* 1962;2:126-129.

105. Simmonds FA. The diagnosis of the ruptured Achilles tendon. *Practitioner.* 1957;179:56-58.

106. Thompson TC. A test for rupture of the tendon Achillis. *Acta Orthop Scand.* 1962;32:461-465.

107. Scott BW, Al Chalabi A. How the Simmonds–Thompson test works. *J Bone Joint Surg.* 1992;74B:314-315.

108. Matles AL. Rupture of the tendon Achilles: another diagnostic sign. *Bull Hosp Joint Dis.* 1975;36:48-51.

Index

Page numbers followed by "*f*" indicate figures, and "*t*" indicate tables.